Smart Healthcare Systems

In recent years, the fields of Artificial Intelligence (AI) and the Internet of Things (IoT) have revolutionized numerous industries, and healthcare is no exception. The convergence of AI and IoT has given birth to smart healthcare systems, transforming the way we deliver, receive, and experience healthcare services. This book explores the profound impact of these technologies on healthcare and presents a comprehensive overview of their applications, challenges, and future prospects.

Smart Healthcare Systems: AI and IoT Perspectives addresses various aspects of how smart healthcare can be used to detect and analyze diseases, the underlying methodologies, and related security concerns. It also discusses healthcare as a multidisciplinary field that involves a range of sectors such as the financial system, social factors, health technologies, and organizational structures that affect the healthcare provided to individuals, families, institutions, organizations, and populations. The book presents the goals of healthcare services which include patient safety, timeliness, effectiveness, efficiency, and equity. An outline of what smart healthcare consists of which is m-health, e-health, electronic resource management, smart and intelligent home services, and medical devices is included along with highlights on how AI- and IoT-enabled healthcare technologies are suitable for remote health monitoring, including rehabilitation, assisted ambient living, etc. Rounding the offers of this book out is that it also covers how healthcare analytics can be applied to the data gathered from different areas to improve healthcare at a minimum expense.

Researchers, academicians, industry, R&D organizations, and students working in the fields of artificial intelligence, the internet of things, healthcare informatics, biomedical engineering, healthcare information systems, medical informatics, and related fields along with researchers, medical professionals, scholars, PG students, and policymakers can use this book to help them make the appropriate decisions regarding these emerging disciplines.

Smart Healthcare Systems
AI and IoT Perspectives

Edited by
Pankaj Bhambri, Rashmi Soni, and Tien Anh Tran

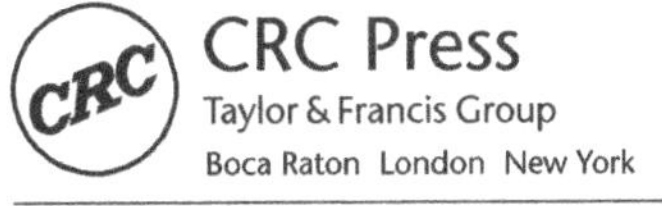

CRC Press is an imprint of the
Taylor & Francis Group, an informa business

Designed cover image: Shutterstock—PopTika

First edition published 2025
by CRC Press
2385 NW Executive Center Drive, Suite 320, Boca Raton FL 33431

and by CRC Press
4 Park Square, Milton Park, Abingdon, Oxon, OX14 4RN

CRC Press is an imprint of Taylor & Francis Group, LLC

Library of Congress Cataloging-in-Publication Data
Names: Bhambri, Pankaj, editor. | Soni, Rashmi (Writer on artificial intelligence), editor. | Tran, Tien Anh, editor.
Title: Smart healthcare systems : AI and IoT perspectives / edited by Pankaj Bhambri, Rashmi Soni, Tien Anh Tran.
Other titles: Smart healthcare systems (Bhambri)
Description: First edition. | Boca Raton : CRC Press, 2025. | Includes bibliographical references and index.
Identifiers: LCCN 2024007983 (print) | LCCN 2024007984 (ebook) | ISBN 9781032698335 (hardback) | ISBN 9781032698502 (paperback) | ISBN 9781032698519 (ebook)
Subjects: MESH: Artificial Intelligence | Internet of Things | Medical Informatics Applications | Medical Informatics Computing
Classification: LCC R855.3 (print) | LCC R855.3 (ebook) | NLM W 26.55.A7 | DDC 610.285—dc23/eng/20240528
LC record available at https://lccn.loc.gov/2024007983
LC ebook record available at https://lccn.loc.gov/2024007984

ISBN: 978-1-032-69833-5 (hbk)
ISBN: 978-1-032-69850-2 (pbk)
ISBN: 978-1-032-69851-9 (ebk)

DOI: 10.1201/9781032698519

Typeset in Times LT Std
by Apex CoVantage, LLC

Contents

Preface

In recent years, the fields of Artificial Intelligence (AI) and Internet of Things (IoT) have revolutionized numerous industries, and healthcare is no exception. The convergence of AI and IoT has given birth to smart healthcare systems, transforming the way we deliver, receive, and experience healthcare services. This book, titled "Smart Healthcare Systems: AI and IoT Perspectives," explores the profound impact of these technologies on healthcare and presents a comprehensive overview of their applications, challenges, and future prospects.

The integration of AI and IoT in healthcare has paved the way for an era of personalized medicine, preventive care, and improved patient outcomes. Through the utilization of machine learning techniques and AI algorithms, healthcare providers have the ability to examine extensive quantities of medical data with unparalleled efficiency and precision. This capability enables the early identification of diseases, accurate diagnostic procedures, and the development of personalized treatment strategies. The IoT enables seamless connectivity among medical devices, wearable, and healthcare systems, facilitating real-time monitoring, remote patient care, and efficient resource management.

This book serves as a roadmap for readers interested in exploring the vast landscape of smart healthcare systems. It begins with a foundational introduction to AI and IoT, providing readers with the necessary background to understand their potential in the healthcare domain. Various applications of AI and IoT in healthcare, along with their role in clinical decision support systems, telemedicine, smart hospitals, digital therapeutics, are delved into. Additionally, ethical and privacy considerations that arise with the adoption of these technologies, emphasizing the need for responsible and secure implementations are also be explored.

Throughout the chapters, leading experts in the fields of AI, IoT, and healthcare share their knowledge, insights, and experiences. Real-world case studies and success stories, highlighting the transformative power of AI and IoT in diverse healthcare settings are also shared in detail. Furthermore, the challenges and limitations that must be addressed to fully realize the potential of smart healthcare systems, including interoperability, data governance, regulatory frameworks, and workforce readiness are also being discussed.

About the Editors

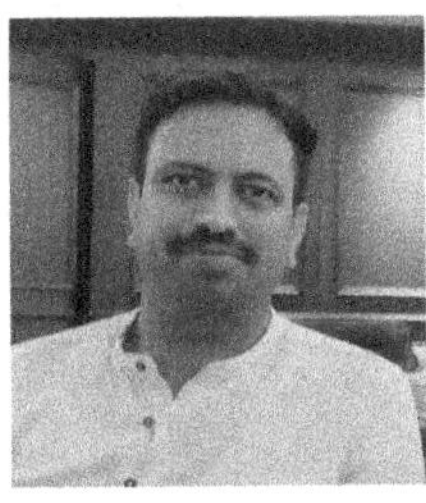

Dr Pankaj Bhambri works in the Department of Information Technology at Ludhiana's Guru Nanak Dev Engineering College. He serves as the institute's coordinator, skill enhancement cell, and has almost two decades of teaching experience. He earned his M.Tech. (CSE) and a B.E. (IT) with honors from the I.K.G. Punjab Technical University, Jalandhar, India, and Dr. B.R. Ambedkar University, Agra, India, respectively. Dr Bhambri earned his doctorate in computer science and engineering from the I.K.G. Punjab Technical University, Jalandhar, India. His research has appeared in a variety of prestigious international/national journals and conference proceedings, and he has contributed to numerous books and has also filed several patents. Dr Bhambri has been awarded the ISTE Best Teacher Award in 2023 and 2022, the I2OR National Award in 2020, the Green ThinkerZ Top 100 International Distinguished Educators in 2020, the I2OR Outstanding Educator Award in 2019, the LCHC Best Teacher Award in 2007, the CIPS Rashtriya Rattan Award in 2008, and the SAA Distinguished Alumni Award in 2012 along with countless other accolades from various government and non-profit organizations. Machine learning, bioinformatics, wireless sensor networks, and network security are his areas of interest.

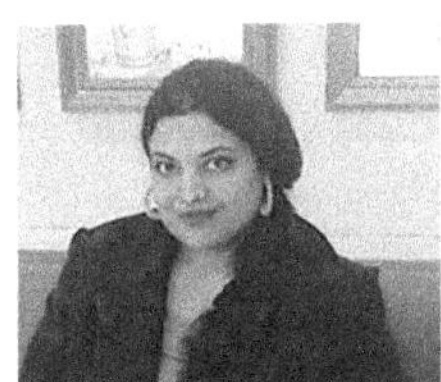

Dr Rashmi Soni is Associate Professor in Information Science and Engineering Department, Dayananda Sagar Academy of Technology and Management, Bengaluru, and Research Supervisor guiding six research scholars in CSE Department of Oriental University, Indore. She has more than 12 years of experience in academic and research. She served as editor for the book "Futuristic Trends in IOT" book series IIPV3EBS08_G13 under IIP USA and India and serving as editor for upcoming book "Personalized Medicine: Navigating Genetics for Tailored Healthcare" AAP Apple Academic Press, Taylor and Francis CRC Book Series. She also served as session chair, advisory and program committee member, and reviewer for 13 international conferences journals of IEEE, Springer USA and India from year 2018–2023. Dr Soni has published seven patents and holds diverse range of professional roles of educator, reviewer, editor and author for various prominent International journals and conferences. Her research interests include cloud computing, IOT, AIOT, bioinformatics, AR and VR, image processing, blockchain. She published papers in 23 journals and conferences. She has supervised many UG/PG/six PhD research projects and dissertations. Dr Soni organized five FDPs, workshops and seminars for different colleges and attended 25 FDPs, workshops, seminars and webinars.

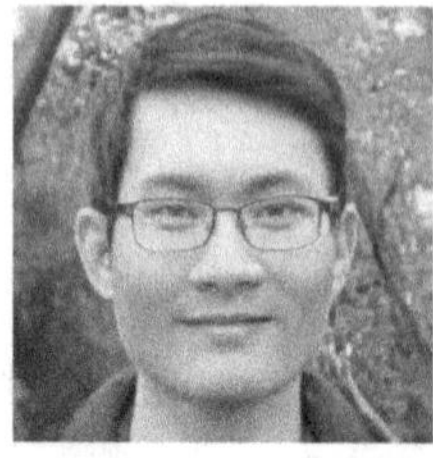

Dr Tien Anh Tran is a research fellow at Seoul National University in South Korea and an assistant professor at the Department of Marine Engineering at Vietnam Maritime University in Vietnam. He is a member of the IEEE and IMarEST. He is an honorary professor at Galgotias University in India, namely in the School of Computing Science and Engineering. Dr Tran obtained his bachelor of engineering (B.Eng) and master of science (M.Sc) degrees from Vietnam Maritime University in 2011 and 2014, respectively. He then successfully finished his doctor of philosophy (Ph.D.) at Wuhan University of Technology in China in 2018, with the support of the Chinese Government Scholarship (CSC). He has made significant contributions by serving as an editor for prestigious journals, including Springer, Wiley, SAGE, Elsevier, and the IEEE Internet of Things Magazine. Having received the prestigious NEPTUNE prize in 2019, he has been put forward as a candidate for the Ta Quang Buu prize in 2022. Dr Tran has been chosen to participate in the postdoctoral fellowship programme offered by the National Research Foundation (NRF) in South Korea. He has made significant contributions to academia through his work as an editor, organizer of conferences, and deliverer of keynote speeches. The papers and research encompass a wide range of topics, including IoT-enabled industrial control systems and the influence of the COVID-19 epidemic on environmentally conscious communities.

Contributors

Surabhi Adhikari
Columbia University
New York, UNITED STATES

Satyam Kumar Agrawal
Chitkara University
Rajpura, Punjab, INDIA

A. Anitha
Vellore Institute of Technology
Vellore, Tamil Nadu, INDIA

Kamaraj Balakrishnan
Madurai Medical College
Madurai, Tamil Nadu, INDIA

Sujit Bebortta
Ravenshaw University
Cuttack, Odhisha, INDIA

Pankaj Bhambri
Guru Nanak Dev Engineering College
Ludhiana, Punjab, INDIA

Mehmet Cem Catalbas
Ankara University
Ankara, TURKEY

N. Chaithra
JAIN (Deemed to be University)
Bengaluru, Karnataka, INDIA

Arkaprava Chakrabarty
Institute of Engineering and Management
Kolkata, West Bengal, INDIA

Harpreet Kaur Channi
Chandigarh University
Mohali, Punjab, INDIA

Satyabrata Dash
GITAM (Deemed to be University)
Visakhapatnam, Andhra Pradesh, INDIA

Atharv Rajesh Gangodkar
JAIN (Deemed to be University)
Bengaluru, Karnataka, INDIA

Soumik Gangopadhyay
Institute of Engineering and Management
Kolkata, West Bengal, INDIA

Kirti Amresh Gautam
GD Goenka University, Gurugram, Haryana, INDIA

P. Geetha
SRM Institute of Science and Technology
Chennai, Tamil Nadu, INDIA

Ahona Ghosh
Maulana Abul Kalam Azad University of Technology, West Bengal
Kolkata, West Bengal, INDIA

Umashankar Ghugar
O.P. Jindal University
Raigarh, Chhatisgarh, INDIA

Bhuvaneshwari Gojanur
Christ (Deemed to be University)
Bengaluru, Karnataka, INDIA

Mohan Sellppa Gounder
Nitte Meenakshi Institute of Technology
Bengaluru, Karnataka, INDIA

Praveen Gupta
GITAM (Deemed to be University)
Visakhapatnam, Andhra Pradesh, INDIA

Sushmita Sunil Jain
Chitkara University
Rajpura, Punjab, INDIA

Janhvi Jha
JAIN (Deemed to be University)
Bengaluru, Karnataka, INDIA

Christian Kaunert
Dublin City University
Dublin, IRELAND

S. Krithika
Sri Venkateswara College of Engineering
Chennai, Tamil Nadu, INDIA

Pulkit Kumar
Chandigarh University
Mohali, Punjab, INDIA

Suresh Kumar
Geeta University
Panipat, Haryana, INDIA

Udhayaranjani Sellappagounder Mohan
Dalhousie University
Halifax, Nova Scotia, CANADA

N. Nandhini
Vellore Institute of Technology
Vellore, Tamil Nadu, INDIA

S. Lakshmi Narayanan
Sri Venkateswara College of Engineering
Chennai, Tamil Nadu, INDIA

Rakesh Nayak
O.P. Jindal University
Raigarh, Chhatisgarh, INDIA

S. Padmapriya
Christ (Deemed to be University)
Bengaluru, Karnataka, INDIA

Thinagaran Perumal
Universiti Putra
Serdang, Selangor, MALAYSIA

Venkata Tulasi Krishna Ponnada
Acharya Nagarjuna University
Guntur, Andhra Pradesh, INDIA

Venkata Tulasi Ramu Ponnada
Acharya Nagarjuna University
Guntur, Andhra Pradesh, INDIA

Rachna Rana
Ludhiana Group of Colleges
Ludhiana, Punjab, INDIA

Ritu
Chandigarh Group of Colleges Jhanjeri
Mohali, Punjab, INDIA

Sriparna Saha
Maulana Abul Kalam Azad University of Technology, West Bengal
Kolkata, West Bengal, INDIA

Azaharuddin Saikh
Maulana Abul Kalam Azad University of Technology, West Bengal
Kolkata, West Bengal, INDIA

Shouvik Sanyal
Dhofar University
Salalah, SULTANATE OF OMAN

Indranil Sarkar
Guru Nanak Institute of Technology
Kolkata, West Bengal, INDIA

Anu Sayal
Taylor's University,
Selangor Darul Ehsan, MALAYSIA

Wasswa Shafik
Universiti Brunei Darussalam
Bandar Seri Begawan, BE1410,
BRUNEI DARUSSALAM

Ankit Singh
United Institute of Medical Sciences
Prayagraj, Uttar Pradesh, INDIA

Bhupinder Singh
Sharda University
Greater Noida, Uttar Pradesh, INDIA

Brij Nandan Singh
United Institute of Medical Sciences
Prayagraj, Uttar Pradesh, INDIA

Manpreet Singh
Lovely Professional University
Jalandhar, Punjab, INDIA

Dhanabalan Thangam
Presidency College
Bengaluru, Karnataka, INDIA

Surendrabikram Thapa
Virginia Tech
Blacksburg, Virginia, UNITED STATES

Tien Anh Tran
Vietnam Maritime University
Haiphong, VIETNAM

Bebesh Tripathy
Chandigarh University
Mohali, Punjab, INDIA

Biswajit Tripathy
Ravenshaw University
Cuttack, Odhisha, INDIA

Subhranshu Sekhar Tripathy
KIIT Deemed to be University
Bhubaneswar
Odhisha, INDIA

Amitava Ukil
Eminent College of Management and
Technology
Barasat, West Bengal,
INDIA

R.K. Kapila Vani
Sri Venkateswara College of
Engineering
Chennai, Tamil Nadu, INDIA

Vani Vasudevan
Nitte Meenakshi Institute of
Technology
Bengaluru, Karnataka, INDIA

1 Artificial Intelligence Enabled Internet of Medical Things for Enhanced Healthcare Systems

Pankaj Bhambri

1.1 INTRODUCTION

The swift progression of technology has created opportunities for significant breakthroughs in healthcare, particularly through the integration of internet of things (IoT) and artificial intelligence (AI), which are crucial in redefining the field. This chapter explores the complex overlap of AI and the IoT in the healthcare field, with a specific emphasis on how these technologies come together in the context of the internet of medical things (IoMT). With an overarching goal of enhancing healthcare systems, this chapter explores the multifaceted ways in which AI and IoT synergize to bring about significant improvements in patient care, diagnostics, treatment methodologies, and overall healthcare delivery (Bose et al., 2021).

In understanding the foundations of this synergy, it is imperative to recognize the profound impact that both AI and IoT individually have had on the healthcare sector. AI, with its ability to analyze vast datasets and derive meaningful insights, has revolutionized diagnostics, treatment planning, and personalized medicine. Simultaneously, the IoT has established a network of networked devices that can collect data in real-time, offering a substantial amount of information for healthcare experts. The significance of these technologies lies in their potential to create a symbiotic relationship, where AI processes the wealth of data generated by IoT devices to derive actionable intelligence for medical decision-making.

The main objective of this chapter is to clarify the complex subtleties of utilizing artificial intelligence in the context of the internet of medical things to improve health care systems (Sumathi et al., 2021). Our objective is to offer a thorough comprehension of the technical landscape by exploring the fundamental principles of AI and IoT in healthcare. Moreover, the chapter will explore the specific applications of AI in healthcare, the emergence of IoMT, and the challenges and opportunities presented by the integration of these technologies. By analyzing real-life examples and examining upcoming developments, our goal is to provide readers with a deep

DOI: 10.1201/9781032698519-1

understanding of the revolutionary capabilities of AI-enabled IoMT and its impact on the future of healthcare.

1.2 FOUNDATIONS OF AI AND IoT IN HEALTHCARE

The foundations of AI and the IoT in healthcare are rooted in their individual capabilities to revolutionize the sector. AI, with its advanced algorithms and machine learning models, has the power to analyze complex medical datasets, aiding in diagnostics, personalized treatment plans, and predictive analytics (Babu et al., 2021). Simultaneously, the IoT introduces a network of interconnected medical devices, wearables, and sensors capable of real-time data collection, fostering a seamless flow of information (Bakshi et al., 2021). Together, these technologies form the backbone of a data-driven healthcare ecosystem, where AI processes the wealth of data generated by IoT devices to derive actionable insights. The integration of AI and IoT in healthcare creates a powerful collaboration that optimizes decision-making, improves patient outcomes, and simplifies healthcare procedures, ultimately establishing a more efficient and patient-focused healthcare model. Figure 1.1 depicts the roles and operations of AI and the IoT within the healthcare industry.

1.2.1 Overview of Artificial Intelligence in Healthcare

The integration of AI in healthcare represents a paradigm shift, revolutionizing traditional approaches to medical diagnosis, treatment, and patient care (Bröring and Strüker, 2019). AI, with its capacity to analyze vast and diverse datasets, offers unprecedented capabilities in pattern recognition, predictive analytics, and decision

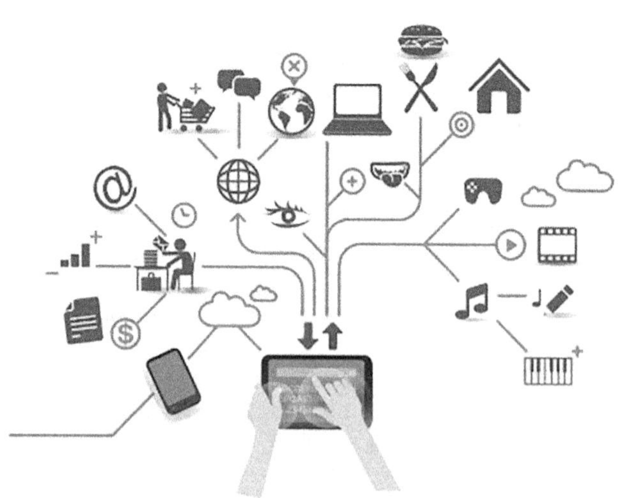

FIGURE 1.1 Role of AI and IoT in healthcare.

support systems. In the healthcare domain, AI applications range from diagnostic imaging interpretation, where algorithms can identify abnormalities in medical images with remarkable accuracy, to personalized treatment plans derived from comprehensive patient data analysis (Car and Sheikh, 2019). Natural Language Processing (NLP) allows AI to extract important information from unstructured medical records and research literature, thereby enhancing decision-making based on evidence (Thilakanathan et al., 2018). The potential of AI for healthcare goes beyond improving efficiency, offering increased diagnostic accuracy, tailored treatment, and eventually, better patient outcomes. Nevertheless, the integration of AI in the healthcare sector also gives rise to ethical dilemmas, issues over data privacy, and the necessity for strong regulatory frameworks to guarantee responsible and secure implementation.

1.2.2 Role of Internet of Things in Healthcare

The role of the IoT in healthcare is integral to the paradigm shift towards more patient-centric, efficient, and data-driven healthcare systems (Pei and Zheng, 2019). IoT devices in healthcare encompass a diverse array of interconnected technologies, ranging from wearable devices and remote patient monitoring tools to smart medical equipment. These devices facilitate the seamless collection and transmission of real-time health data, enabling healthcare providers to monitor patients remotely, track vital signs, and gain valuable insights into patient health (Chen et al., 2019). By fostering continuous, unobtrusive monitoring, IoT contributes to preventive healthcare, early detection of anomalies, and personalized treatment plans. The deployment of IoT in healthcare not only enhances patient outcomes but also streamlines healthcare operations, optimizing resource utilization and reducing costs. Nevertheless, as the IoT network in the healthcare sector grows, it is crucial to address challenges related to data security, interoperability, as well as ethical concerns. This is necessary to ensure the responsible and efficient integration of these advancements into the healthcare system (Kuzhaloli et al., 2020).

1.2.3 Integration of AI and IoT in Healthcare Systems

The incorporation of AI and the IoT into healthcare systems signifies a fundamental change in the manner in which medical services are provided and supervised. This integration comprises the seamless connectivity of intelligent gadgets, wearables, and sensors that gather real-time health information, which is subsequently processed and evaluated by artificial intelligence algorithms. This convergence enables healthcare providers to access a wealth of patient information, leading to more informed decision-making, timely interventions, and personalized treatment plans. Challenges in interoperability, data security, and privacy considerations come to the forefront during this integration, requiring robust frameworks and protocols to ensure the ethical and secure use of sensitive health data (Rachna et al., 2022). Despite these challenges, the integration of AI and IoT holds immense potential to enhance diagnostics, enable proactive healthcare management, and ultimately contribute to more efficient and patient-centric healthcare systems.

1.3 INTERNET OF MEDICAL THINGS

The IoMT is a transformative development in the healthcare sector, which involves a network of interlinked medical equipment and apps that gather, transmit, and interpret health-related information (Devadutta et al., 2020). At its core, IoMT extends the principles of the broader IoT into the realm of healthcare, fostering connectivity among various medical devices, wearables, and sensors. These devices are equipped with the capability to capture and share a diverse array of health metrics, ranging from vital signs and medication adherence to patient activity and environmental factors.

The scope of IoMT is expansive, encompassing a wide array of medical devices and technologies that contribute to the digitization and connectivity of healthcare systems (Arora and Patel, 2018). These devices include wearable fitness trackers, smart insulin pumps, remote patient monitoring systems, smart inhalers, and a host of other sensor-laden technologies. The data generated by these devices offer valuable insights into patient health and enable healthcare providers to make more informed decisions regarding diagnosis, treatment, and ongoing care.

One of the key aspects defining the scope of IoMT is its ability to facilitate remote patient monitoring, allowing healthcare professionals to access real-time data and track patient conditions outside traditional healthcare settings (World Health Organization, 2018). This is particularly beneficial for individuals with chronic conditions, as continuous monitoring can lead to early detection of potential issues and personalized interventions. Additionally, IoMT supports the concept of personalized medicine by tailoring treatment plans based on individual health data, thereby optimizing outcomes and minimizing adverse effects.

As IoMT continues to evolve, its scope extends beyond individual patient care to encompass broader healthcare system improvements (Miotto et al., 2018). Enhanced connectivity and data sharing among medical devices contribute to the development of smart hospitals and healthcare ecosystems, where seamless communication between devices streamlines operations, reduces errors, and improves overall efficiency. The potential of IoMT to revolutionize healthcare delivery makes it a dynamic and influential force in the ongoing transformation of the medical landscape.

1.3.1 IoMT Applications in Healthcare

The applications of the IoMT in healthcare are diverse and impactful, ushering in a new era of patient-centric and data-driven healthcare delivery. IoMT integrates a myriad of smart, interconnected medical devices and sensors, fostering seamless communication and data exchange (Bhambri et al., 2021). These applications range from remote patient monitoring and wearable health devices that continuously collect and transmit vital signs to healthcare providers, enabling real-time tracking of patient health, to smart medication dispensers that enhance medication adherence. IoMT also facilitates the creation of smart hospital environments through interconnected medical equipment, optimizing resource utilization and workflow efficiency (Singh et al., 2021). Furthermore, IoMT plays a pivotal role in preventive care, allowing for early detection of health issues through continuous monitoring, thus empowering healthcare professionals to intervene proactively. The transformative impact of IoMT applications extends beyond the clinical setting, influencing healthcare management, reducing costs, and ultimately contributing to improved patient outcomes.

1.3.2 Challenges and Opportunities in Implementing IoMT

IoMT in healthcare presents a dichotomy of challenges and opportunities. On one hand, the integration of IoMT devices into existing healthcare systems introduces complex interoperability issues, necessitating standardized protocols for seamless communication among diverse devices. Privacy and security concerns loom large, demanding robust measures to safeguard sensitive patient data and protect against potential cyber threats (Arora et al., 2019). Moreover, the large amount of data produced by IoMT devices presents difficulties in terms of conserving information, administration, and analysis. On the other hand, these challenges open avenues for innovation and improvement. Standardization efforts can foster a more cohesive IoMT ecosystem, facilitating collaboration among different manufacturers and ensuring compatibility. Addressing privacy and security concerns can result in the development of advanced encryption and authentication mechanisms, enhancing overall data security. Moreover, the wealth of data generated by IoMT devices provides unprecedented opportunities for predictive analytics, personalized medicine, and more informed decision-making in healthcare delivery (Rana et al., 2021). Balancing these challenges and opportunities is crucial for unlocking the full potential of IoMT in revolutionizing patient care and healthcare systems.

1.4 AI APPLICATIONS IN HEALTHCARE

AI applications in healthcare have ushered in a paradigm shift by revolutionizing various facets of the industry. From diagnostic tools that can analyze medical images with unprecedented accuracy to predictive analytics models that aid in forecasting patient outcomes, AI has become a powerful ally in augmenting healthcare delivery (Charitos et al., 2019). Treatment recommendations and decision support systems leverage machine learning algorithms to process vast datasets, providing healthcare professionals with personalized and evidence-based insights. The use of AI in the healthcare sector not only improves the effectiveness of medical procedures but also facilitates the progress of precision medicine, which involves customizing treatment strategies based on specific patient characteristics (Bhambri et al., 2022). As AI applications continue to evolve, the healthcare sector is witnessing a transformation in disease detection, risk assessment, and therapeutic approaches, ultimately leading to improved patient care and outcomes.

1.4.1 Diagnostic Applications

Diagnostic applications represent a cornerstone in the realm of AI applications in healthcare, revolutionizing the accuracy and efficiency of medical diagnoses

(Kuo et al., 2018). Through advanced machine learning algorithms, AI systems can analyze vast datasets comprising patient records, medical imaging, and clinical data, providing healthcare professionals with unprecedented insights. These apps demonstrate exceptional proficiency in identifying anomalies, patterns, and subtle indications that may go unnoticed by humans, therefore improving the accuracy of diagnostic procedures. From early detection of diseases such as cancer to predicting the likelihood of various health conditions, AI-driven diagnostic tools empower medical practitioners to make more informed decisions (Rajkomar et al., 2018). Additionally, these applications contribute to the optimization of workflows by expediting the diagnostic timeline, enabling timely interventions and personalized treatment plans. As diagnostic accuracy is pivotal for successful patient outcomes, the integration of AI in this domain exemplifies its potential to significantly elevate the standard of healthcare delivery.

1.4.2 Predictive Analytics for Patient Care

Predictive analytics in patient care represents a groundbreaking application of AI in healthcare, revolutionizing how medical professionals anticipate, prevent, and manage illnesses. By harnessing the power of machine learning algorithms and data analytics, healthcare systems can analyze vast datasets encompassing patient records, diagnostic information, and treatment outcomes (Vijayalakshmi et al., 2021). This enables the identification of patterns and trends that might go unnoticed through traditional methods. Predictive analytics enables the timely identification of possible health problems, enabling preemptive interventions and customized treatment strategies (Banaee et al., 2015). By enabling healthcare practitioners to anticipate disease onset and identify patients susceptible to problems, these technologies equip them to administer focused and preemptive therapy, thereby enhancing patient outcomes and alleviating strain on healthcare resources. Predictive analytics integration improves healthcare delivery efficiency and supports the transition from reactive to proactive patient care methods, aligning with the goal of increasing personalized medicine in the dynamic healthcare landscape.

1.4.3 Treatment Recommendations and Decision Support

AI algorithms, fueled by vast datasets and machine learning capabilities, play a pivotal role in assisting healthcare professionals in making informed decisions about treatment plans (Niazi et al., 2019). These systems analyze patient data, including medical histories, diagnostic images, and genomic information, to generate personalized treatment recommendations. By discerning patterns and correlations that might elude human observation, AI facilitates precision medicine, tailoring interventions to individual patient characteristics (Smith, 2018). This not only enhances the efficacy of treatments but also contributes to minimizing adverse effects. Moreover, AI-driven decision support systems provide clinicians with real-time insights, aiding in the identification of optimal treatment pathways and ensuring that medical interventions align with the latest advancements in medical research (Chung et al., 2018). The incorporation of AI into treatment recommendations enhances the effectiveness of healthcare delivery and has the potential to enhance patient outcomes and promote a patient-centered approach to medical care.

1.4.4 AI-Driven Personalized Medicine

AI-Driven personalized medicine stands at the forefront of healthcare innovation, offering a paradigm shift from traditional one-size-fits-all approaches to tailored and precise patient care (Esteva et al., 2017). This application of artificial intelligence utilizes advanced algorithms to analyze extensive datasets, encompassing genetic information, clinical records, and even lifestyle factors. By discerning unique patterns and correlations within this vast array of data, AI empowers healthcare providers to predict individual patient responses to specific treatments, optimize drug regimens, and even forecast disease risks with unprecedented accuracy. This transformative approach not only enhances treatment efficacy but also minimizes adverse effects, fostering a more patient-centric healthcare model. AI-driven personalized medicine holds immense promise for ushering in an era where medical interventions are finely tuned to the genetic makeup and distinctive characteristics of each patient, ultimately maximizing therapeutic outcomes and improving overall health outcomes.

1.5 INTEGRATION OF AI AND IoT IN HEALTHCARE SYSTEMS

The incorporation of AI and the IoT into healthcare systems signifies a fundamental change, completely transforming the methods by which medical data is gathered, analyzed, and applied. This synergy enables the creation of interconnected healthcare ecosystems where AI algorithms analyze real-time data generated by IoT devices, ranging from wearables to remote monitoring sensors (Istepanian and Sungoor, 2019). This integration enhances diagnostic accuracy, facilitates predictive analytics for proactive patient care, and streamlines treatment strategies (Greenspan et al., 2016). However, challenges such as data security, interoperability, and scalability need to be carefully addressed to fully realize the potential of this integration (Alkhodre et al., 2019). The seamless collaboration of AI and IoT not only empowers healthcare professionals with timely and actionable insights but also lays the foundation for personalized and patient-centric healthcare delivery, ultimately improving outcomes and the overall efficiency of healthcare systems.

1.5.1 Interconnected Devices and Data Flow

Interconnected devices, ranging from wearable health monitors to medical imaging equipment, create a network that continuously collects and transmits valuable health-related data (Chen et al., 2018). This interconnectedness enables real-time monitoring of patient vitals, medication adherence, and other relevant health parameters. The data flow from these devices is instrumental in fueling AI algorithms, providing them with a constant stream of information for analysis (Hsieh and Chen, 2018). This dynamic collaboration enables the prompt identification of health problems, individualized treatment strategies, and timely treatments. Nevertheless, the task of handling the vast amount of data produced by interconnected devices has difficulties pertaining to data security, privacy, and interoperability. Achieving an optimal equilibrium between leveraging the advantages of networked devices and tackling these obstacles is crucial for maximizing the possibilities of IoT and artificial intelligence integration in health care systems.

1.5.2 Data Security and Privacy Considerations

The integration of AI and IoT in healthcare systems brings forth a myriad of benefits, but it also raises critical concerns, particularly in the realm of data security and privacy. The vast amount of sensitive patient data collected by IoT devices and processed by AI algorithms necessitates stringent measures to safeguard against unauthorized access and potential breaches (Abiodun et al., 2018). Implementing robust encryption protocols, secure data transmission channels, and adopting privacy-preserving techniques are imperative to uphold the confidentiality and integrity of healthcare data. Maintaining a careful equilibrium between utilizing AI for data-driven analysis and safeguarding patient confidentiality is of utmost importance. The ethical responsibility of healthcare providers and technology developers is underscored in establishing frameworks that not only comply with regulatory standards but also go beyond to prioritize the protection of patient information, fostering trust in the integration of AI and IoT for the betterment of healthcare systems.

1.5.3 Scalability and Interoperability Challenges

The integration of AI and the IoT in healthcare systems introduces significant challenges, particularly in terms of scalability and interoperability (Dey et al., 2019). As healthcare infrastructures adopt increasingly complex networks of interconnected devices and AI-driven applications, ensuring scalability becomes a critical concern. The ability to seamlessly accommodate the growing volume of data generated by IoT devices and the computational demands of AI algorithms is essential for sustaining efficient and responsive healthcare systems. Additionally, interoperability challenges arise due to the diverse range of devices, platforms, and standards within the healthcare ecosystem (Gartner, 2019). Achieving seamless communication and data exchange between various AI applications and IoT devices is crucial for harnessing the full potential of these technologies. Addressing scalability and interoperability issues is imperative for creating a cohesive and integrated healthcare environment that maximizes the benefits of AI and IoT while minimizing disruptions to patient care and medical workflows.

1.6 CASE STUDIES AND EXEMPLARY IMPLEMENTATIONS

Below examples showcase the diverse applications of AI-enabled IoMT in healthcare, ranging from diagnostics and personalized medicine to remote patient monitoring and predictive maintenance of medical equipment:

- IBM Watson Health: IBM Watson Health has been a pioneer in leveraging AI and IoT in healthcare. Their studies entail utilizing AI algorithms to scrutinize medical imaging, genomic data, and clinical records in order to aid healthcare practitioners in formulating more precise diagnoses and tailored treatment strategies. Integrating IoT devices for real-time patient monitoring enhances the data available for AI analysis, contributing to more proactive and personalized healthcare interventions.
- Google's DeepMind in Healthcare: Google's DeepMind has been involved in various healthcare projects, including collaborations with hospitals and research institutions. One notable example is the use of AI for analyzing retinal scans to detect signs of eye diseases like diabetic retinopathy. The integration of IoT devices, such as smart sensors for continuous patient monitoring, further enriches the dataset used by AI algorithms, leading to more precise diagnostics and timely interventions.
- Siemens Healthineers: Siemens Healthineers has explored the integration of AI and IoT to enhance diagnostic imaging. Their projects involve incorporating AI algorithms into medical imaging devices like MRI and CT scanners. The synergy of AI with IoT enables these devices to collect and analyze real-time data during imaging procedures, allowing for adaptive imaging techniques and personalized treatment plans.
- GE Healthcare: GE Healthcare has implemented AI and IoT technologies to improve medical equipment performance and enhance patient care. Their focus includes predictive maintenance of medical devices through AI-driven analytics, ensuring optimal functionality and reducing downtime. Integrating IoT sensors within medical equipment enables continuous monitoring, allowing for early detection of potential issues.
- Startups in Remote Patient Monitoring: Several startups are leveraging AI-enabled IoMT for remote patient monitoring. These solutions frequently entail wearable devices outfitted with sensors that consistently gather health data, which is subsequently analyzed by AI algorithms. This method enables prompt identification of health problems and permits appropriate actions, hence enhancing patient outcomes and decreasing healthcare expenses.

1.6.1 Real-World Examples of AI and IoT Integration in Healthcare

Following real-world examples highlight the diverse applications of AI and IoT integration in healthcare, showcasing how these technologies work synergistically to improve patient outcomes, streamline healthcare operations, and enhance the overall quality of care:

- Early Detection of Sepsis with AI: Hospitals have implemented AI algorithms in conjunction with IoT devices to detect early signs of sepsis. These systems continuously monitor patients' vital signs, such as heart rate and temperature, using IoT sensors. AI algorithms analyze the data in real-time, providing healthcare professionals with alerts and early warnings of potential sepsis, enabling prompt intervention.

- Smart Wearables for Chronic Disease Management: IoT sensors and AI analytics are integrated into wearable devices to monitor and control chronic diseases like diabetes and cardiovascular problems. These gadgets monitor essential signs, physical activity, along with other pertinent health parameters. AI algorithms process this data to generate insights into the health of patients and deliver tailored recommendations to manage their illnesses.
- Remote Patient Monitoring with IoT: Various healthcare providers are adopting IoT-enabled devices for remote patient monitoring. These devices, ranging from smart home health monitors to wearable gadgets, collect patient data and transmit it to healthcare systems. AI algorithms then analyze the data to identify trends, anomalies, or potential health issues, allowing for timely interventions and reducing the need for frequent hospital visits.
- AI-Assisted Radiology Imaging: Radiology departments in hospitals are integrating AI algorithms with imaging devices such as MRI and CT scanners. These AI systems can assist radiologists in interpreting medical images more efficiently and accurately. The combination of IoT sensors within the imaging equipment and AI analysis enhances diagnostic capabilities, leading to improved patient outcomes.
- Predictive Analytics for Patient Admissions: Hospitals and healthcare systems are using AI-driven predictive analytics in combination with IoT data to forecast patient admission rates. By analyzing historical patient data, environmental factors, and other relevant parameters, these systems can predict periods of high patient influx. This helps healthcare facilities allocate resources effectively, optimize staffing levels, and enhance overall operational efficiency.
- Medication Adherence Monitoring: IoT-enabled pill dispensers and smart medication packaging, combined with AI algorithms, are employed to monitor and improve medication adherence. These systems track when patients take their medications and can send reminders or alerts to both patients and healthcare providers. AI analysis of adherence patterns can contribute to personalized medication management plans.

1.7 CHALLENGES AND ETHICAL CONSIDERATIONS

The integration of AI into the IoMT presents a myriad of challenges and ethical considerations within the realm of enhanced healthcare systems (Rajkomar et al., 2019). One major challenge revolves around data security and privacy, as the vast amount of sensitive health data collected by IoMT devices and processed by AI algorithms necessitates robust measures to protect patient confidentiality (Topol, 2019). Interoperability issues arise due to the diversity of devices and standards in healthcare, hindering seamless communication and data exchange. Additionally, the transparency and interpretability of AI algorithms pose challenges, as complex machine learning models may operate as "black boxes," making it difficult to comprehend their decision-making processes. Ethical concerns include issues related to informed consent, the responsible use of patient data, and the potential for bias in AI algorithms, which may lead to disparities in healthcare outcomes. Balancing the promise of enhanced healthcare through AI-enabled IoMT with these challenges requires a comprehensive approach that addresses technological, legal, and ethical dimensions to ensure the responsible and equitable deployment of these transformative technologies.

1.7.1 Ethical Concerns in AI and IoT Applications in Healthcare

The integration of AI and the IoT in healthcare brings about several ethical concerns that need careful consideration. One primary concern revolves around data privacy and security, given the highly sensitive nature of health information (Jabeen et al., 2021). As IoT devices collect and transmit vast amounts of patient data, ensuring robust measures to safeguard this information from unauthorized access or breaches becomes paramount. Informed consent is another ethical consideration, as patients may not always fully understand how their data is being used or may not have sufficient control over its dissemination. Moreover, the potential for biases in AI algorithms poses ethical challenges, as these systems may inadvertently perpetuate or exacerbate existing disparities in healthcare outcomes, particularly if the training data used for AI models reflects existing biases in the healthcare system. The openness and comprehensibility of AI judgments are crucial to enable healthcare providers and patients to fully understand and have confidence in the suggestions generated by AI systems. Moreover, there are apprehensions over the enduring consequences on the doctor-patient rapport, as dependence on AI could modify the dynamics of interpersonal communication in healthcare environments. To tackle these ethical concerns, a comprehensive approach involving experts from various fields such as technology, ethics, policymaking, and healthcare is necessary. This approach aims to develop guidelines as well as frameworks that give priority to patient well-being, privacy, and fairness when implementing IoT and artificial intelligence technologies in healthcare.

1.7.2 Legal and Regulatory Challenges

The integration of AI into the internet of medical things IoMT within healthcare systems is accompanied by significant legal and regulatory challenges. One key challenge is the lack of comprehensive and standardized regulations governing AI and IoMT in many jurisdictions (Shickel et al., 2018). The rapidly evolving nature of these technologies often outpaces the development of appropriate legal frameworks, leading to uncertainty regarding liability, accountability, and compliance with existing healthcare laws. The question of ownership and control over the vast amount of health data generated by IoMT devices is another legal challenge. Clarifying the rights and responsibilities of various stakeholders, including healthcare providers, technology developers, and patients, is crucial. Moreover, issues related to medical device regulations and certification standards for AI-driven healthcare applications need careful consideration. Striking a balance between fostering innovation and ensuring patient safety through regulatory measures remains a complex task. Legal frameworks also need to address data protection and privacy concerns, especially in light of stringent regulations like the General Data Protection Regulation (GDPR) in Europe. As these legal and regulatory challenges continue to evolve, collaboration between policymakers, legal experts, industry stakeholders, and healthcare professionals becomes essential to create frameworks that facilitate the responsible development and deployment of AI-enabled IoMT while upholding patient rights and safety.

1.7.3 Patient Consent and Data Ownership

Obtaining meaningful and informed consent from patients for the collection, sharing, and utilization of their health data is a complex challenge. The interconnected nature of IoMT devices and the extensive data processing involved in AI applications demand a clear and comprehensive understanding from patients about how their data will be utilized. Patients should have the autonomy to decide whether they are comfortable with their health information being used for AI analysis, personalized medicine, or other purposes.

Data ownership is closely tied to consent, raising questions about who ultimately owns and controls the health data generated by IoMT devices (Ozdemir and Tumerdem, 2019). While patients are the primary sources of this data, the involvement of various stakeholders, including healthcare providers, technology companies, and researchers, complicates the landscape. Striking a balance between ensuring patients' rights to ownership and control over their health data and facilitating responsible data sharing for research and healthcare improvements is a delicate ethical challenge.

To address these concerns, healthcare systems and AI/IoMT developers must prioritize transparency in communicating with patients about data usage, implement robust consent mechanisms that go beyond mere legal compliance, and establish clear policies regarding data ownership and access. Ethical frameworks that emphasize patient empowerment, privacy, and the fair and responsible use of health data are crucial in navigating the evolving landscape of AI-enabled IoMT in healthcare.

1.8 FUTURE TRENDS AND INNOVATIONS

Predicting future trends and innovations in the dynamic field of AI enabled IoMT for enhanced healthcare systems involves anticipating the evolution of emerging technologies (Bhambri et al., 2023). Some of the potential future trends and innovations are:

- Advancements in Telemedicine and Remote Patient Monitoring: The integration of AI and IoMT is expected to further enhance telemedicine and remote patient monitoring capabilities. Advanced wearables and sensors will enable continuous health monitoring, allowing for real-time data collection and analysis. This trend can lead to more personalized and proactive healthcare interventions, reducing the need for hospital visits and improving overall patient outcomes.

- Edge Computing for Real-Time Processing: Edge computing entails the processing of data in proximity to its origin, specifically IoMT devices, instead of depending exclusively on central cloud servers. Implementing this method can decrease the time delay and improve the ability to analyze data in real-time. Accelerated examination of health information at the periphery can result in expedited decision-making, particularly in urgent circumstances, and may contribute to more prompt and effective healthcare systems.
- Blockchain for Secure Health Data Exchange: Blockchain technology is gaining traction for its potential to ensure secure and transparent health data exchange. It can enhance data integrity, privacy, and interoperability in AI and IoMT applications. Improved security and trust in health data transactions can encourage greater collaboration among healthcare entities and foster the responsible sharing of patient information.
- Explainable AI for Healthcare Decision Support: As AI systems become more complex, the need for explainable AI (XAI) is growing. Future innovations will likely focus on making AI algorithms more interpretable, providing clearer insights into their decision-making processes. Explainable AI is crucial in healthcare settings, where trust and understanding of AI recommendations are essential for gaining acceptance among healthcare professionals and patients.
- Personalized Medicine and Treatment Plans: AI algorithms, fueled by extensive patient data and genomic information, will contribute to the advancement of personalized medicine (Ravi et al., 2017). Treatment plans can be tailored to individual patient profiles, optimizing therapeutic outcomes. Personalized health care has the capacity to transform healthcare by optimizing treatment effectiveness, avoiding negative effects, and enhancing overall patient contentment.
- AI-Driven Drug Discovery and Development: The utilization of AI in drug discovery is on the rise, facilitating the rapid identification of promising molecules and streamlining clinical trial procedures. Accelerated and economically efficient drug development procedures can result in the identification of innovative medicines and therapies, effectively fulfilling unfulfilled medical requirements.
- Human Augmentation Technologies: Integrating AI and IoMT into human augmentation technologies, such as smart prosthetics and brain-computer interfaces, holds promise for enhancing the quality of life for individuals with disabilities or chronic conditions. This trend may lead to breakthroughs in rehabilitation, neurology, and assistive technologies, fostering a more inclusive and supportive healthcare environment.

1.8.1 Prospects for AI and IoT in the Future of Healthcare

The prospects for AI and the IoT in the future of healthcare are promising and transformative. AI's ability to analyze vast datasets, coupled with the real-time data collection capabilities of IoT devices, is expected to revolutionize diagnostics, treatment strategies, and overall healthcare delivery. Predictive analytics powered by AI can enable early detection of diseases, personalized treatment plans, and efficient resource allocation. The integration of AI and IoT in wearable devices and medical sensors is likely to foster a shift towards proactive and preventive healthcare, with continuous monitoring and data-driven insights. Moreover, the collaborative potential of AI and IoT can enhance interoperability, leading to more seamless communication between healthcare systems and devices (Ritu and Bhambri, 2022). As these technologies continue to mature, the future healthcare landscape holds the promise of improved patient outcomes, cost-effectiveness, and a more patient-centric, data-driven approach to healthcare management. However, these advancements must be accompanied by robust ethical frameworks and privacy measures to ensure responsible and secure implementation in the evolving healthcare ecosystem.

1.8.2 Potential Impact on Healthcare Delivery and Patient Outcomes

The seamless synergy of AI and IoMT can streamline and optimize healthcare processes, leading to more efficient and personalized care. Real-time data collection through interconnected devices enables continuous patient monitoring, facilitating early detection of health issues and allowing for timely interventions. AI-driven analytics contribute to more accurate diagnostics, treatment planning, and the development of personalized medicine, ultimately enhancing the precision and effectiveness of healthcare interventions. Additionally, the potential for predictive analytics can revolutionize preventive care by identifying and addressing health risks before they escalate. This transformative impact on healthcare delivery, characterized by improved efficiency, accuracy, and personalization, has the potential to result in better patient outcomes, reduced hospitalization rates, and an overall enhancement of the quality of healthcare services.

1.9 CONCLUSION

In conclusion, this chapter has explored the intricate intersection of AI and the IoMT to enhance healthcare systems. Key points have been elucidated, including the foundational aspects of AI and IoT in healthcare, real-world applications, challenges, and ethical considerations. The integration of AI with IoMT presents unparalleled opportunities for revolutionizing healthcare delivery, from personalized medicine and early disease detection to optimizing healthcare operations. The emphasis on patient consent, data ownership, and ethical considerations underscores the importance of responsible deployment, ensuring that the transformative potential of AI-enabled IoMT aligns with patient welfare, privacy, and equitable access to healthcare resources.

Looking ahead, the implications for the future of healthcare are profound. The convergence of AI and IoMT is poised to redefine patient care, making it more proactive, personalized, and accessible. Continuous advancements in telemedicine, remote patient monitoring, and personalized treatment plans are likely to become standard practices. However, to fully realize these benefits, further research and development are essential. Future efforts should focus on addressing existing challenges, such as scalability, interoperability, and ethical concerns. Moreover, exploring the potential of emerging technologies like blockchain for secure health data exchange and advancing explainable AI will be crucial. Collaborative efforts among researchers, healthcare professionals, policymakers, and technology developers are essential to shape a future where AI-enabled IoMT not only transforms healthcare systems but does so responsibly, ethically, and in a manner that prioritizes the well-being of patients.

REFERENCES

Abiodun, O. I., Jantan, A., & Omolara, A. E. (2018). Datasets for machine learning with IoT applications: A survey. *Information Fusion*, 42, 34–46.

Alkhodre, F., Alameh, M. G., Alasaad, A., & AL-Dhalaan, M. (2019). Towards IoT-based health informatics: Implementation of a framework for developing a diabetes monitoring system. *IEEE Access*, 7, 76451–76462.

Arora, R., Saini, R., & Jain, P. (2019). A review of internet of things (IoT) based health care system. In *Proceedings of the international conference on inventive communication and computational technologies (ICICCT)*. IEEE (pp. 1–5).

Arora, S., & Patel, N. (2018). Internet of Things (IoT): A new era of healthcare service delivery. *Advances in Human-Computer Interaction*, 2018, Article ID 4592805.

Babu, G. C. N., Gupta, S., Bhambri, P., Leo, L. M., Rao, B. H., & Kumar, S. (2021). A semantic health observation system development based on the IoT sensors. *Turkish Journal of Physiotherapy and Rehabilitation*, 32(3), 1721–1729.

Bakshi, P., Bhambri, P., & Thapar, V. (2021). A review paper on wireless sensor network techniques in internet of things (IoT). In *Proceedings of the international conference on contemporary issues in engineering & technology*. GNA University, Phagwara.

Banaee, H., Ahmed, M. U., & Loutfi, A. (2015). Data mining for wearable sensors in health monitoring systems: A review of recent trends and challenges. *Sensors*, 15(10), 26472–26504.

Bhambri, P., Singh, M., Dhanoa, I. S., & Kumar, M. (2022). Deployment of ROBOT for HVAC duct and disaster management. *Oriental Journal of Computer Science and Technology*, 15.

Bhambri, P., Singh, M., Jain, A., Dhanoa, I. S., Sinha, V. K., & Lal, S. (2021). Classification of the GENE expression data with the aid of optimized feature selection. *Turkish Journal of Physiotherapy and Rehabilitation*, 32(3), 1158–1167.

Bhambri, P., Singh, S., Sangwan, S., Devi, J., & Jain, S. (2023). Plants recognition using leaf image pattern analysis. *Journal of Survey in Fisheries Sciences*, 10(2S), 3863–3871. Green Wave Publishing of Canada.

Bose, M. M., Yadav, D., Bhambri, P., & Shankar, R. (2021). Electronic customer relationship management: Benefits and pre-implementation considerations. *Journal of Maharaja Sayajirao University of Baroda*, 55(01(VI)), 1343–1350. The Maharaja Sayajirao University of Baroda.

Bröring, A., & Strüker, J. (2019). An IoT based system architecture for personalized and preventive healthcare. In *Proceedings of the IEEE European conference on networks and communications (EuCNC)*. IEEE (pp. 341–345).

Car, J., & Sheikh, A. (2019). Wearing sensors to monitor the elderly. *The New England Journal of Medicine*, 381(26), 2586–2587.

Charitos, T., Koutkias, V., Stalidis, G., & Maglaveras, N. (2019). IoT-based biomedical data collection and monitoring: Review on physiological signals. *Computers in Biology and Medicine*, 111, 103346.

Chen, M., Hao, Y., & Hwang, K. (2018). Artificial intelligence in healthcare: A comprehensive survey. *Artificial Intelligence Review*, 49(1), 1–30.

Chen, M., Masse, F., & Lalla-Ruiz, E. (2019). Artificial intelligence and the internet of things. *IEEE Internet of Things Journal*, 6(1), 1.

Chung, K., Park, J. Y., & Lee, J. (2018). Security and privacy issues in health data and mobile health apps. In *Proceedings of the international conference on information networking (ICOIN)*. IEEE (pp. 530–533).

Devadutta, K., Bhambri, P., Gountia, D., Mehta, V., Mangla, M., Patan, R., Kumar, A., Agarwal, P. K., Sharma, A., Singh, M., & Gadicha, A. B. (2020). Method for cyber security in email communication among networked computing devices [Patent application number 202031002649]. India.

Dey, N., Ashour, A. S., Shi, F., & Bejleri, I. (Eds.). (2019). *Internet of things and big data technologies for next generation healthcare*. Springer.

Esteva, A., Kuprel, B., Novoa, R. A., Ko, J., Swetter, S. M., Blau, H. M., & Thrun, S. (2017). Dermatologist-level classification of skin cancer with deep neural networks. *Nature*, 542(7639), 115–118.

Gartner. (2019). *Gartner says worldwide spending on the internet of things to reach $1.2 trillion in 2022*. Retrieved from www.gartner.com/en/newsroom/press-releases/2019-11-13-gartner-says-worldwide-spending-on-the-internet-of-things-to-reach-1-point-2-trillion-in-2022

Greenspan, H., van Ginneken, B., & Summers, R. M. (2016). Guest editorial deep learning in medical imaging: Overview and future promise of an exciting new technique. *IEEE Transactions on Medical Imaging*, 35(5), 1153–1159.

Hsieh, J. C., & Chen, Y. C. (2018). A systematic review of utilizing internet of things for healthcare. *Computers, Materials & Continua*, 57(2), 249–266.

Istepanian, R. S., & Sungoor, A. (2019). Introduction to the special section on internet of medical things. *IEEE Journal of Biomedical and Health Informatics*, 23(3), 935–937.

Jabeen, A., Pallathadka, H., Pallathadka, L. K., & Bhambri, P. (2021). E-CRM successful factors for business enterprises CASE STUDIES. *Journal of Maharaja Sayajirao University of Baroda*, 55(01(VI)), 1332–1342. The Maharaja Sayajirao University of Baroda.

Kuo, A. M. H., Borycki, E., & Kushniruk, A. W. (2018). A model for smart homes for managing health care services: A qualitative study of design and functionality. *JMIR mHealth and uHealth*, 6(6), e140.

Kuzhaloli, S., Devaneyan, P., Sitaraman, N., Periyathanbi, P., Gurusamy, M., & Bhambri, P. (2020). IoT based smart kitchen application for gas leakage monitoring [Patent application number 202041049866A]. India.

Miotto, R., Wang, F., Wang, S., Jiang, X., & Dudley, J. T. (2018). Deep learning for healthcare: Review, opportunities, and challenges. *Briefings in Bioinformatics*, 19(6), 1236–1246.

Niazi, M., Parwani, A. V., Gurcan, M. N., & Ghose, S. (2019). An overview of deep learning in medical imaging focusing on MRI. *Journal of the American College of Radiology*, 16(11), 1585–1592.

Ozdemir, S., & Tumerdem, Y. (2019). Healthcare IoT security issues and perspectives. *Procedia Computer Science*, 155, 458–465.

Pei, L., & Zheng, Y. (2019). Challenges and opportunities: From big data to knowledge in AI-based personalized medicine. *IEEE Access*, 7, 35349–35357.

Rajkomar, A., Dean, J., & Kohane, I. (2019). Machine learning in medicine. *New England Journal of Medicine*, 380(14), 1347–1358.

Rajkomar, A., Oren, E., Chen, K., Dai, A. M., Hajaj, N., Hardt, M., . . . Dean, J. (2018). Scalable and accurate deep learning with electronic health records. *NPJ Digital Medicine*, 1(1), 1–10.

Rana, R., Bhambri, P., & Chhabra, Y. (2022). Deployment of distributed clustering approach in WSNs and IoTs. In *Cloud and fog computing platforms for internet of things*. Chapman and Hall/CRC (pp. 85–98).

Rana, R., Chhabra, Y., & Bhambri, P. (2021). Design and development of distributed clustering approach in wireless sensor network. *Webology*, 18(1), 696–712.

Ravi, D., Wong, C., Deligianni, F., Berthelot, M., Andreu-Perez, J., Lo, B., & Yang, G. Z. (2017). Deep learning for health informatics. *IEEE Journal of Biomedical and Health Informatics*, 21(1), 4–21.

Ritu, & Bhambri, P. (2022). A CAD system for software effort estimation. Paper presented at the International Conference on Technological Advancements in Computational Sciences, 140–146. IEEE. DOI: 10.1109/ICTACS56270.2022.9988123.

Shickel, B., Tighe, P. J., Bihorac, A., & Rashidi, P. (2018). Deep EHR: A survey of recent advances in deep learning techniques for electronic health record (EHR) analysis. *IEEE Journal of Biomedical and Health Informatics*, 22(5), 1589–1604.

Singh, M., Bhambri, P., Lal, S., Singh, Y., Kaur, M., & Singh, J. (2021). Design of the effective technique to improve memory and time constraints for sequence alignment. *International Journal of Applied Engineering Research (Netherlands)*, 6(2), 127–142. Roman Science Publications and Distributions.

Smith, A. (2018). Internet of things applications in healthcare: A comprehensive review. *Journal of Healthcare Informatics Research*, 2(1), 17–33.

Sumathi, N., Thirumagal, J., Jagannathan, S., Bhambri, P., & Ahamed, I. N. (2021). A comprehensive review on bionanotechnology for the 21st century. *Journal of the Maharaja Sayajirao University of Baroda*, 55(1), 114–131.

Thilakanathan, D., Chen, S., Nepal, S., Calvo, R., & Chen, J. (2018). Blockchain-based system for secure data storage with private-key only retrieval. *IEEE Transactions on Industrial Informatics*, 14(6), 2581–2589.

Topol, E. J. (2019). High-performance medicine: The convergence of human and artificial intelligence. *Nature Medicine*, 25(1), 44–56.

Vijayalakshmi, P., Shankar, R., Karthik, S., & Bhambri, P. (2021). Impact of work from home policies on workplace productivity and employee sentiments during the Covid-19 pandemic. *Journal of Maharaja Sayajirao University of Baroda*, 55(01(VI)), 1314–1331. The Maharaja Sayajirao University of Baroda.

World Health Organization. (2018). *Ethics and governance of artificial intelligence for health.* Retrieved from www.who.int/health-topics/artificial-intelligence/ethics

2 Internet of Medical Things with Artificial Intelligence for Improved Healthcare Systems

N. Chaithra, Janhvi Jha, Anu Sayal and Atharv Rajesh Gangodkar

2.1 INTRODUCTION

The rapid and exponential growth of connectivity, intelligent devices, and AI is transforming healthcare. These advances culminate on the internet of medical things (IoMT), a hardware component that will change events. Interconnected medical devices on different networks monitor patient care as part of the internet of things (IoT). Machine learning-based artificial intelligence, interfacial sensors, and automation enable continuous patient health monitoring with minimal human intervention in healthcare IoT devices. It connects patients and healthcare professionals by remotely retrieving, examining, and transferring medical data via medical devices over a secure network (Razdan and Sharma, 2021). IoMT technologies enable wireless health monitoring, reducing hospitalization and costs. The internet of medical things market includes stationary and wearable health monitoring devices for hospitals and clinics and real-time wearables for homes. Smart wristbands, smartphone-integrated devices, electronic textiles and garments, and sports watches can track fitness and health (Manimurugan et al., 2020). AI in IoMT systems automates and transforms processes. IoMT solutions using AI improve healthcare access, delivery, and cost. Artificial intelligence and advanced connectivity enable real-time vital sign monitoring and disease detection through scan analysis. The technology allows proactive, predictive, and accurate healthcare. This chapter examines the integration of AI and the IoMT in critical healthcare sectors and their effects (Gupta et al., 2023).

First, we explain the framework and examine the key components that make IoMT systems work. Then, we examine cutting-edge AI technologies like quantum computing, machine learning, and natural language processing. These technologies boost interconnected medical devices and data networks, causing exponential

 DOI: 10.1201/9781032698519-2

growth. Many examples of AI-assisted IoMT improvements in remote patient monitoring, diagnosis, and treatment planning are in the paper.

AI-facilitated healthcare ecosystems require security, which this chapter addresses. Furthermore, it sheds light on effective privacy measures (Qiu et al., 2021). In conclusion, we will analyze emerging trends and make evidence-based predictions about these rapidly advancing technologies' futures. This chapter combines academic, industry, and policy perspectives to show how integrating AI and IoMT can transform global healthcare.

2.2 BASICS OF INTERNET OF MEDICAL THINGS (IoMT)

Cloud computing, wireless body area networks (WBANs), edge computing, fog computing, autonomic computing, communication technology advances, and sensor integration within the IoT create many benefits and opportunities in various fields (Rahman and Hossain, 2021). Many IoT healthcare applications use widely adopted technologies. WBANs connect patient sensors and other communication or data processing devices like routers and gateways. Fog computing processes data quickly, while cloud computing stores and analyzes data. The IoMT has promising clinical and non-clinical applications (Dalal et al., 2020).

Medical IoT systems, advancing telemedicine and diagnostics, rely on efficient data exchange. IoT's network of sensors and devices facilitates remote monitoring and precision healthcare. Data visualization, processing, and intelligent modules incorporating deep learning are essential. IoMT's data acquisition involves biosensors, both wearable (e.g., fitness trackers, cancer cell detectors) and non-wearable (e.g., intelligent medication dispensers), requiring signal amplification for analysis. IoT gateways connect these sensors to the cloud, with CPUs and wireless connectors playing a pivotal role in data management.

In healthcare, the IoMT monitors body temperature, ECG readings, blood pressure, and oxygen saturation. Dashboards help doctors monitor patients' vital signs. Wearable devices use customized sensors to collect data (Naresh et al., 2020). These tiny sensors can be discreetly attached to clothing using expert sewing or seamless integration. Famous wearables include Fitbit, Apple Watch, and Samsung Galaxy Gear. Wearable devices use sensors to continuously monitor physiological parameters like body temperature, respiration rate, pulse oximetry, and blood pressure (Baker et al., 2017).

Huang and their research group published a comprehensive study in 2014 on their IoT-based Medical Nursing System (MNS). This advanced system seamlessly integrates 2G-3G, WSN, RFID, sensors, ZigBee, Wi-Fi, and Bluetooth data transfer technologies. These technologies also improve pharmaceutical administration precision (Huang and Cheng, 2014). Kumar introduced an innovative OSA and related condition monitoring method in a 2016 study. Shanin and colleagues also developed an e-health system to continuously monitor electrocardiogram (ECG), body temperature, foot pressure, and heart rate (Adamis et al., 2020). They say this system is adaptable and energy efficient. Fog computing and IoT were seamlessly integrated into Sood and Mahajan's healthcare system to detect chikungunya outbreaks. Fog nodes collect sensor data and analyze it using the fuzzy c-means algorithm (Sood and Mahajan, 2017). Kumar also proposed an IoT-based architectural framework for mental healthcare applications in 2017. This architectural design includes sensors that detect vital signs of health and send data to the Intel Qurie hardware platform (Kumar, 2017).

2.3 REVOLUTIONARY AI TECHNOLOGIES IN IoMT

2.3.1 Deep Learning and Neural Networks

Health records, especially disease prevention, healing, and treatment, depend on medical images. In computerized diagnostics, image classification is difficult (Singh et al., 2004). Researchers proposed using optimal deep learning to classify brain imaging, lung cancer, and Alzheimer's disease. The researchers created a Deep Learning (DL) model for medical image classification that includes preprocessing, feature selection, and classification. This study aims to create a reliable medical image classification feature selection model. The Opposition-based Crowd Search (OCS) approach aims to improve the DL classifier. The OCS algorithm chooses the best preprocessed image features. The analyzed attributes include many textures and grayscale levels. To conclude, ideal attributes improved medical image diagnosis precision, selectivity, and responsiveness, improving classification (Raj et al., 2020).

Deep learning enhances medical image classification and reduces reliance on medical professionals. Generative Adversarial Networks (GANs) create synthetic medical images, supplementing training data for CNNs. The Firefly Algorithm (FA) selects optimal elements for data-based learning, improving model performance (Gupta et al., 2023). IoT and deep learning innovate elderly cardiac care, with portable devices and algorithms enabling remote healthcare (Mahmoud et al., 2018). Body Sensor Networks (BSNs) monitor vital signs, advancing healthcare infrastructure.

The IoMT's integration in cardiac disease screening enables self-examination for heart abnormalities. Deep learning and skin temperature monitoring enhance valvular disease screening and heart blood supply assessment (Su et al., 2021; Jha et al., 2023). Lung CT image segmentation using transfer learning and machine learning shows high accuracy (Birckhead et al., 2019; Wang et al., 2017). AFD-UNet and DeepEDN (Ding et al., 2021) advance image segmentation and encryption. EDCNN improves heart disease prognosis, outperforming several models with a 99.1% accuracy (Pan et al., 2020). AHDCNN diagnoses chronic kidney disease, leveraging CNNs and CRFs for enhanced detection and segmentation (Chen et al., 2020).

2.3.2 Quantum Computing in Drug Discovery

Quantum computing works well with many computationally demanding healthcare applications in the IoT digital healthcare framework, including interconnected medical devices like medical sensors that can be linked to the Internet or cloud (Singh et al., 2004). The improved processing capabilities benefit the internet of things in healthcare and could lead to groundbreaking advances in quantum computing (Jain and Bhambri, 2005). Using qubits instead of classical bits could improve healthcare and pharmaceutical research. This transition could speed up clinical trials, measure the affinity between a biomolecule (like DNA or protein) and its ligand or binding partner (like a medicine), help develop new pharmaceuticals and enzymes, and enable protein folding studies. The following are brief examples of possible uses. Fast DNA sequencing with a quantum computer allows for personalized treatment plans (Banchi et al., 2020). Using extensive modeling techniques can speed up drug development (Fedorov and Leonov, 2018). Quantum computing may help medical professionals develop real-time imaging systems with higher resolution and speed. It can also solve complex optimization problems like creating a radiation plan that kills cancer cells without harming healthy tissue. Quantum computing (QC) will enable molecular interaction analysis at the fundamental level, opening new avenues for drug development and medical research (Sayal et al., 2023a). Whole-genome sequencing and analysis are time-consuming, but qubits may help. Real-time computation, medical data security, chronic disease prediction, and drug discovery can revolutionize the healthcare system with QC (Ur Rasool et al., 2023).

Quantum computing, leveraging quantum mechanics, is transformative in computational chemistry and pharmaceutical research. It synergizes with advanced machine learning techniques and IoMT for quantum data processing. Quantum biology, particularly quantum-based mRNA technology, aligns with IoMT's focus on biological data (Rattan et al., 2005a). The internet of viral things (IoVT), using biological networks for information transmission, presents bioethical and safety challenges, underscoring the need for robust security in IoMT. This paradigm shift emphasizes interconnectedness and data-driven value creation in IoMT and IoVT ecosystems (Virolle et al., 2020; Gupta et al., 2023).

2.3.3 Natural Language Processing for Patient Records Analysis

NLP is crucial in IoMT for healthcare, enhancing patient outcome prediction, hospital triage systems, and early-stage chronic disease diagnostics. It processes unstructured medical data, aiding in communication through NLG and NLU, and is instrumental in chatbot interactions (Lin et al., 2019). CogStack and other tools facilitate data organization and clinical categorization (Shi et al., 2019). Despite the move towards structured EHRs, NLP remains essential in IoMT, demonstrated by chatbots in apps like Health Tap and Babylon Health, and has been particularly valuable during the COVID-19 pandemic (Locke et al., 2021).

2.3.4 Case Study: AI-Powered Predictive Analytics for Early Disease Detection

In a pioneering study, (Vaccari et al., 2021) explored the use of IoMT devices in integrated healthcare, focusing on patient monitoring. CompuGroup Medical's Health Platform v3, a cloud platform proof-of-concept, adhered to GDPR and medical device certification standards, excelling in data accessibility and aggregation (Kumar et al., 2021). The study involved monitoring vital signs and respiratory rates using interconnected devices like spirometers, ECG patches, and pulse meters, with plans to integrate patient questionnaires and advanced Bluetooth Low Energy sensor communication.

Environmental monitoring systems were installed in both residential and commercial areas to track atmospheric variables, contributing to a comprehensive understanding of health factors. The dataset, combining environmental and health data, is crucial for AI-driven analytics to detect complex patterns and guide medical interventions.

The study utilized a large dataset of biometric data collected over three months, including measurements like oxygen saturation, body temperature, heart rate, blood pressure, and pulmonary function, using various medical devices (Martinez-Martin et al., 2020). This extensive data collection allowed for continuous monitoring of the patient's cardiovascular and respiratory health.

The dataset, structured as 43-element pandas DataFrame, included twelve columns of health indicators (Lu and Mao, 2021). Despite some missing data due to device malfunctions or non-compliance, key columns like FEV1 and PEF were largely complete, essential for pulmonary function assessment (Sayal et al., 2023b). The pandas 'describe().T' function provided a statistical summary of each health metric, aiding in initial data analysis.

Data preprocessing involved excluding certain columns with significant missing values and translating column headers from Italian to English (Riva et al., 2020). A SimpleImputer from the sklearn library was used for mean value imputation to handle missing values. Risk assessment was added to the dataset, calculating a risk score for each patient based on clinically significant thresholds for health metrics.

Exploratory Data Analysis (EDA) included visualizing correlations between health metrics using a heatmap (referring to Figure 2.1 and Figure 2.2) and differentiating patients at risk for pulmonary conditions through various charts. Histograms and boxplots (refer Figure 2.3) were used for a detailed examination of the dataset, revealing the distribution characteristics of each metric.

For predictive modeling, the dataset was split into training and test datasets, with the 'At_Risk' column as the dependent variable. A stratified splitting strategy ensured equitable distribution of the target variable, and feature normalization was performed using z-scores (Rattan et al., 2005b).

Model evaluation involved testing various machine learning models like Logistic Regression, Random Forest classifier, K-Neighbors classifier, Decision Tree classifier, Gradient Boosting classifier, Support Vector Machine, and Gaussian Naive Bayes. Each model's predictive performance was assessed using accuracy scores and confusion matrices. The evaluation highlighted the need for additional validation to ensure the models' relevance to new data (refer Figure 2.4 and Figure 2.5).

2.4 APPLICATIONS OF AI-ENABLED IoMT IN HEALTHCARE

2.4.1 Remote Health Monitoring

2.4.1.1 Next-Gen Wearable Devices with AI Integration

Wearable biosensing devices are advancing rapidly, featuring improved data collection, wireless communication, and interactive interfaces. These AI-assisted

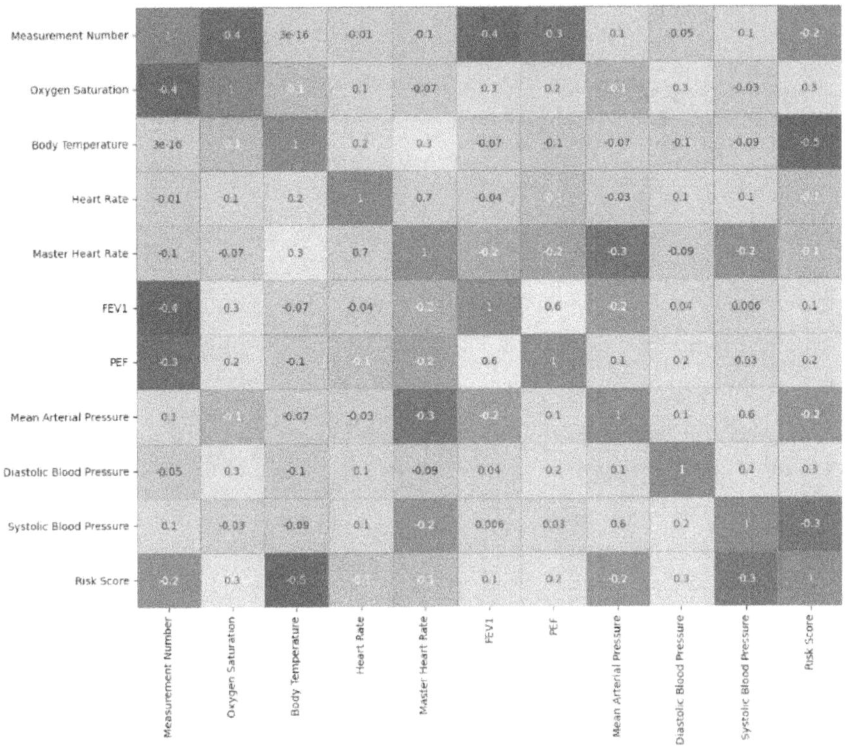

FIGURE 2.1 Heatmap of the dataset.

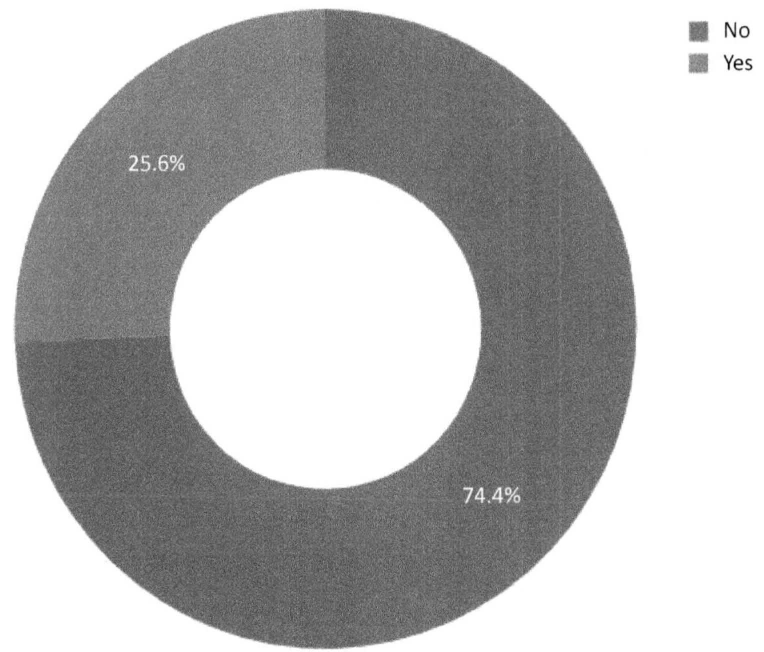

FIGURE 2.2 Pie chart for 'at risk' and 'not at risk'.

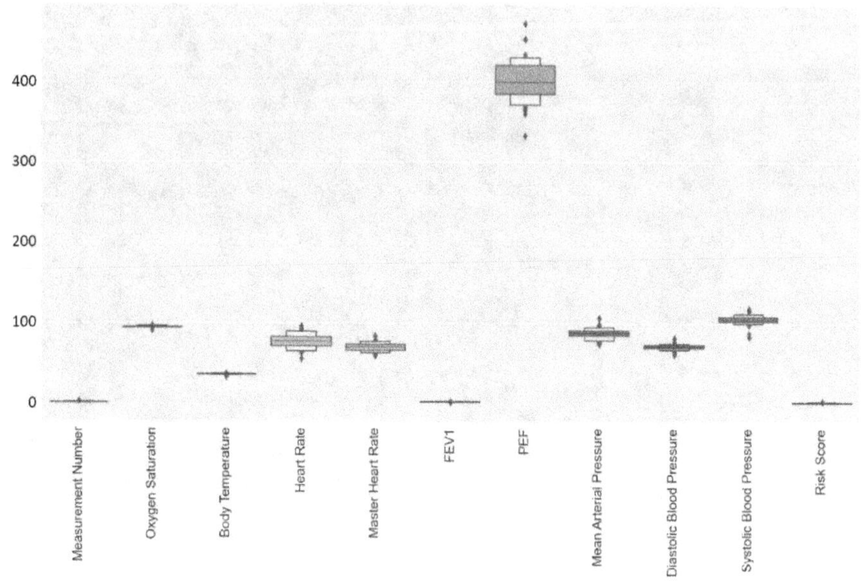

FIGURE 2.3 Boxenplot for different parameters.

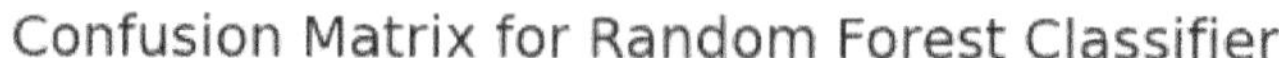

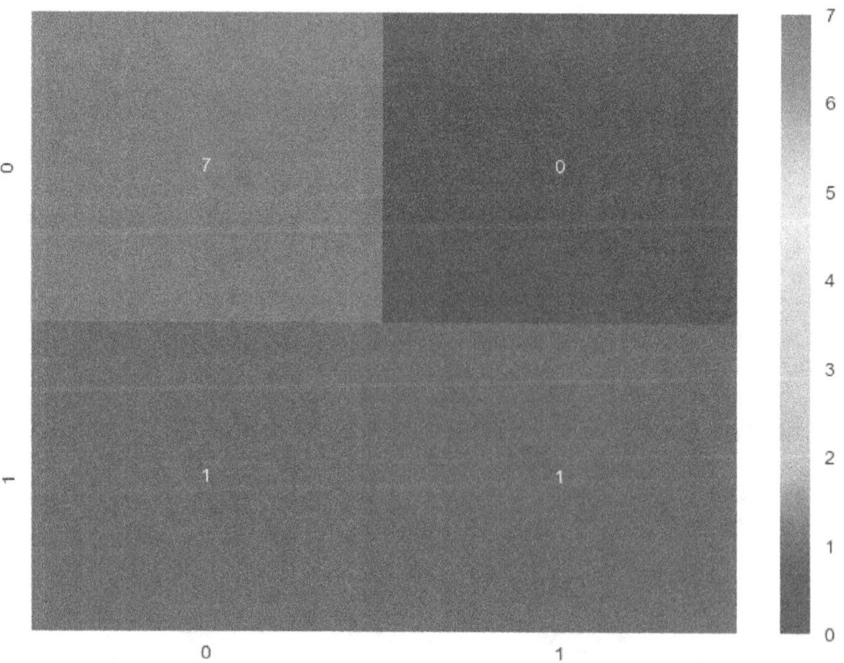

FIGURE 2.4 Confusion matrix for random forest classifier.

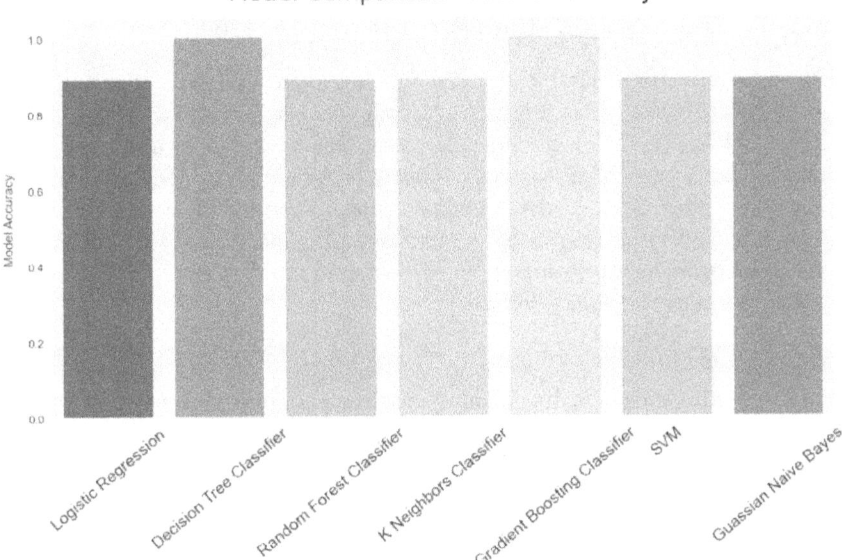

FIGURE 2.5 Bar chart for model comparison.

biosensors, including sensing modules and wireless components, gather extensive physiological data from body fluids using bioreceptors and transducers. They adapt to various forms like wristbands and electronic skin, transmitting data wirelessly for processing and storage. This integration of sensing technology, wireless communication, and AI transforms diagnostics, making non-invasive health monitoring more accessible (Jeong et al., 2021).

2.4.1.2 Case Study

Researchers have explored using Amazon Echo's ultrasonic sensors for fall detection and remote health monitoring. Wrist-worn accelerometers have also been studied for continuous monitoring and fall prediction (Nath et al., 2018). Smart socks with integrated nanogenerators collect user data and transmit it to AI systems for health analysis. Wearable sensors enable monitoring without extensive patient effort. Brain-computer interfaces allow those with disabilities to control appliances using neural signals. However, these require significant cognitive effort. An alternative system uses eye movements for hands-free control (Jafri et al., 2019; Khan et al., 2020).

Wireless EEG headsets, computer vision techniques, and accelerometers provide inexpensive in-home health monitoring to improve care for elderly and disabled patients. Machine learning categorizes patient motion and physiological signals (Sapci and Sapci, 2019). Overall, advances in wearable sensors, wireless communication, and AI analysis facilitate accessible remote health monitoring and assisted living applications to address growing needs.

2.4.2 Assisted Living and Rehabilitation

2.4.2.1 Robotics and AI in Physical Rehabilitation

Smart buildings and wearable devices enable remote patient monitoring, while robotics in healthcare offers physical and cognitive support across various settings (Sharma and Juglan, 2018). Robots, guided by sensors and algorithms, range from autonomous to teleoperated, easing healthcare providers' workloads and enhancing patient independence. They adapt to human behavior, promoting collaborative rehabilitation. Socially assistive robots like Paro and Milo aid in caring for patients with dementia, autism, and other conditions, demonstrating the evolving role of robotics in healthcare (Sayal et al., 2023b).

2.4.2.2 Case Study

Cognitive dysfunction, including memory loss and poor responsiveness, affects daily life following stroke and increases dementia risk. Computer-assisted cognitive rehabilitation uses VR and wearables for personalized, flexible, and affordable programs. VR improves neurorehabilitation and trains episodic memory.

Mild Cognitive Impairment (MCI) increases Alzheimer's disease risk. VR-based interventions are cost-effective alternatives to drug therapies for MCI. Embodied cognition is essential to cognitive rehabilitation and motor function recovery. As embodied technology, VR affects cognition (Cotelli et al., 2019).

In severe brain injury patients, tailored VR interventions can improve cognitive and motor recovery, showing neurorehabilitation potential (Zhang et al., 2020). More implementation studies across diverse populations are needed to maximize VR's cognitive rehabilitation potential. A 17-year-old woman with severe brain injuries from an accident showed improved visual, motor, and cognitive function after personalized VR training during intensive rehabilitation.

2.4.3 Personalized Treatment and Medication

2.4.3.1 AI Algorithms for Personalized Medicine

AI is rapidly evolving in clinical applications, with a focus on ophthalmology. Deep learning, which uses neural networks inspired by biological systems, has revolutionized image analysis. Convolutional neural networks (CNNs) have been crucial in retinal image classification. Due to large datasets, retinal analysis was the initial AI focus. With diverse datasets, AI applications will expand across clinical domains. Ophthalmology image analysis has improved greatly with deep learning, especially CNNs. Early work focused on classifying retinal images using abundant data (Ting et al., 2019). AI applications in many clinical fields are expected to expand as datasets diversify (Budak et al., 2020). Emerging technologies like generative adversarial networks and reinforcement learning should enhance healthcare AI applications. Importantly, automated platforms are democratizing AI, allowing non-specialists to study its healthcare applications. These platforms enable innovation by providing advanced AI tools (Sadda et al., 2018). AI system development relies on use case identification. Patients, clinicians, regulators, and payers have different expectations.

Thus, these perspectives must be considered when shaping AI applications to meet diverse and complex needs (Chaithra et al., 2023).

2.4.3.2 Case Study

Artificial intelligence is transforming healthcare through technologies that can outperform clinicians at certain tasks like pattern recognition and data management. However, AI should collaborate with providers as 'augmented intelligence' rather than fully replacing human roles. AI excels at data processing but lacks human creativity and empathy (Ting et al., 2019).

AI decision-support systems reduce errors, improve clinical decision-making, and analyze complex electronic health records. Advances in natural language processing also enable understanding of unstructured medical data. These innovations have proven useful in areas like oncology, medical imaging, and primary care (Ting et al., 2019).

Precision medicine leverages AI, genetics, and diverse health data to provide individualized care. It allows early disease identification, tailored treatments, and personalized drug dosing. AI-enabled molecular analysis also facilitates targeted cancer therapies. However, successful implementation requires overcoming data biases and respecting privacy (Wang and Preininger, 2019).

Overall, AI augments clinician expertise and enhances data-driven care. But human collaboration remains essential, as empathy and creativity are irreplaceable human skills. Ongoing challenges include algorithmic bias and data limitations affecting diverse groups.

2.5 CUTTING-EDGE HEALTHCARE ANALYTICS

The healthcare industry has many electronic data acquisition, examination, appraisal, conservation, and dissemination obligations. Cloud computing has proven its benefits in telemedicine, healthcare management systems, and bioinformatics. The IoMT, a subset of the IoT, is relevant in today's healthcare landscape (Singh and Singh, 2017). Healthcare apps, the IoMT, smart medical devices, and fast networks working together seamlessly have strengthened medical systems. This has improved disease diagnosis, treatment, monitoring, and management efficiency. Healthcare services and remote monitoring efficiency depend on staying current on technology. To maximize the potential of these technological innovations, it is crucial to accurately identify and address critical requirements. A reliable internet connection, accurate data, high-speed network capabilities, and long-lasting battery performance are essential for smooth operations. The scalability and dependability of 5G technology have proven to be highly effective in meeting market demands (Sutradhar et al., 2023).

In 2021, Dilibal et al., introduced a machine learning method to enhance IoMT medical device development, simplifying AI deficiency diagnosis. Rehman and Hossain developed an IoMT strategy for distinguishing COVID-19 symptoms. Qiu et al., presented a system for healthcare service in fog-computing-based IoMT, raising privacy concerns. Kumar et al., used fuzzy c-means clustering and genetic optimization for emotion detection, and testing on the WESAD dataset. Schmidt et al., (2018) and Indikawati and Winiarti (2020) explored machine learning algorithms for stress detection with high accuracy (Dilibal et al., 2021; Indikawati and Winiarti, 2020).

2.6 ENSURING PATIENT SAFETY AND PRIVACY IN AI-ENABLED IoMT

Securing IoMT systems is crucial due to their susceptibility to cyber threats, as over 70% of IoMT devices are vulnerable (CyberMDX, 2020). Healthcare data, highly valued on the black market, requires comprehensive security infrastructure and adherence to CIANA standards. These standards encompass authentication, data confidentiality, non-repudiation, availability, and integrity.

2.6.1 Security

IoT device security necessitates robust measures like unique identity tokens, security keys, and X.509 certificates for secure gateway connections, with authentication being crucial (Hatzivasilis et al., 2019). IoT devices face connectivity risks, requiring encryption and secure protocols like AMQP, MQTT, and HTTP to mitigate threats like DDoS. In IoMT, cloud computing security challenges include preventing unauthorized data access, necessitating a coordinated defense against multi-host attacks.

2.6.2 Privacy

2.6.2.1 Data Privacy

IoMT security protocols address privacy concerns in transmitting personal information. Data encryption and access control are key (Hatzivasilis et al., 2018). Focus on both intentional and accidental threats, reducing data and using edge computing for protection. User privacy requires concealed zones and k-anonymity (Yamaguchi et al., 2012). Manimurugan et al.'s IDS detects online security breaches effectively (Manimurugan et al., 2020). DNN and DAL methods are used for intrusion detection (Soderi et al., 2017).

2.7 FUTURE TRENDS AND PERSPECTIVES

The AI-IoMT convergence is revolutionizing healthcare with technologies like NLP and predictive analytics. The rise of 5G and developments in sensors enhance medical information exchange. Deep learning advancements facilitate complex health data analysis, leading to autonomous IoMT and home-based health management. This shift towards personalized healthcare necessitates diverse training datasets to minimize biases. Addressing ethical and legal implications, ensuring data privacy, and balancing human cognition with AI are vital in this data-driven era (Naresh et al., 2020).

2.8 CONCLUSION

The AI-IoMT combination promises to revolutionize healthcare, providing individualized care through technologies like wearable devices, chatbots, and machine learning algorithms. This chapter covers AI applications in various healthcare areas, including the challenges in security, privacy, and algorithmic bias. It explores edge computing, 5G, deep learning, and quantum computing, emphasizing patient-centricity and flexibility for evolving healthcare research, with a focus on ethical principles and collaborative frameworks.

REFERENCES

Adamis, A. P., Brittain, C. J., Dandekar, A., & Hopkins, J. J. (2020). Building on the success of anti-vascular endothelial growth factor therapy: A vision for the next decade. *Eye, 34*(11), 1966–1972.

Baker, S. B., Xiang, W., & Atkinson, I. (2017). Internet of things for smart healthcare: Technologies, challenges, and opportunities. *IEEE Access, 5*, 26521–26544.

Banchi, L., Fingerhuth, M., Babej, T., Ing, C., & Arrazola, J. M. (2020). Molecular docking with gaussian boson sampling. *Science Advances, 6*(23). doi:10.1126/sciadv.aax1950

Birckhead, B., Khalil, C., Liu, X., Conovitz, S., Rizzo, A., Danovitch, I., . . . Spiegel, B. (2019). Recommendations for methodology of virtual reality clinical trials in health care by an international working group: iterative study. *JMIR Mental Health, 6*(1), e11973.

Budak, Ü., Guo, Y., Tanyildizi, E., & Şengür, A. (2020). Cascaded deep convolutional encoder-decoder neural networks for efficient liver tumor segmentation. *Medical Hypotheses, 134*, 109431.

Chaithra, N., Jha, J., Sayal, A., Gupta, V., & Gupta, A. (2023). A paradigm shift towards computer vision. In *2023 International Conference on Device Intelligence, Computing and Communication Technologies, (DICCT)*. doi:10.1109/dicct56244.2023.10110300

Chen, G., Ding, C., Li, Y., Hu, X., Li, X., Ren, L., . . . Xue, W. (2020). Prediction of chronic kidney disease using adaptive hybridized deep convolutional neural network on the internet of medical things platform. *IEEE Access, 8*, 100497–100508. doi:10.1109/access.2020.2995310

Cotelli, M., Manenti, R., Brambilla, M., Gobbi, E., Ferrari, C., Binetti, G., & Cappa, S. F. (2019). Cognitive telerehabilitation in mild cognitive impairment, Alzheimer's disease and frontotemporal dementia: A systematic review. *Journal of Telemedicine and Telecare, 25*(2), 67–79.

CyberMDX. (2020). Retrieved from www.healthcareinfosecurity.com/whitepapers/2020-vision-review-major-cybersecurity-issues-affecting-healthcare-w-6017

Dalal, P., Aggarwal, G., & Tejasvee, S. (2020, April). Internet of things (IoT) in healthcare system: IA3 (idea, architecture, advantages and applications). In *Proceedings of the International Conference on Innovative Computing & Communications (ICICC)*. doi:10.2139/ssrn.3566282

Dilibal, C., Davis, B. L., & Chakraborty, C. (2021, June). Generative design methodology for internet of medical things (IoMT)-based wearable biomedical devices. In *2021 3rd International Congress on Human-Computer Interaction, Optimization and Robotic Applications (HORA)* (pp. 1–4). IEEE.

Ding, Y., Wu, G., Chen, D., Zhang, N., Gong, L., Cao, M., & Qin, Z. (2021). DeepEDN: A deep-learning-based image encryption and decryption network for internet of medical things. *IEEE Internet of Things Journal, 8*(3), 1504–1518. doi:10.1109/jiot.2020.3012452

Fedorov, V. V., & Leonov, S. L. (2018). Combinatorial and model-based methods in structuring and optimizing cluster trials. *Platform Trial Designs in Drug Development*, 265–286. doi:10.1201/9781315167756-18

Gupta, A., Chaithra, N., Jha, J., Sayal, A., Gupta, V., & Memoria, M. (2023). Machine learning algorithms for disease diagnosis using medical records: A comparative analysis. In *2023 4th International Conference on Intelligent Engineering and Management (ICIEM)*. doi:10.1109/iciem59379.2023.10165850

Hatzivasilis, G., Fysarakis, K., Soultatos, O., Askoxylakis, I., Papaefstathiou, I., & Demetriou, G. (2018). The industrial internet of things as an enabler for a circular economy Hy-LP: A novel IIoT protocol, evaluated on a wind park's SDN/NFV-enabled 5G industrial network. *Computer Communications*, *119*, 127–137.

Hatzivasilis, G., Soultatos, O., Ioannidis, S., Verikoukis, C., Demetriou, G., & Tsatsoulis, C. (2019, May). Review of security and privacy for the internet of medical things (IoMT). In *2019 15th International Conference on Distributed Computing in Sensor Systems (DCOSS)* (pp. 457–464). IEEE.

Huang, C. H., & Cheng, K. W. (2014). RFID technology combined with IoT application in medical nursing system. *Bulletin of Networking, Computing, Systems, and Software*, *3*(1), 20–24.

Indikawati, F. I., & Winiarti, S. (2020, March). Stress detection from multimodal wearable sensor data. In *IOP Conference Series: Materials Science and Engineering* (Vol. 771, No. 1, p. 012028). IOP Publishing.

Jafri, S. R. A., Hamid, T., Mahmood, R., Alam, M. A., Rafi, T., Ul Haque, M. Z., & Munir, M. W. (2019). Wireless brain computer interface for smart home and medical system. *Wireless Personal Communications*, *106*, 2163–2177.

Jain, V. K., & Bhambri, P. (2005). *Fundamentals of Information Technology & Computer Programming*. KATSONS.

Jeong, H., Lee, J. Y., Lee, K., Kang, Y. J., Kim, J. T., Avila, R., . . . Rogers, J. A. (2021). Differential cardiopulmonary monitoring system for artifact-canceled physiological tracking of athletes, workers, and COVID-19 patients. *Science Advances*, *7*(20), eabg3092.

Jha, J., Vishwakarma, A. K., N, C., Nithin, A., Sayal, A., Gupta, A., & Kumar, R. (2023). Artificial intelligence and applications. In *2023 1st International Conference on Intelligent Computing and Research Trends (ICRT)*. doi:10.1109/icrt57042.2023.10146698

Khan, Z. H., Siddique, A., & Lee, C. W. (2020). Robotics utilization for healthcare digitization in global COVID-19 management. *International Journal of Environmental Research and Public Health*, *17*(11), 3819.

Kumar, A., Sharma, K., & Sharma, A. (2021). Genetically optimized Fuzzy C-means data clustering of IoMT-based biomarkers for fast affective state recognition in intelligent edge analytics. *Applied Soft Computing*, *109*, 107525.

Kumar, N. (2017, August). IoT architecture and system design for healthcare systems. In *2017 International Conference on Smart Technologies for Smart Nation (SmartTechCon)* (pp. 1118–1123). IEEE.

Lin, S. Y., Mahoney, M. R., & Sinsky, C. A. (2019). Ten ways artificial intelligence will transform primary care. *Journal of General Internal Medicine*, *34*(8), 1626–1630. doi:10.1007/s11606-019-05035-1

Locke, S., Bashall, A., Al-Adely, S., Moore, J., Wilson, A., & Kitchen, G. B. (2021). Natural language processing in medicine: A review. *Trends in Anaesthesia and Critical Care*, *38*, 4–9. doi:10.1016/j.tacc.2021.02.007

Lu, W., & Mao, Q. (2021). The effects of family follow-up nursing on elderly cognitive impairment patients' Barthel index scores and mental statuses. *American Journal of Translational Research*, *13*(6), 6702.

Mahmoud, M. M., Rodrigues, J. J., Ahmed, S. H., Shah, S. C., Al-Muhtadi, J. F., Korotaev, V. V., & De Albuquerque, V. H. (2018). Enabling technologies on cloud of things for smart healthcare. *IEEE Access*, *6*, 31950–31967. doi:10.1109/access.2018.2845399

Manimurugan, S., Al-Mutairi, S., Aborokbah, M. M., Chilamkurti, N., Ganesan, S., & Patan, R. (2020). Effective attack detection in internet of medical things smart environment using a deep belief neural network. *IEEE Access*, *8*, 77396–77404.

Martinez-Martin, E., Escalona, F., & Cazorla, M. (2020). Socially assistive robots for older adults and people with autism: An overview. *Electronics*, *9*(2), 367.

Naresh, V. S., Pericherla, S. S., Murty, P. S. R., & Reddi, S. (2020). Internet of things in healthcare: Architecture, applications, challenges, and solutions. *Computer Systems Science & Engineering*, *35*(6).

Nath, R. K., Bajpai, R., & Thapliyal, H. (2018, January). IoT based indoor location detection system for smart home environment. In *2018 IEEE International Conference on Consumer Electronics (ICCE)* (pp. 1–3). IEEE.

Pan, Y., Fu, M., Cheng, B., Tao, X., & Guo, J. (2020). Enhanced deep learning assisted convolutional neural network for heart disease prediction on the internet of medical things platform. *IEEE Access*, *8*, 189503–189512. doi:10.1109/access.2020.3026214

Qiu, Y., Zhang, H., & Long, K. (2021). Computation offloading and wireless resource management for healthcare monitoring in fog-computing-based internet of medical things. *IEEE Internet of Things Journal*, *8*(21), 15875–15883.

Rahman, M. A., & Hossain, M. S. (2021). An internet-of-medical-things-enabled edge computing framework for tackling COVID-19. *IEEE Internet of Things Journal*, *8*(21), 15847–15854.

Raj, R. J., Shobana, S. J., Pustokhina, I. V., Pustokhin, D. A., Gupta, D., & Shankar, K. (2020). Optimal feature selection-based medical image classification using deep learning model in internet of medical things. *IEEE Access*, *8*, 58006–58017. doi:10.1109/access.2020.2981337

Rattan, M., Bhambri, P., & Shaifali. (2005a). Information retrieval using soft computing techniques. In *National Conference on Bio-informatics Computing* (pp. 58–60). TIET.

Rattan, M., Bhambri, P., & Shaifali. (2005b, February). Institution for a sustainable civilization: Negotiating change in a technological culture. In *National Conference on Technical Education in Globalized Environment-Knowledge, Technology & The Teacher* (p. 45). SBBSIET.

Razdan, S., & Sharma, S. (2021). Internet of medical things (IoMT): Overview, emerging technologies, and case studies. *IETE Technical Review*, *39*(4), 775–788.

Riva, G., Mancuso, V., Cavedoni, S., & Stramba-Badiale, C. (2020). Virtual reality in neurorehabilitation: A review of its effects on multiple cognitive domains. *Expert Review of Medical Devices*, *17*(10), 1035–1061.

Sadda, S. R., Tuomi, L. L., Ding, B., Fung, A. E., & Hopkins, J. J. (2018). Macular atrophy in the HARBOR study for neovascular age-related macular degeneration. *Ophthalmology*, *125*(6), 878–886.

Sapci, A. H., & Sapci, H. A. (2019). Innovative assisted living tools, remote monitoring technologies, artificial intelligence-driven solutions, and robotic systems for aging societies: Systematic review. *JMIR Aging*, *2*(2), e15429.

Sayal, A., Jha, J., & Chaithra, N. (2023a). Blockchain: A digital breakthrough in healthcare. *Blockchain for Healthcare*, *4.0*, 1–25. doi:10.1201/9781003408246-1

Sayal, A., Jha, J., Chaithra, N., Gupta, V., Gupta, A., & Memoria, M. (2023b). Blockchain: Its applications and challenges. In *2023 International Conference on Computational Intelligence, Communication Technology and Networking (CICTN)*. doi:10.1109/cictn57981.2023.10140202

Schmidt, P., Reiss, A., Duerichen, R., Marberger, C., & Van Laerhoven, K. (2018, October). Introducing WESAD, a multimodal dataset for wearable stress and affect detection. In *Proceedings of the 20th ACM International Conference on Multimodal Interaction* (pp. 400–408). ACM Digital Library. doi:10.1145/3242969.3242985

Sharma, V., & Juglan, K. C. (2018). Automated classification of fatty and normal liver ultrasound images based on mutual information feature selection. *IRBM*, *39*(5), 313–323. doi:10.1016/j.irbm.2018.09.006

Shi, J., Liu, S., Pruitt, L. C., Luppens, C. L., Ferraro, J. P., Gundlapalli, A. V., . . . Bucher, B. T. (2019). Using natural language processing to improve EHR structured data-based surgical site infection surveillance. In *AMIA Annual Symposium Proceedings* (Vol. 2019, p. 794). American Medical Informatics Association.

Singh, P., Singh, M., & Bhambri, P. (2004, November). Interoperability: A problem of component reusability. In *International Conference on Emerging Technologies in IT Industry* (p. 60). PCTE.

Singh, P., Singh, M., & Bhambri, P. (2005, January). Embedded systems. In *Seminar on Embedded Systems* (pp. 10–15). KMV.

Singh, S., & Singh, N. (2017). Object classification to analyze medical imaging data using deep learning. In *2017 International Conference on Innovations in Information, Embedded and Communication Systems (ICIIECS)*. doi:10.1109/iciiecs.2017.8276099

Soderi, S., Mucchi, L., Hämäläinen, M., Piva, A., & Iinatti, J. (2017). Physical layer security based on spread-spectrum watermarking and jamming receiver. *Transactions on Emerging Telecommunications Technologies*, *28*(7), e3142.

Sood, S. K., & Mahajan, I. (2017). Wearable IoT sensor based healthcare system for identifying and controlling chikungunya virus. *Computers in Industry*, *91*, 33–44.

Su, Y.-S., Ding, T.-J., & Chen, M.-Y. (2021). Deep learning methods in internet of medical things for valvular heart disease screening system. *IEEE Internet of Things Journal*, *8*(23), 16921–16932. doi:10.1109/jiot.2021.3053420

Sutradhar, S., Karforma, S., Bose, R., & Roy, S. (Accepted 2023, April). A dynamic stepwise tiny encryption algorithm with fruit fly optimization for quality of service improvement in healthcare. *Healthcare Analytics*, *3*, 100177. doi:10.1016/j.health.2023.100177

Ting, D. S. W., Pasquale, L. R., Peng, L., Campbell, J. P., Lee, A. Y., Raman, R., . . . Wong, T. Y. (2019). Artificial intelligence and deep learning in ophthalmology. *British Journal of Ophthalmology*, *103*(2), 167–175.

Ur Rasool, R., Ahmad, H. F., Rafique, W., Qayyum, A., Qadir, J., & Anwar, Z. (2023). Quantum computing for healthcare: A review. *Future Internet*, *15*(3), 94. doi:10.3390/fi15030094

Vaccari, I., Orani, V., Paglialonga, A., Cambiaso, E., & Mongelli, M. (2021). A generative adversarial network (GAN) technique for internet of medical things data. *Sensors*, *21*(11), 3726. doi:10.3390/s21113726

Virolle, C., Goldlust, K., Djermoun, S., Bigot, S., & Lesterlin, C. (2020). Plasmid transfer by conjugation in gram-negative bacteria: From the cellular to the community level. *Genes*, *11*(11), 1239. doi:10.3390/genes11111239

Wang, F., & Preininger, A. (2019). AI in health: State of the art, challenges, and future directions. *Yearbook of Medical Informatics*, *28*(01), 016–026.

Wang, S., Zhou, M., Liu, Z., Liu, Z., Gu, D., Zang, Y., . . . Tian, J. (2017). Central focused convolutional neural networks: Developing a data-driven model for lung nodule segmentation. *Medical Image Analysis*, *40*, 172–183. doi:10.1016/j.media.2017.06.014

Yamaguchi, R. S., Hirota, K., Hamada, K., Takahashi, K., Matsuzaki, K., Sakuma, J., & Shirai, Y. (2012, October). Applicability of existing anonymization methods to large location history data in urban travel. In *2012 IEEE International Conference on Systems, Man, and Cybernetics (SMC)* (pp. 997–1004). IEEE.

Zhang, Z., He, T., Zhu, M., Shi, Q., & Lee, C. (2020, January). Smart triboelectric socks for enabling artificial intelligence of things (AIoT) based smart home and healthcare. In *2020 IEEE 33rd International Conference on Micro Electro Mechanical Systems (MEMS)* (pp. 80–83). IEEE.

3 Blockchain for Transparent, Privacy Protected and Secure Health Data Management

Rachna Rana and Pankaj Bhambri

3.1 INTRODUCTION

The utilization of blockchain has dispersed in various commercial enterprise in new years, including healthcare. Since blockchain is a changeless, crystal clear, localized apportioned information that can be used to make a trustworthy series, this is not shocking. Medical information systems are developing as a result of the digitization of the healthcare industry. A person's life depends on welfare, as well as the accompanying data that help diagnose the disease and guide treatment decisions. In the past, a message was located and stored on an information bearer service that could be easily deleted or manipulated (Aggarwal et al., 2019).

3.1.1 Blockchain and Blockchain Engineering

Blockchain: Blockchain became famous due to the success of Bitcoin and can be utilized to make assured and dependable proceedings on a trustworthy system without the help of a centered third organization. Now let's talk about the main ingredients of blockchain. Social process is the most crucial feature above all; data is stored and managed through a system of connections, which eliminates the need for a key control constituent. In addition, decipherable hash engineering ensures data integrity, as each block contains the previous decipherable hash, making it very hard to modify the information. Agreement mechanisms facilitate the addition of extra collection, while sharp system changes and immediate path adjustments.

Blockchain is a reliable source of verifiable information because to its immutability and reliance on cryptographic technology, which guarantees the security and transfer of transactions. Blockchain has the potential to completely transform the healthcare industry by improving efficiency and prioritizing the patient inside the system (Bhambri et al., 2019). Deliberate and methodical, it can independently allow

DOI: 10.1201/9781032698519-3

or reject entry to their medical data and has enhanced control over it due to localized information storage and natural security measures. It enhances patient-concentrated aid by rising secrecy and facilitating the sharing of surgical information between accredited organizations (Akhai, 2023).

As blockchain engineering is dispensed, this geographical area may modification. This gives you the ability to withstand setbacks and attacks in a disjointed and unwavering manner. It also includes data authenticity and ownership. Consequently, blockchain technology is gaining recognition as a versatile technical solution with applications in several industries and use cases, including identity verification, supply chain management, healthcare, security, and contract management. Blockchain's unique features include decentralization, traceability, transparency and reliability. Blockchain can therefore solve interoperability, security and secrecy issues. Blockchain allows unlimited parties to conduct various online transactions. Blockchain engineering can be used to record and store information from a network of distributed devices (Andreina et al., 2022).

3.1.2 Types of Blockchain Technology

There are three types of blockchain engineering which are based on the rights acknowledged to connections and how they differentiate (Dash et al., 2021):

3.1.2.1 Private Blockchain: Access control governs the operation of the private blockchain network and requires authority or asking before users can join.

3.1.2.2 Unrestricted Book of Account System: The unconstrained blockchain is accessible to anybody at any time, whether they wish to participate as a base node or get monetary benefits.

3.1.2.3 Blockchain Consortium: A consortium that operates on both a public and private blockchain is referred to as a semi-private blockchain. Accredited make is commonly awarded in establishments to promote commercial concerns.

3.1.3 Benefits of Blockchain Technology

3.1.3.1 Patient Ad Hoc Benefits: Protection and legal instrument is one of the patient benefits of blockchain application (Sharma et al., 2020). The studies of research papers display that the utilization of blockchain can modify the medical information by protecting patient messaging through with localized peer-to-peer system and putting the patient in the middle of the group. The studies of research papers report that blockchain can understate incidents of information breaks since the system does not sustain from an individual component of occurrence.

Furthermore, blockchain technology has been acknowledged for its ability to authenticate individuals, ensuring that healthcare information may be accessed with a single personal identity, as demonstrated in various research publications. Furthermore, research articles have indicated that blockchain technology can facilitate personalized healthcare by allowing healthcare providers to access shared patient data and develop tailored healthcare plans for each individual. The following study paper examines the potential of blockchain technology to facilitate the tracking of patient information by physicians using pre-recorded timestamps for each case (Singh et al., 2005). In addition, the research paper studies concluded that the engineering modifies watching of patients' welfare, where this function is also essential for critically ill patients, as doctors can intimately monitor patients and act immediately in an exigency, according to the research paper studies.

3.1.3.2 Organizational Benefits: In summation to patient ad hoc benefits, blockchain engineering is also best known for its organizational benefits (Bhambri and Singh, 2006). Research papers suggest that blockchain technology can facilitate secure sharing of patient information among healthcare companies. Other research publications focused on the social process purpose, which was found to be a crucial element in facilitating effective communication of health information among healthcare organizations. For example, a study demonstrates the use of a blockchain to securely and accurately transfer healthcare data along with surgical images within a blockchain network.

As the research paper studies have reported, blockchain engineering has also helped organizations by serving the governance of medical institution trials for dose experiments. In specific, the research paper studies recovered that the security needs that must be well-advised when managing medical institution trials can be handily met using a secluded blockchain. In summation to the research paper studies that recovered blockchain traceability to assist dose indefinite quantity chain establishment, the utilization of blockchain was recovered to preclude cases of assumed doses, as shown by the research paper studies.

The research paper studies show that blockchain has non-medical institution benefits, such as health insurance management, in addition to clinical benefits. Previous research has considered immutability as the most crucial characteristic of blockchain that has assisted in the healthcare security commercial enterprise being more reliable. Furthermore, the research article found that blockchain technology enabled enterprises to securely keep and maintain healthcare security records, as duplicates of the shared ledger are stored on users' PCs.

3.2 BLOCKCHAIN FOR TRANSPARENT, PRIVACY PROTECTED AND SAFE HEALTH DATA MANAGEMENT (HDM)

3.2.1 Blockchain for Transparent HDM

The physical phenomena of blockchain is essential as it enables private and consortium blockchains to regulate network permissions and ensure that only authorized entities can access the system. Blockchain can help address several challenges in healthcare and play a crucial role in prioritizing patients inside the system. This improves capacity, safety, and confidentiality and can prioritize patients inside the system. Blockchain can be employed for remote monitoring, portable applications, and surgical data storage systems that grant patients ownership of their records and access and sharing of patient surgical data.

The application of blockchain in healthcare could overturn the keeping and mutuality of patient information, making processes safer and more expeditious (Kaur et al., 2019). However, there are concerns about blockchain security and secrecy in healthcare, peculiarly when it comes to protecting erogenous patient information. The motive of this literary study's review is to provide an overview of existing research on blockchain security and secrecy in healthcare.

The generator evaluated the potential applications of blockchain technology in the healthcare industry. The creators contemplated that blockchain has the capacity to improve health security and confidentiality, but emphasized that obstacles like as capability and the legal situation still need to be overcome (Khatoon et al., 2019).

The developers contended that in this era of analog technology, the utmost importance is in maintaining the confidentiality and security of patient data in the healthcare industry, necessitating a transition to analog methods. Health data may be effectively monitored by employing blockchain technology. This facilitates the attainment of the desired ultimate goal of authenticity, accountability, and efficacy (Liu et al., 2022). The study paper explored the use of aid blockchains to ensure secure information exchange in the help industry.

The investigation explored several technology solutions, including nameless manners and stenography know-how, to tackle issues related to privacy and security. The written content additionally examined the potential use of engineering in assistance and classified the basis for utilizing blockchain (Esposito et al., 2018).

3.2.2 Blockchain for Privacy Protected HDM

In general, the information shown in blockchain has the capacity to improve the security and confidentiality of patient information storage and communication. Nevertheless, there are still obstacles to overcome, such as capability, limited solutions, and the need for suitable access control methods. Additional research is required to thoroughly explore the potential of blockchain in the field of aid and to assure its responsible use in order to safeguard patient privacy and safety (Dandoush et al., 2023).

Blockchain technology has been identified as a potential solution for various healthcare issues, particularly in enhancing the security and confidentiality of patient data. Due to the sensitive nature of patient data records, which must be kept confidential, ensuring isolation is a crucial challenge in the healthcare industry.

Patients may suffer from the unauthorized use of excessive information, and healthcare providers may face legal consequences (Uma Maheswari et al., 2023). Blockchain engineering provides a distinct advantage that makes it a highly sought-after choice for enhancing privacy in the field of aid. It is a book of account that is specific to a certain area or region, and the information it contains is shared among multiple connections on the web. Consequently, there is a reduced likelihood of a focused occurrence or a clear starting point of reference. Furthermore, blockchain technology enhances the development of smart systems by automating data processes and ensuring compliance with privacy regulations (Guo et al., 2022).

The capacity to encode and decipher pseudonymous data accumulation on the blockchain enables the safeguarding of personal information while granting authorized entities the power to access crucial information (Suganthi and Sree Kala, 2023). Blockchain engineering has the potential to enhance patient privacy, but there are several important issues that need to be addressed. The interoperability of various blockchain platforms poses a significant challenge since it hinders communication amongst aid suppliers who may be using different networks. Another issue pertains to the efficacy of employing blockchain technology, since it necessitates the presence of both generator and technical skills, which may not be universally accessible in all help facilities. Blockchain engineering combines many privacy-enhancing advances to enhance the security of sensitive patient information.

Healthcare information can be securely transferred and stored using encoding, and access is restricted to individuals who possess the necessary decipherable devices and have proper authorization. Permission establishment in intelligent systems allows patients to accurately determine who can access their information by combining reliable information establishment with patient orientation. The utilization of zero-information proofs in the blockchain provides a new manner to formalize information without showing the fundamental information, thus increasing data confidentiality (Rachamalla, 2021).

The intellectual content of unsatisfactory unit information storage is very important for highly crucial information, ensuring that important data is stored off-chain for reference only (crypto-decentralization), reducing the risk of data disclosure. Blockchain further improves obscurity by knowingly proceedings with decipherable addresses instead of real individuality and works with various privacy-enhancing innovation. This algorithm improves patient simplicity by addressing the issue of how exclusive data is linked to a restricted blockchain transaction. Blockchain improves security and accountability in healthcare data management through the modification of permission establishment and information access rights.

This not only ensures restrictive balance, but also supplies agreeable processing information. In the end, blockchain engineering has the possibility to improve privacy in healthcare by giving a localized and safe structure to store and exchange patient data. Different solutions must be resolved before blockchain engineering can be widely utilized in healthcare facilities (Li et al., 2023).

3.2.3 Blockchain for Safe HDM

This chapter explores the security and privacy aspects of blockchain technology in the healthcare industry. By meticulously categorizing the current written material, this analysis provides a clear understanding of the current situation, focusing on relevant issues and disputes. This study provides valuable information about effective research methods and advancements by offering a critical appraisal. Healthcare information security is accomplished through various methods. Various examinations have successfully achieved this through the implementation of social control, physical measures, and specialized concepts.

These regulations consist of various security approaches employed by healthcare institutions to enhance the protection of nonhazardous patient information contained in analogue healthcare records (Qammar et al., 2023). The approach to patient information is constrained by a safety communications protocol that safeguards against unauthorized access. The structural criterion of the bastion instrument can be employed for this purpose. Blockchain technology has the potential to revolutionize the healthcare business by securely storing and managing sensitive patient data (McGhin et al., 2019).

Intelligent interior schemes can offer healthcare services to individuals with specific needs in the comfort of their own homes. Simply put, an intelligent home utilizes advanced technology in the field of physical science to enable remote management of automated devices primarily designed for healthcare purposes. This ensures the safety and well-being of both the patient and the household. The sensors are connected to a specific ability component responsible for processing sensor data, detecting emergencies, and facilitating communication between the patient at home and the others involved in their care, such as doctors, healthcare providers, emergency workers, and paraprofessionals. An intelligent interior can improve the quality of patient life and provide protection through the inventive use of advanced technology (Forward-Secure Customizable data Sharing in Block Chain-Based EHR Systems, 2023).

Extreme medicine and distant establishment are the traveling force behind the execution of the intelligent home. Tel-medicine information systems (TMIS) have advantage intercontinental attraction over the previous twenty years as contemporary ex-cogitation have made the distant delivery of healthcare a realism. Enhancing multidisciplinary investigation and applications, TMIS clutches sophisticated conception in engineering, discipline, biosensors and unreal intelligence information, including intelligent conception. TMIS utilization the latest motorized and radio-communication engineering and widely acquirable cyberspace structure to supply superior services to domestic patients to distant access their wellness content, as well as get tel-medicine services. TMIS offers the possibility to supply healthcare employment to patients for $24 as well as $7. Its cognitive content is to supply patients with easy and fast tel-wellness employment that significantly enhance the superior and inefficiency of wellness employment. Nevertheless, the unfastened and shaky causal agency of the computer network presents an amount of legal document dangers to patient confidentiality and privacy.

TMIS security planning is important. Centralized security and privacy are ensured by shared hallmark and centralized contract rules and regulations. The author of the paper predicts the development of a cost-effective and secure two-lane binding using connectionless mutual authentication and the TMIS core contract protocol. The suggested methodology employs fuzzy classification, utilizing biometric data, to accurately identify patients (Singh et al., 2023). The security of the proposed laws and regulations relies on the intractability of the Elliptic Curve Discrete Logarithm Problem (ECDLP) and the Elliptic Curve Computational Diff-Hellman Problem (ECCDHP) to maintain individual privacy. A detailed analysis of safety measures is conducted, and the outcomes of the comparison are discussed.

Data security is crucial in the healthcare industry as it protects sensitive patient information, including medical history, healthcare provider details, and psychometric test results (Rizwan et al., 2021). The potential compromising of this data could have a negative impact on patients. Healthcare companies find blockchain engineering appealing due to its implementation of a secure and decentralized system for sharing and storing information. Blockchain is a secure and encrypted ledger that records transactions. The term "blockchain" is a combination of the phrases "blocks" and "chains". Data is kept in blocks, and each block is part of a chain. The following features of blockchain engineering make it suitable for safe healthcare information:

3.2.3.1 Decentralized Storage: Information stored in standard information storage is centralized, making it vulnerable to hackers. Blockchain technology distributes and stores information online in a decentralized fashion, making it difficult for inexperienced individuals to code.

3.2.3.2 Immutability: Data stored in the blockchain cannot be transformed or withdrawn once contributed. This properly defends information by assuring its unity.

3.2.3.3 Encryption: Data is protected by state-of-the-art encryption methods in blockchain engineering, which ensures that only authorized parties can access it.

3.2.3.4 Smart systems: These self-executing legal systems can be used to automate information dealing and recover restraint processes. This property adds an extra layer of safety by assuring that only accredited users can recover information.

3.2.3.5 Transparency: Blockchain engineering enhances transparency by disseminating information to all network participants. This attribute has the potential to enhance accountability and diminish criminal activity. Security must be a paramount concern when implementing blockchain technology in the healthcare sector. Given the physical nature and simplicity of wellness content, it is crucial to emphasize the implementation of important safety precautions and the usage of high-quality resources.

3.2.3.6 Encryption: Innovation is required to maintain information confidentiality and integrity and enable information encryption and digital signatures. Regaining power and uniqueness inside an establishment can be achieved through the implementation of security measures such as role-based access control (RBAC) and multi-factor authentication (MFA). These measures enhance the security of user credentials and restrict access to information.

In addition, regular information security audits and continuous monitoring are necessary so that information security problems can be quickly discovered and corrected. Blockchain technology has the potential to revolutionize the healthcare business by offering a safe and decentralized method for storing and sharing sensitive medical data.

There are still problems to be solved before general adoption is achieved. These consist of judicial and regulative needs, ability and the demand for joint rules and regulations (Saluja, 2023). The concept of sensory activity as a service was developed to address the challenges that future smart cities will face in managing a large number of sensors. A smart city must find a solution to the complex cognitive aspects of economic interdependence among users, ensuring the confidentiality of information without compromising its integrity, communication, or noninterference. Advancements in blockchain technology have the potential to address these challenges more effectively.

However, present models are constrained by issues such as the need for extensive storage capacity, limited customization options for blockchains, high transaction costs, and expensive processing requirements. The proposed AH-LO-PrivPresKey Gen model is described as a secure network based on blockchain technology, utilizing a smart contract in a smart city. Blockchain intelligent groups utilize a highly advanced centralized configuration technology that reduces user involvement. The planned group implements many safety measures, such as information encryption protocols, content partitioning, biometric authentication, and one-time passwords. To summarize, the safety pace is strengthened by many functions, including deuce commodity, polynomial, and keys that are ideally generated using AHLO.

The projected AHLO is obtained with the combination of compounding, middling, arithmetic operation-based improvement, and intercrossed comptroller-based improvement. The projected exemplar possesses a minimum mental representation capacity of 0.0305GB, a minimum engineering time requirement of 28.467GB, a superior cryptography rating of 0.808, a high perception magnitude ratio of 0.898, a minimum outcome of 41,679, and a minimum information measure of 95, surpassing the conventional counterpart. The 6G networks are designed to provide artificial intelligence data to various devices by utilizing machine learning in base stations. However, in the context of information security, it is not necessary to transfer raw data to a black box for machine learning training (Ma et al., 2023).

United Learning (UL) is a probable framework that enhances distributed machine learning while ensuring information privacy through the collaboration of artificial intelligence models without sharing raw data. However, traditional UL requires an intermediary device to enhance the global model, making traditional UL a single-component critique. In summary, traditional UL cannot facilitate efficient communication amongst unreliable inclinations, resulting in low training proficiency among inclinations. Blockchain is a promising approach to solve the aforementioned problems, as it can create a safe decentralized and shared environment for entrusted devices.

In this chapter, the authors combine blockchain technology with UL (Ultra-Low) to establish a decentralized framework for planning and communication. In this framework, remote devices execute advanced planning tasks while sink stations provide communication based on building blocks. To summarize, it will establish a nonessential agreement framework backed by a recognized non-governmental organization to enhance the development of blockchain technology. The system employs a diverse algorithm based on robust machine learning to choose high-quality candidates for an ambassadorial committee. Quantitative analysis demonstrates that the proposed theoretical model can achieve superior quality compared to traditional UL. Additionally, the proposed DRL selection method can significantly reduce the waiting time for agreements.

3.3 LITERATURE SURVEY ON BLOCKCHAIN FOR TRANSPARENT, PRIVACY PROTECTED AND SAFE HDM

This work presents an improved GGS-YOLO model based on YOLOv5. The model enhances the capacity to distinguish the original network and features by using an ordered care chemical mechanism and a BiFPN characteristic unification method to boost identification accuracy. In addition, the model becomes lighter and more accurate thanks to the newly developed GGS convolution module. The model achieves a reduced number of parameters of 0.34 × 107, but still achieves a higher recognition accuracy of 85.6%. We combine the model with blockchain engineering for road sign recognition on the internet of vehicles (IoV), with the aim of expanding its use. This approach proves to be feasible and robust in real-world applications, showing exceptional performance in vehicular online traffic sign recognition tasks (Liu et al., 2023).

This study discusses the latest security and secrecy solutions for CAV. It explores the difficulties, disadvantages and effectiveness of integrating them with decentralized engineering such as blockchain. In addition, it included a list of several cyberattacks that are being investigated for security and privacy features of CAVs (Khan et al., 2023). This report recommends a framework for health system and BC protection, information security and privacy information so that PHRs can be safely and properly stored. This system provides open access to PHRs, collaborative data and comprehensive patient registration. It also protects patient privacy and maintains PHR continuity.

The patient can self-manage, collect and share their PHR using this architecture. The framework provides participants with reliable information validated by experimental results. The ability of the framework's access control method to protect essential PHRs from external threats is critical. In addition, the frame structure offers a lightweight PHRS with low time consumption compared to traditional thematic centralized information storage. In this study, only the health sector used this BC safety framework. As expected, we take advantage of this system. (Hossain et al., 2021)

3.4 CONCLUSION AND FUTURE SCOPE OF BLOCKCHAIN FOR TRANSPARENT, PRIVACY PROTECTED AND SAFE HDM

The chapter describes how blockchain engineering can be used in healthcare to solve some of the industry's long-standing problems. Blockchain is regarded as a cutting-edge technology for aggregating medical data, facilitating medical processes, and organizing and managing medical information in a decentralized and uninterrupted healthcare network. Despite the lack of attention given to the blockchain in terms of support, the utilization of this technology in data transfer still elicits worries over privacy and security. This chapter contains a study on blockchain for transparent, privacy preservation and safe health information management, 2018–2023.

The goal of the investigation survey is to evaluate the circulating state of affairs, mostly focusing on applicable applications and efforts. The literature survey notes that blockchain engineering has applicable applications for addressing privacy and safety problems. Blockchain engineering enables enhanced safety and privacy of EHRs and PHRs by giving a localized place to accumulate and exchange crucial patient information. In addition, blockchain can give patients more control over who has access to their information through patient authentication.

However, healthcare organizations and experts need to carefully assess the suitability of implementing blockchain solutions in their operations to ensure compliance with privacy regulations and feasibility.

Contempt can be felt, but blockchain engineering is not an outstanding answer and may require customization to fulfill specific objectives. Overall, the survey provides a comprehensive overview of the current state of blockchain utilization in healthcare, highlighting specific areas that require additional investigation and enhancement in order to advance the technology and its applications in the healthcare sector.

REFERENCES

Aggarwal, S., Chaudhary, R., Aujla, G. S., Kumar, N., Choo, K. R., & Zomaya, A. Y. (2019). Block chain for smart communities: Applications, challenges and opportunities. *Journal of Network and Computer Applications*, 144, 13–48. https://doi.org/10.1016/j.jnca.2019.06.018

Akhai, S. (2023). Healthcare record management for healthcare 4.0 via block chain: A review of current applications, opportunities, challenges, and future potential. *Block Chain for Healthcare*, 4.0, 211–223. https://doi.org/10.1201/9781003408246-11

Andreina, S., Bohli, J., Karame, G. O., Li, W., & Marson, G. A. (2022). PoTS: A secure proof of TEE-stake for permissionless block chains. *IEEE Transactions on Services Computing*, 15(4), 2173–2187. https://doi.org/10.1109/tsc.2020.3038950

Bhambri, P., & Singh, M. (2006). Artificial intelligence. In *Seminar on E-Governance—Pathway to Progress* (p. 14). SSIET.

Bhambri, P., Sinha, V. K., Dhanoa, I. S., & Kaur, J. (2019). Genome DNA sequence matching using HBM algorithm. *International Journal of Control and Automation*, 12(5), 531–539.

Dandoush, A., Gouissem, A., & Ciftler, B. (2023). Secure and privacy-preserving federated learning-based resource allocation for next generation networks. https://doi.org/10.36227/techrxiv.22591852

Dash, S., Gantayat, P. K., & Das, R. K. (2021). Block chain engineeringin healthcare: Opportunities and challenges. *Intelligent Systems Reference Library*, 97–111. https://doi.org/10.1007/978-3-030-69395-4_6

Esposito, C., Palmieri, F., & Choo, K. R. (2018). Cloud message queueing and notification: Challenges and opportunities. *IEEE Cloud Computing*, 5(2), 11–16. https://doi.org/10.1109/mcc.2018.022171662

Forward-Secure Customizable data Sharing in Block Chain-Based EHR Systems. (2023). 2023 20th Annual International Conference on Privacy, Security and Trust (PST). https://doi.org/10.1109/pst58708.2023.10320178

Guo, C., Zhang, W., Dong, N., Liu, Z., & Xiang, Y. (2022). Qos-aware diversified service selection. *IEEE Transactions on Services Computing*, 1–15. https://doi.org/10.1109/tsc.2022.3210658

Hossain, M. J., Wadud, M. A., & Alamin, M. (2021). HDM-chain: A secure block chain-based healthcare data management framework to ensure privacy and security in the health unit. 2021 5th International Conference on Electrical Engineering and Information Communication Engineering (ICEEICT). https://doi.org/10.1109/iceeict53905.2021.9667820

Kaur, J., Bhambri, P., & Kaur, S. (2019). SVM Classifier based method for software defect prediction. *International Journal of Analytical and Experimental Model Analysis*, 11(10), 2772–2776.

Khan, R., Mehmood, A., Maple, C., Curran, K., & Song, H. H. (2023). Performance analysis of block chain-enabled security and privacy algorithms in connected and autonomous vehicles: A comprehensive review. *IEEE Transactions on Intelligent Transportation Systems*, 1–12. https://doi.org/10.1109/tits.2023.3341358

Khatoon, S., Rahman, S. M., Alrubaian, M., & Alamri, A. (2019). Privacy-preserved, provable secure, mutually authenticated key agreement protocol for healthcare in a smart city environment. *IEEE Access*, 7, 47962–47971. https://doi.org/10.1109/access.2019.2909556

Li, J., Wang, T., Yang, B., Yang, Q., Zhang, W., & Hong, K. (2023). Undefined. *IEEE Transactions on Services Computing*, 16(5), 3182–3195. https://doi.org/10.1109/tsc.2023.3292498

Liu, J., Dong, H., & Xue, Y. (2022). A secure and privacy-preserved delegate-based block chain and federated learning for 6G networks. *International Journal of Communication Systems*. https://doi.org/10.1002/dac.5367

Liu, Y., Qian, Q., Zhang, H., Li, J., Zhong, Y., & Xiong, N. N. (2023). Application of sustainable block chain technology in the internet of vehicles: Innovation in traffic sign detection systems. *Sustainability*, 16(1), 171. https://doi.org/10.3390/su16010171

Ma, Y., Ma, Y., Liu, Y., & Cheng, Q. (2023). A secure and efficient certificateless authenticated key agreement protocol for smart healthcare. *Computer Standards & Interfaces*, 86, 103735. https://doi.org/10.1016/j.csi.2023.103735

McGhin, T., Choo, K. R., Liu, C. Z., & He, D. (2019). Block chain in healthcare applications: Research challenges and opportunities. *Journal of Network and Computer Applications*, 135, 62–75. https://doi.org/10.1016/j.jnca.2019.02.027

Qammar, A., Naouri, A., Ding, J., & Ning, H. (2023). Block chain-based optimized edge node selection and privacy preserved framework for federated learning. *Cluster Computing*. https://doi.org/10.1007/s10586-023-04145-0

Rachamalla, S. (2021). Secure data sharing based on block chain technology. *International Journal of Forensic Sciences*, 5(2). https://doi.org/10.23880/ijfsc-16000230

Rizwan, M., Sohail, M. N., Asheralieva, A., Anjum, A., & Angin, P. (2021). SAID: ECC-based secure authentication and incentive distribution mechanism for block chain-enabled data sharing system. 2021 IEEE International Conference on Block Chain (Block Chain). https://doi.org/10.1109/Block Chain53845.2021.00080

Saluja, P. (2023). Securing clinical trials data with block chain. *Block Chain Technology in Healthcare—Concepts, Methodologies, and Applications*, 34–53. https://doi.org/10.2174/9789815165197123010005

Sharma, R., Bhambri, P., & Sohal, A. K. (2020). Energy bio-inspired for MANET. *International Journal of Recent Technology and Engineering*, 8(6), 5580–5585.

Singh, M. B., Singh, H., & Pratap, A. (2023). Energy-efficient and privacy-preserving block chain based federated learning for smart healthcare system. *IEEE Transactions on Services Computing*, 1–12. https://doi.org/10.1109/tsc.2023.3332955

Singh, P., Singh, M., & Bhambri, P. (2005). Security in virtual private networks. In *Seminar on Network Security and Its Implementations* (p. 11). Doaba College.

Suganthi, S., & Sree Kala, T. (2023). A novel secure aware privacy preserved data sharing framework in an e-government system based on a consortium block chain. *Journal of Control and Decision*, 1–19. https://doi.org/10.1080/23307706.2023.2211071

Uma Maheswari, J., Somasundaram, S. K., & Sivakumar, P. (2023). Hybrid optimization enabled secure privacy preserved data sharing based on block chain. *Wireless Networks*. https://doi.org/10.1007/s11276-023-03588-y

4 SPSHS
Security and Privacy Concerns in Smart Healthcare Systems

Umashankar Ghugar, Rakesh Nayak, Praveen Gupta and Satyabrata Dash

4.1 INTRODUCTION

The development of intelligent healthcare systems has completely changed the way healthcare is provided, providing creative answers to enhance patient care and outcomes. This summary gives a general overview of the idea of smart healthcare systems, emphasizing its main characteristics, advantages, and potential drawbacks. Smart healthcare systems leverage state-of-the-art innovations using technologies such as the internet of things (IoT), artificial intelligence (AI), and big data analytics to make the delivery of medical care more effective and individualized than ever before. The applications for these systems are extensive, spanning from wearables to telemedicine to EHRs to remote patient monitoring. There are many benefits to using a smart healthcare system. They improve access to healthcare services, allow for real-time monitoring and early health issue diagnosis, promote individualized treatment programs, and provide patients the capacity to take an active role in their care. These solutions can also assist healthcare professionals in streamlining workflows, enhancing diagnosis precision, and maximizing resource allocation [1].

The framework's design for scalable healthcare is shown in Figure 4.1. This design has four layers: network, data, analysis, and presentation. Merging hospital, laboratory, X-ray, and pharmacy prescription databases from multiple contexts is necessary.

4.1.1 Smart Healthcare System Concept

Smart healthcare systems integrate cutting-edge technologies and data-driven strategies to improve the provision of healthcare services. The internet of things (IoT), artificial intelligence (AI), big data analytics, and wearable gadgets are all used to monitor and improve people's health in real-time. Smart healthcare systems seek to optimize efficiency, enable tailored treatment regimens, and improve patient care. Thus, healthcare practitioners may remotely monitor patients' vital signs, medication compliance, and health. This allows early detection and treatment of health issues.

 DOI: 10.1201/9781032698519-4

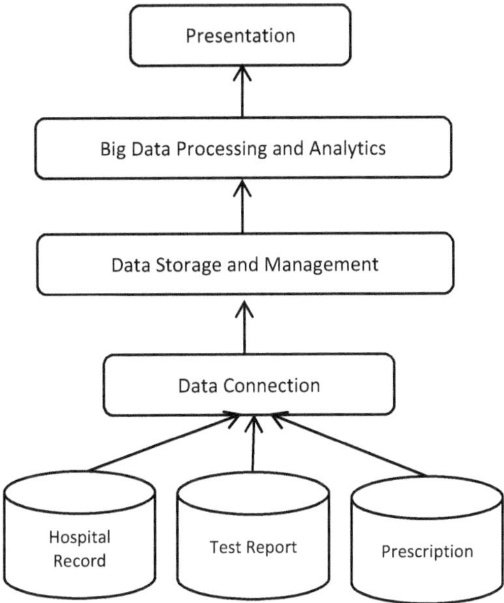

FIGURE 4.1 Architecture.

Smart healthcare systems also make it possible for patients, healthcare professionals, and medical equipment to seamlessly exchange information. Access to medical information, consultations, and follow-up treatment is made safe and practical using electronic health records (EHRs) and telehealth services. The use of machine learning and AI algorithms to evaluate vast amounts of healthcare data is also included in the idea of a smart healthcare system. The idea of a smart healthcare system, which relies on technology and data-driven methods to improve patient outcomes, boost efficiency, and revolutionize the healthcare experience, marks a paradigm shift in the way healthcare is delivered [2].

4.1.2 Smart Healthcare Benefits

Smart healthcare systems offer numerous benefits that can significantly improve patient care and healthcare outcomes. Some of the key benefits include:

- **Enhanced Patient Care**: Real-time monitoring of patient's vital signs, medication compliance, and general health state is made possible through smart healthcare systems. This enhances patient care and results by enabling healthcare professionals to identify health concerns early and administer prompt treatments.
- **Reduced Error Rates**: Smart healthcare systems can aid in lowering mistakes in procedures related to medicine administration, diagnosis, and treatment by utilizing technology and automation. As a result, healthcare is delivered in a safer and more precise manner.

- **Efficient Time Usage**: Smart healthcare technologies automate mundane processes and simplify workflows so that healthcare professionals may better manage their time and concentrate on providing high-quality care. By lowering wait times and raising patient satisfaction, can increase efficiency in healthcare settings.
- **Personalized Treatment Plans**: Smart healthcare systems can evaluate vast amounts of patient data using AI algorithms and big data analytics to produce individualized treatment regimens. This makes it possible for medical professionals to customize therapies based on unique patient traits, resulting in more efficient and focused care.

It is crucial to remember that while smart healthcare systems have many advantages, some difficulties and issues must be taken into account regarding data security, privacy, and ethical implications to ensure their responsible and successful adoption.

4.1.3 Smart Healthcare Solutions

The term "smart healthcare solutions" refers to the application of data analytics, networking, and technology to enhance patient care, healthcare delivery, and overall healthcare results. These systems employ IoT, AI, big data analytics, mobile applications, and remote patient care to deliver real-time monitoring and individualized therapy [3].

Several instances of intelligent healthcare options include:

- **Remote Patient Monitoring**: Healthcare professionals may remotely monitor patients' vital signs, medication compliance, and general health state thanks to smart healthcare systems. This lessens the need for hospital visits and enhances patient convenience by enabling early diagnosis of health concerns and prompt treatments.
- **Telemedicine**: Through video conferencing or mobile applications, smart healthcare solutions enable virtual consultations between healthcare practitioners and patients. For patients who live in remote locations or have restricted mobility, this enables remote diagnosis, treatment, and monitoring.
- **Electronic Health Records (EHR)**: EHR systems digitalize patient medical records so that healthcare professionals can conveniently access them [4]. The ability to combine smart EHR systems with other healthcare technologies allows for seamless data exchange, decision assistance, and enhanced care coordination.
- **Health Monitoring Apps**: Numerous elements of health, such as nutrition, exercise, sleep, and mental well-being, may be tracked and monitored using mobile applications. These applications offer individualized advice, health advice, and insights to assist users in making well-informed health decisions.

These are only a handful of the many intelligent healthcare solutions that are readily available. These ideas aim to improve patient care, boost healthcare productivity, and improve people's ability to manage their health.

4.1.4 Smart Healthcare Devices

The term "smart healthcare devices" refers to medical equipment that uses connectivity, data analytics, and sophisticated technology to enhance patient monitoring, healthcare delivery, and overall health results. These gadgets are made to gather, process, and communicate health-related data, empowering medical practitioners to decide wisely and deliver individualized treatment [5].

Here are some instances of smart medical equipment:

- **Smart Pill Dispensers**: By distributing the appropriate pills at the appropriate time, these devices assist patients in managing their medication schedules. They can warn caregivers or healthcare providers if a dosage is missed, issue reminders, and monitor adherence.
- **Smart Blood Pressure Monitors**: With the use of these gadgets, people may check their blood pressure at home and communicate the results with

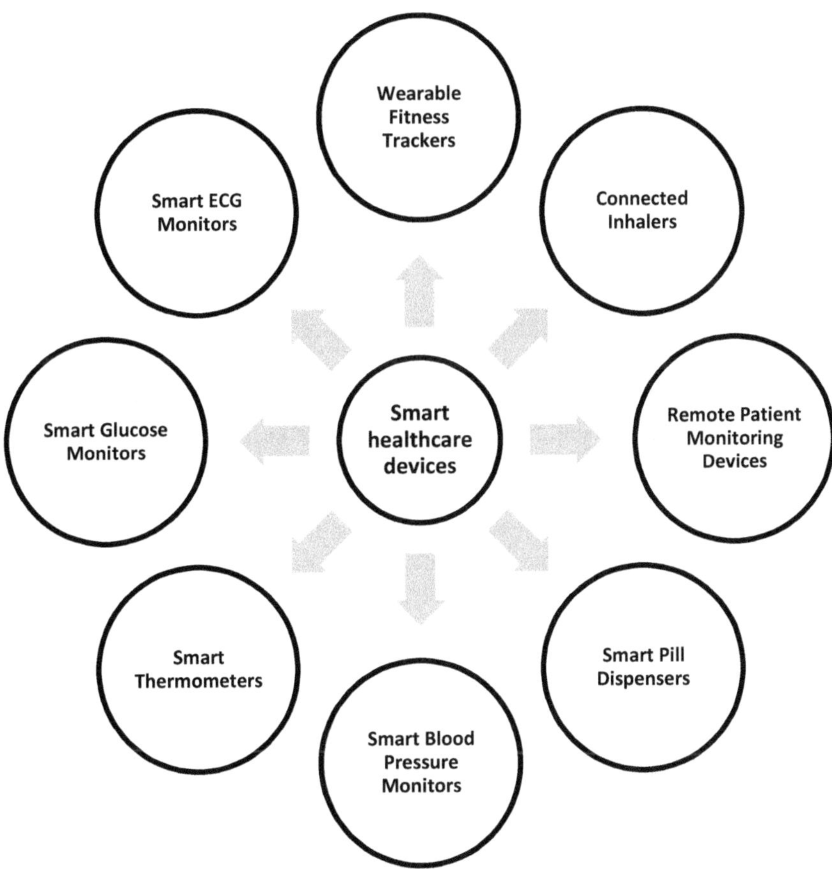

FIGURE 4.2 Smart healthcare devices.

medical specialists. They give precise measurements, monitor trends, and support hypertension management.

- **Smart Thermometers**: These smart thermometers offer precise temperature readings and may be connected to mobile applications. They can communicate information with healthcare professionals, guide patients on drug doses, and monitor trends of fever.
- **Smart Glucose Monitors**: These tools make it easier for diabetics to keep an eye on their blood sugar levels. Real-time readings, trend tracking, and alarms for hypo- or hyperglycemic episodes are all capabilities of these devices.
- **Smart ECG Monitors**: Electrocardiograms (ECGs) can be performed using these portable devices at home or while travelling. They can help with the early detection of cardiac diseases, transfer data to healthcare professionals, and identify abnormal heart rhythms.

Section 4.1 of this chapter, which essentially consists of four sections, elaborates on the establishment of a Smart Healthcare System (SHS). The application of the security and privacy concept to SHS is covered in Section 4.2 of this article. Section 4.3 covers the SHS's vulnerability, and Section 4.4 wraps up all of the SHS principles.

4.2 DISCUSSION ON SHS

Smart healthcare systems, which make use of IoT and telemedicine technology, provide several advantages in terms of ease and enhanced patient care [6]. They do, however, carry some hazards that must be properly controlled. Following are some salient details from the search results:

- Smart healthcare systems' telemedicine technology enables remote patient monitoring and consultations. They can increase access to care, particularly for people living in distant locations. However, obstacles including a lack of infrastructure and privacy issues must be dealt with.
- The capabilities of smart healthcare may be improved further by incorporating artificial intelligence (AI) into healthcare systems. AI can help with patient monitoring, therapy planning, and diagnosis. However, it's important to address ethical issues and the possibility of prejudice in AI systems.

Some procedures are developed by adhering to standards. Confidentiality can be maintained, for example, by using encryption algorithms so that only the intended recipients can read encoded messages. Access to "editing" functions is typically limited to administrators only by authorization requirements. Finding the right balance between convenience and risk in SHS requires the implementation of robust cybersecurity safeguards. These measures should include encryption, access limitations, and periodic security assessments. Privacy rules, such as HIPAA, are severely affected.

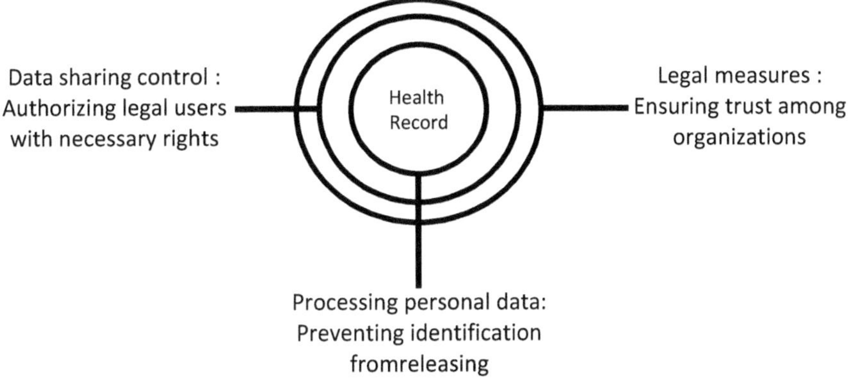

FIGURE 4.3 Health information confidentiality and security principles.

4.2.1 The Growing Concerns in SHS

The healthcare industry has benefited greatly from the incorporation of smart healthcare equipment and technologies, including better patient monitoring, individualized care, and improved health outcomes. The rising use of connection and digital technology in healthcare does, however, bring up questions regarding security and privacy [7].

- **Privacy Concerns:** Privacy issues may arise from the gathering, storing, and communication of sensitive health information via smart healthcare equipment. Patients worry about their personal health information being accessed, used, or disclosed without their permission. To preserve patient privacy, it is necessary to have strict privacy rules and secure data handling procedures.
- **Data Security:** Secure data transmission and storage are essential components of smart healthcare systems. However, because of their interconnectedness, these systems are susceptible to hacker assaults and data breaches. Malicious actors may seek to get illegal access to private medical records, endangering patients and medical professionals.
- **Data Ownership and Control:** There are concerns regarding who owns and controls the data produced by smart healthcare devices as their use increases. Patients could worry about the possible exploitation or exploitation of their health information by third parties. To solve the ownership and management of data concerns, clear rules and laws are required.

4.2.2 Privacy Challenges in Healthcare

With the digitalization of medical records and the deployment of technology in healthcare systems, privacy issues have risen to the forefront of the industry.

Following are some salient details from the search result [8]:

- Concerns regarding potential data breaches and privacy violations have been raised by the proliferation of digital health systems. The hazards related to privacy and securities are increased by the extensive gathering and storage of health data.
- Healthcare businesses may find it difficult to embrace electronic health records (EHRs) due to privacy and security worries [9]. To build confidence and promote the broad use of EHR systems, patient information must be protected.
- Big healthcare data is becoming more and more prevalent, which has raised worries about security and privacy. Healthcare institutions must handle these issues if they are to safeguard private patient data.

Organizations should use encryption, access restrictions, and security audits to protect healthcare privacy. Privacy laws like GDPR and HIPAA must be followed. Raising awareness among healthcare workers and patients about privacy hazards and appropriate practices may help resolve privacy issues.

4.2.3 Security Risks in SHS

Security flaws in SHSs can jeopardize patient privacy and the integrity of healthcare data. These risks can include [10]:

- **Data Breaches:** Hackers are drawn to smart healthcare systems because they store and communicate sensitive patient data. Unauthorized access, theft, or modification of patient information can occur as a result of data breaches.
- **Malware and Ransomware Attacks**: Malicious malware can infiltrate smart healthcare equipment and systems, interfering with their operation or encrypting data until a ransom is paid. These assaults have the potential to interrupt patient treatment and jeopardize the security of healthcare data.
- **Denial of Service (DoS) Attacks:** Attackers can flood smart healthcare systems with requests, making them unreachable to genuine users. This can interrupt patient care and cause vital healthcare treatments to be delayed.
- **Insider Threats:** Employees or authorized personnel with access to smart healthcare systems may abuse or divulge sensitive patient data, either purposefully or accidentally. Data breaches or unauthorized access to patient information can be caused by insider threats.
- **Insecure Device and Network Configurations:** Misconfigured smart healthcare equipment or network settings might expose vulnerabilities to attackers. Weak passwords, unpatched software, and unsecured network connections might jeopardize the whole system's security.

Healthcare firms should establish robust security measures, such as tight access restrictions, encryption methods, frequent software upgrades, and employee training on cybersecurity best practices, to prevent these security concerns [11]. Furthermore, compliance with privacy legislation and standards such as HIPAA in the United States is critical for securing patient data in smart healthcare systems.

4.3 THE VULNERABILITIES OF SHS

While smart healthcare systems provide several benefits, they also have weaknesses that might lead to data breaches. Here are some key points from the search results [12]:

- Smart healthcare systems rely on the internet of things (IoT) and cloud services, which might expose them to cyber threats. Malicious actors can exploit these flaws to get unauthorized access to sensitive patient data.
- Data breaches, smart home gadgets, smart cities, and the usage of blockchain technology can all cause security and privacy difficulties in smart healthcare systems. These concerns must be addressed to preserve patient information.
- Artificial intelligence (AI) integration in smart healthcare systems may provide extra privacy problems. AI algorithms may have access to sensitive healthcare data; therefore, it is critical that these algorithms be safe and do not jeopardize patient privacy.

It is critical to adopt effective security measures in smart healthcare systems to reduce vulnerabilities and breaches of privacy. To safeguard patient data from cyber risks, this includes encryption, access limits, and regular security assessments.

4.3.1 Managing Security in Healthcare Systems

Managing security in healthcare systems is crucial to guaranteeing the confidentiality of sensitive patient data and the integrity of healthcare operations. Here are some key considerations and strategies for managing security in healthcare systems [13]:

- **Risk Assessment and Management**: Regular risk assessments aid in the identification of possible weaknesses and threats to the security of healthcare systems. Physical security, network infrastructure, data storage, and access restrictions are all evaluated. Risk management solutions like as encryption, firewalls, and intrusion detection systems can aid in mitigating recognized hazards.
- **Data Protection and Privacy**: Healthcare systems deal with massive volumes of sensitive patient data, such as medical records, personal information, and financial information [14]. Encryption, access restrictions, and secure data storage are critical to protecting patient privacy and compliance with relevant requirements such as HIPAA (Health Insurance Portability and Accountability Act).
- **Security Awareness and Training**: Employee security awareness and training initiatives should be prioritized by healthcare firms. This involves

training employees on typical security risks, recommended practices for data security, and how to identify and report possible security problems. Employee security awareness may be reinforced through regular training sessions and simulated phishing activities.

Healthcare businesses may successfully manage security risks and secure patient data in their systems by applying these techniques and regularly assessing and updating security measures.

4.3.2 Preventing Medical Data Breaches

It is critical to prevent medical data breaches to ensure patient privacy and the integrity of healthcare systems. Here are some key strategies to prevent medical data breaches [15]:

- **Conduct Regular Security Risk Assessments:** Assessing security threats in your healthcare system aids in the identification of weaknesses and potential entry sites for attackers. Physical security, network infrastructure, and access restrictions are all evaluated.
- **Implement Strong Access Controls**: Make certain that only authorized people have access to patient information. To limit access to sensitive information based on employment duties and responsibilities, use role-based access controls (RBAC). To validate user identities, utilize robust authentication mechanisms such as multi-factor authentication.

Implementing these techniques can dramatically lower the danger of medical data breaches while also protecting patient privacy and confidence.

4.3.3 Data Protection in Medicine

In medicine, data protection refers to the policies and procedures in place to secure patient data and maintain its privacy and security. It entails safeguarding sensitive medical information from illegal access, use, or disclosure. Here are some key aspects of data protection in medicine [16]:

- **Legal and Regulatory Frameworks**: HIPAA in the United States and GDPR in the European Union control medical data protection. These frameworks govern patient data collection, storage, and exchange.
- **Patient Consent and Privacy**: Before collecting and utilizing patients' personal health information, healthcare practitioners must acquire their informed consent. Patients have the right to know how their data will be used and shared, and they have the right to seek access to their information and, if required, adjustments.
- **Secure Data Storage and Transmission**: Medical data should be securely kept and transferred to avoid unwanted access or breaches. This involves

encrypting data at rest and in transit, building secure storage systems, and employing secure communication methods.
- **Incident Response and Breach Management**: To address data breaches or security events as soon as possible, healthcare companies should have an incident response strategy in place. This involves containment measures, notifying impacted persons, and making efforts to reduce the consequences of the breach.

Healthcare businesses may preserve patient data, retain confidence, and comply with legal and regulatory obligations by establishing strong data protection procedures. It is critical to keep current on growing data security standards and react to new threats in the healthcare business.

4.3.4 Ensuring Privacy and Security in Healthcare

Compliance with HIPAA (Health Insurance Portability and Accountability Act) is critical for healthcare businesses to maintain patient privacy and secure sensitive health information [17]. Here are some key requirements for HIPAA compliance:

- **Privacy Rule:** The HIPAA Privacy Rule outlines guidelines for safeguarding medical records and other sensitive health information. It necessitates the implementation of rules and processes to preserve this information and restrict its use and dissemination.
- **Security Rule:** The HIPAA Security Rule establishes guidelines for the protection of electronic protected health information (ePHI). Administrative, physical, and technological measures must be implemented by covered organizations to prevent unauthorized access, use, and disclosure of ePHI.
- **Risk Assessment:** Covered entities must undertake frequent risk assessments to identify possible vulnerabilities and adopt steps to protect the confidentiality, integrity, and availability of electronic protected health information (ePHI).

Healthcare businesses must assess and update their HIPAA compliance plans regularly to react to changing technology and growing risks to patient privacy and data security.

4.3.5 The Role of Regulations and Policies

Regulations and policies play a crucial role in safeguarding privacy in the digital age. Here are some key points from the search results [18]:

- Medical information in the digital era, privacy laws such as the Health Insurance Portability and Accountability Act (HIPAA) are critical. HIPAA is concerned with the protection of health information and the privacy and security of electronic health data. It includes provisions for breach reporting, noncompliance fines, and patient rights.

- Regulations should focus not just on safeguarding individuals' privacy, but also on balancing the advantages of data-driven technology. It is critical to strike a balance that allows for innovation and economic progress while also protecting individuals' privacy rights.

Overall, rules and policies are critical in protecting privacy in the digital age. They provide a framework for companies to use personal data ethically while still protecting individuals' privacy rights. However, keeping legislation up to speed with fast-expanding technology and rising privacy issues is a continual struggle.

4.3.6 Building Trust: Enhancing Security and Privacy in SHS

Building trust and improving security and privacy in SHS is critical to ensuring the technology's acceptance and success. Here are some key points from the search results [19]:

- **Blockchain Technology** has the potential to enhance security and privacy in smart healthcare systems. Blockchain technology enables a decentralized, tamper-resistant ledger for securely storing and sharing health care data. It can make transactions safer and more transparent, increase data integrity, and protect patient privacy.
- **Internet of Things (IoT)** plays a significant role in smart healthcare systems. Wearable sensors and remote monitoring devices, for example, capture and send sensitive health data. Maintaining confidence in these systems requires ensuring the security and privacy of this data.

Building trust and improving security and privacy in smart healthcare systems necessitates the use of technologies such as blockchain, stringent data protection measures, openness, stakeholder engagement, and continual education and awareness campaigns. By resolving these issues, we can establish a safe and private environment in which to deploy smart healthcare technology.

4.3.7 The Future of Smart Healthcare Systems

Smart healthcare systems have the potential to revolutionize the way we give and receive medical care. However, ensuring the security and privacy of these technologies is important for their effective implementation and general adoption. Here are some key points from the search results [20]:

- 5G-based smart healthcare networks that integrate IoT and enhanced wireless connectivity may improve the healthcare business. However, preserving sensitive patient data and sustaining network trust requires addressing security and privacy issues.
- The integration of AI and IoT in smart healthcare systems introduces new security and privacy challenges. To maintain patient privacy and prevent data breaches, the adoption of AI-driven IoT devices and cloud technologies necessitates careful evaluation of data protection measures.

- Cloud computing plays a significant role in smart healthcare systems, but it also introduces security and privacy risks. To preserve patient information and retain confidence in these systems, it is critical to ensure the security and privacy of data stored and processed in the cloud.

Addressing security and privacy concerns is critical to the development of smart healthcare systems. This involves establishing strong security measures, tackling the particular issues posed by AI, IoT, and cloud technologies, and encouraging stakeholder engagement. We can increase trust in these technologies and realize their full potential for enhancing healthcare delivery by emphasizing security and privacy.

4.4 CONCLUSION

Smart healthcare systems may change medical delivery and reception. To protect sensitive patient data and maintain trust in these technologies, these systems must be secure and private. IoT, AI, and cloud computing in smart healthcare systems present security and privacy problems. Strong security, encryption, and data protection are needed to prevent data breaches. In complex smart healthcare systems, security and privacy require collaboration. Working together to protect patient privacy and use new technologies can design and implement best practices, standards, and laws. COVID-19 has underlined the need for safe, private smart healthcare systems. The rapid adoption of these technologies during the outbreak has highlighted security risks and the need for ongoing research. Finally, promoting security and privacy can boost confidence in smart healthcare systems and realize their potential to improve healthcare delivery. Addressing technology challenges and fostering stakeholder engagement are essential to the successful deployment and widespread adoption of smart healthcare systems.

REFERENCES

1. Carlos A. Moreno-Camacho, Jairo R. Montoya-Torres, Anicia Jaegler and Natacha Gondran, Sustainability metrics for real case applications of the supply chain network design problem: A systematic literature review, *J Clean Prod.* 2019; 231: 600–618,
2. Ramesh Rajagopalan, Smart and pervasive health systems—challenges, trends, and future directions. In *Advances in Information and Communication: Proceedings of the 2019 Future of Information and Communication Conference (FICC)* (Vol. 1). Springer International Publishing, 2020.
3. Jaimon T. Kelly, BHlthSc, Mast Nutr & Diet, PhD, Katrina L. Campbell, Enying Gong and Paul Scuffham, The internet of things: Impact and implications for health care delivery, *J Med Internet Res.* 2020 Nov; 22(11): e20135.
4. C. Rachna and P. Bhambri, Various approaches and algorithms for monitoring energy efficiency of wireless sensor networks. In *Lecture Notes in Civil Engineering* (Vol. 113, pp. 761–770). Springer, 2021.
5. Elvira Ismagilova, Laurie Hughes, Nripendra Rana and Yogesh Dwivedi, Security, privacy and risks within smart cities: Literature review and development of a smart city interaction framework. *Inf Syst Front.* 2022; 24. https://doi.org/10.1007/s10796-020-10044-1
6. P. Bakshi, P. Bhambri and V. Thapar, A review paper on wireless sensor network techniques in internet of things (IoT). *Wesleyan Journal of Research* 2021; 14(7): 147–160. http://www.wesleyanjournal.in/.

7. C. Lee Ventola, Mobile devices and apps for health care professionals: Uses and benefits, *PubMed Central.* 2014 May; 39(5): 356–364.
8. U. Ghugar and J. Pradhan, ML-IDS: MAC layer trust-based intrusion detection system for wireless sensor networks. In *Computational Intelligence in Data Mining: Proceedings of the International Conference on ICCIDM 2018.* Springer, 2020.
9. G. Singh and P. Bhambri, Simulation analysis of AODV and DSDV routing protocols for secure and reliable service in mobile adhoc networks (MANETs). In *Integration of AI-Based Manufacturing and Industrial Engineering Systems with the Internet of Things* (pp. 205–216). CRC Press, 2023.
10. Mohammad Mehrtak, Seyed Ahmad Seyed Alinaghi, Mehrzad Mohsseni Pour, Tayebeh Noori, Amirali Karimi, Ahmadreza Shamsabadi, Mohammad Heydari, Alireza Barzegary, Pegah Mirzapour, Mahdi Soleymanzadeh, Farzin Vahedi, Esmaeil Mehraeen and Omid Dadras, Security challenges and solutions using healthcare cloud computing, *J Med Life.* 2021 Jul-Aug; 14(4): 448–461.
11. R. Rana, P. Bhambri and Y. Chhabra, Evolution and the future of industrial engineering with the IoT and AI. In *Integration of AI-Based Manufacturing and Industrial Engineering Systems with the Internet of Things* (pp. 19–37). CRC Press, 2024.
12. Mohammad Mehrtak, Seyed Ahmad Seyed Alinaghi, Mehrzad Mohsseni Pour, Tayebeh Noori, Amirali Karimi, Ahmadreza Shamsabadi, Mohammad Heydari, Alireza Barzegary, Pegah Mirzapour, Mahdi Soleymanzadeh, Farzin Vahedi, Esmaeil Mehraeen and Omid Dadras, Security challenges and solutions using healthcare cloud computing, *J Med Life.* 2021 Jul-Aug; 14(4): 448–461.
13. Umashankar Ghugar and Jayaram Pradhan, NL-IDS: Trust-based intrusion detection system for network layer in wireless sensor networks. In *2018 Fifth International Conference on Parallel, Distributed and Grid Computing (PDGC).* IEEE, 2018.
14. P. Bhambri, S. Singh, S. Jain and S. I. Dhanoa, Plants recognition using leaf image pattern analysis with focus on advanced smart computing technologies, *AIP Conf. Proc.* 2023; 2916, 020003.
15. Adil Hussain Seh, Mohammad Zarour, Mamdouh Alenezi, Amal Krishna Sarkar, Alka Agrawal, Rajeev Kumar and Raees Ahmad Khan, Healthcare data breaches: Insights and implications, *Healthcare (Basel).* 2020 Jun; 8(2): 133.
16. S. Shi, D. He, L. Li, N. Kumar, M.K. Khan and K.R. Choo, Applications of blockchain in ensuring the security and privacy of electronic health record systems: A survey, *Comput Secur.* 2020; 97: 101966. https://doi.org/10.1016/j.cose.2020.101966
17. Metty Paul, Leandros Maglaras, Mohamed Amine Ferrag and Iman Almomani, Digitization of healthcare sector: A study on privacy and security concerns, *ICT Express.* 2023; 9(4): 571–588. ISSN 2405-9595. https://doi.org/10.1016/j.icte.2023.02.007.
18. Rijwan Ratta Khan, Pranav Kaur Amanpreet Sharma and Sparsh Dhiman Gaurav, Application of blockchain and internet of things in healthcare and medical sector: Applications, challenges, and future perspectives, *J Food Qual.* https://doi.org/10.1155/2021/7608296
19. Nishant Kumar and Geetika Jain, Use of blockchain technology for smart health-care services: A critical perspective of ethnic minority group, *J. Sci. Technol. Policy Manag.* 2023. Emerald Publishing Limited. https://doi.org/10.1108/JSTPM-09-2022-0147
20. Y. Sun, J. Zhang, Y. Xiong and G. Zhu, Data security and privacy in cloud computing, *J. Distrib. Sens. Netw.* 2014; 10(7). https://doi.org/10.1155/2014/190903

5 Transforming Healthcare Engagement in the Med-Tech Industry through Digital Marketing

Bhuvaneshwari Gojanur, S. Padmapriya, Shouvik Sanyal and Dhanabalan Thangam

5.1 INTRODUCTION

The healthcare sector has experienced a significant transformation in favor of digital marketing, with the growth of internet populations and social media platforms providing more valuable ways for healthcare providers to connect with patients. With 75% of patients expressing interest in using technology to manage their health, there is an increasing demand for digital healthcare solutions. A survey by Healthcare IT News revealed that 87% of healthcare marketers utilize digital marketing strategies to reach their patient base (webmdignite.com, 2023). Digital marketing has significantly expanded the reach and engagement of healthcare providers with their patients, enabling them to interact with a larger audience and provide important information about their offerings. These channels facilitate real-time interaction, enabling healthcare providers to address patient queries and offer support. This enhanced communication has the potential to yield better patient outcomes and overall satisfaction (Stoumpos et al., 2023). Healthcare communication on social media is tailored to make it easily comprehensible to a diverse audience, with complex messages presented in plain language to ensure relevance and educate the public. Bite-sized, captivating videos are used to convey intricate topics in a simplified manner (Hermes et al., 2020). Conventional marketing techniques, including print and television advertisements, can be expensive and only reach a small audience (Bhambri et al., 2019). Digital marketing is a cost-effective option for healthcare providers, as it is relatively inexpensive and allows for precise targeting of specific demographics (Raju, 2023).

Digital marketing has also enhanced the patient's experience, making healthcare more convenient and accessible. Patients can schedule appointments online, access medical records, and contact healthcare practitioners via messaging apps, contributing to higher patient satisfaction. Healthcare providers can become recognized as authorities in their professions and build a solid reputation for providing top-notch treatment by utilizing digital marketing (webmdignite.com, 2023). Increased

DOI: 10.1201/9781032698519-5

patient referrals may result from this, which would eventually bring in more money for healthcare providers. Digital marketing is also data-driven, helping healthcare professionals track the effectiveness of their campaigns and make wise choices. Analytics tools help track website traffic, engagement rates, and conversion rates, empowering healthcare providers to fine-tune their strategies for better outcomes (Herrmann et al., 2018).

Furtner et al. (2022) mentioned that Covid-19 pandemic has accelerated the need for healthcare stakeholders to place patient desires and concerns at the forefront of every decision. Healthcare professionals (HCPs) are increasingly recognizing the importance of embracing a consumer-centric digital engagement model to bolster their visibility and reputation. As HCPs become increasingly comfortable with these changes, MedTech companies have recognized the critical importance of adapting to the digital landscape to enhance their engagement with HCPs (Raju, 2023).

This transition to digital marketing has fundamentally reshaped the operations and marketing strategies of the medical technology industry (Anand and Bhambri, 2018). Digital channels offer a more efficient and personalized approach to marketing for MedTech companies, transforming an industry traditionally focused on in-person interactions. By adopting digital marketing technologies and workflows, MedTech organizations can forge stronger relationships with HCPs and customers, ultimately enhancing the patient experience (Pandey and Pal, 2020). With this backdrop, this chapter aims to elucidate the expanding role of digital marketing, its significance, applications, digital marketing strategies within the MedTech industry, and the potential for industry growth and future opportunities.

Chapter 5 was created by reviewing scientific journals from reputable sources, including Google Scholar, Wiley Online Library, Science Direct, and Springer Link. It is entirely based on secondary data sources. In addition to these sources, the terms "digital marketing," "digital transformation in healthcare," "importance of digital marketing in healthcare," and "healthcare marketing strategies" has also been used in online sources (Bhambri and Gupta, 2018). The most recent data about the function of digital marketing in the healthcare industry was gathered through a search. This data was then further filtered to identify the several ways that digital marketing could benefit the contemporary healthcare industry.

5.2 IMPORTANCE OF DIGITAL MARKETING IN MEDTECH INDUSTRY

Digital marketing is a crucial aspect of the MedTech industry, as it integrates technology into conventional operations. The primary driving force behind this transformation is competition, and businesses are leveraging technological integrations to improve their operations and decision-making through advanced data analytics (Lo Presti et al., 2019). The main opportunities for effectively applying digital marketing in the MedTech industry revolve around pricing and strategy, workforce and collaboration, and product delivery. Understanding where a specific MedTech product stands among available offerings is crucial for determining its value proposition and distinctive features (Seattle New Media, 2023). Data can be collected from potential or current users of wearable tech to understand their needs better, which can then be included in product positioning and marketing plans. Customer feedback can also help set appropriate price points for products, aligning the purpose and price to drive more purchases (airtank.com, 2022). This leads to more efficient development pipelines based on the popularity and necessity of product features. Digital marketing within a company itself leads to a more effective and productive workforce and development pipeline. As the healthcare industry becomes increasingly digital, industries connected to healthcare are adopting digital practices (Rayner, 2023). Digitization promotes collaboration and innovation, resulting in better products and business outcomes. A solid foundation of digital integration allows employees to work more effectively and plan for the future. The importance of digital marketing is evident during global crises, such as the Covid-19 pandemic, where many aspects of MedTech work shifted to remote and virtual environments (Perzynska, 2023). Companies that had already embraced digital marketing were better equipped to navigate the pandemic because they had a solid foundation for productive digital work. The most complex but highly effective aspect of digital marketing for MedTech companies is the digitization of the supply chain. Shifting to a digitally driven supply chain enables companies to track data across various areas and analyze it for higher efficiency (Bartlett et al., 2021). In a digital supply chain, these areas can communicate and support each other more effectively through a shared digital core of data. Digital data allows for a holistic view of the entire supply network, driving informed business decisions and growth.

5.3 CONTRIBUTION OF DIGITAL MARKETING TO THE HEALTHCARE SECTOR

Healthcare organizations in the United States are facing a fiercely competitive landscape, with consumers demanding ease of access, expediency, and an enhanced enduring journey (innoservdigital.com, 2022). Online marketing can assist healthcare entities maintain a competitive edge by connecting, informing, and swaying consumers through strategies tailored to their core audience via digital channels such as social media, user-friendly apps, and the organization's website. A strong online presence can not only engage current patients but also attract new ones (itrobes.com, 2023).

Digital marketing helps medical professionals build a closer, more intimate relationship with their patients, as they can easily obtain information about their health conditions and available treatments at any time and from any location (Kaur and Bhambri, 2019). This enhanced accessibility results in improved patient engagement and satisfaction, ultimately leading to better patient outcomes (Haleem et al., 2021). By focusing on particular patient groups, healthcare organizations can customize their advertising contents and services to improve with their unique needs, leading to increased income by pull towards hospital more patients attracted in their support, ultimately contributing to higher productivity and augmentation (Bernstein, 2021).

The endemic has underscored the importance of online marketing in health sector, as it has highlighted the significance of healthcare accessibility. More clients are whirling to online platforms to access medicinal information, calendar appointments, be trained about a practice's services, and even obtain digital care (mymarketing.io, 2023). It is more important than ever for healthcare leaders to investigate how digital healthcare strategies can help them achieve their business objectives, given the growing competition in the industry and the increasing reliance on digital platforms for medical information, whether through websites or user-friendly apps (colorwhistle.com, 2023).

5.3.1 Targeted Advertising: It is a highly effective strategy for healthcare providers, but they must navigate marketing fulfillment under the centralized Health Insurance Portability and Accountability Act of 1996 (HIPAA). To safeguard their practice and patients, it is advisable to engage a digital marketing partner well-versed in HIPAA compliance to guide them. The U.S. division of Health and Human Services offers valuable resources on HIPAA solitude canon and promotion, which allow targeted marketing to the specific collection of people who are most expected to require particular products/services or products (Lutkevich, 2022).

5.3.2 Social Media Marketing: It has surfaced as a potent instrument for connecting with and appealing probable patients. Social media sites like Facebook, Instagram, and Twitter offer a plethora of chances for medical professionals to impart their knowledge and enlighten the public on a range of health-related subjects. By sharing relevant and captivating content, healthcare suppliers can institute them as consideration leaders and cultivate confidence among current and prospective patients (sproutsocial.com, 2023).

5.3.3 Email and SMS Marketing: This has materialized as a commanding instrument for observing patients up to date about their engagements and the innovative services available at a practice. By sending modified emails or text messages, healthcare suppliers can enhance the long-suffering care experience and foster patient loyalty to the organization. Regular communications can focus on well-timed wellness information or service-specific details, such as instructions on nutritious, kid-friendly school lunches or engaging developmental activities based on the child's age (River Cartie, 2022).

5.3.4 Search Engine Optimization (SEO): It stands as a powerful digital marketing approach for healthcare suppliers to enhance their digital presence and draw probable patients (Kuzhaloli et al., 2020). By regulating their website using keywords associated with their fields of expertise, healthcare suppliers can enhance their rankings in explore engine results, securing superior positions on search engine outcome pages (Frankel, 2022). Healthcare facilities can enhance their online visibility and credibility by implementing SEO tactics such as acquiring backlinks from other websites linking to their website. This not only strengthens their online authority but also attracts individuals actively seeking their services, resulting in highly targeted web traffic (outlookindia.com, 2023). SEO is an enduring online marketing approach that yields lasting benefits, allowing healthcare providers to sustain high search engine rankings and attract a growing patient base over time.

5.3.5 Price-per-click (PPC) Advertising: It is another non-organic method of enhancing SEO, where business people pay search engine platforms like Google, Yahoo, or Bing to display their advertisement at the pinnacle of search outcome pages (Gandolf, 2023). This non-organic approach can be effective for healthcare facilities, as it can augment website visitors by indenting the individuals searching for keywords related to their services. PPC campaigns generate immediate results, allowing the facility to present tailored ads emphasizing its expertise in treating anxiety and depression (webfx.com, 2023).

5.4 ADVANTAGES OF DIGITAL MARKETING FOR DOCTORS AND CLINICS

The advent of digitalization has significantly transformed various industries, including healthcare, and has reshaped the global business landscape. Traditional marketing practices are no longer sufficient to sustain a business, and healthcare digital marketing has become crucial as patients now base their choices on online reviews and recommendations (Digidotes, 2023). In today's digitally connected world, doctors and clinics can leverage digital marketing techniques such as SEO and social media to reach large audiences, create a favorable brand image, and attract new clients (innoservdigital.com, 2023). For doctors, digital marketing offers five comprehensive advantages: Enhanced visibility, increased patient engagement, enhanced reputation management, cost-effectiveness, and enhanced patient data collection. They are as follows:

5.4.1 Enhanced Visibility: It is achieved through strategic optimization of their online presence for search engines, ensuring that patients can easily locate them when searching for relevant keywords and phrases (itrobes.com, 2023). Utilizing SEO techniques like keyword research, optimizing meta tags, titles, and descriptions, and establishing reputable backlinks to their website from other credible sources can help doctors secure top positions in search results, augmenting visibility and attracting more patients (Josh, 2021).

5.4.2 Increased Patient Engagement: it is another significant benefit of digital marketing for doctors. By leveraging social media, email marketing, and various online platforms, doctors can foster deeper connections with patients, providing valuable information, answering inquiries, and nurturing enduring relationships over time. This helps establish their practice as a trusted authority in their field, fostering long-lasting relationships with patients (futurionic.com, 2023).

5.4.3 Reputation Management: In the digital era patients can easily share their experiences and opinions about doctors and their practices on online review platforms like Yelp and Google My Business. Digital marketing strategies enable doctors to proactively oversee their online reputation, address reviews, and engage with patients to resolve any concerns (Josh, 2021).

5.4.4 Cost-Effectiveness: It is another advantage of digital marketing for physicians. Digital advertising ventures like Google Advertisement, and Facebook Advertisement allow doctors to mark definite spectators based on demographics, common interests, and behavior, yielding a superior return on investment (ROI) for their marketing endeavors (Josh, 2021).

5.4.5 Enhanced Patient Data Collection: It is another advantage of digital marketing tools, as it provides doctors with valuable insights into patient behavior, preferences, and requirements. By scrutinizing this data, doctors can detect trends, make informed decisions, and customize their services to meet their patients' specific needs (futurionic.com, 2023).

5.5 FOR HOSPITALS

The healthcare industry is currently undergoing a significant transformation, and the sole way for businesses to endure the challenges and remain viable is by embracing healthcare digital marketing. Here are a few ways in which digital marketing can benefit a healthcare brand or business.

5.5.1 Reaching the Target Audience: The increasing competition in healthcare has led to a need for businesses to differentiate themselves through effective digital marketing. Google reports that 44% of internet users schedule appointments with clinics or healthcare professionals after visiting their websites or seeking contact details online. Without proper marketing efforts, your website or contact information may not appear in search results, highlighting the importance of reaching your target audience (Prasad, 2023).

5.5.2 Lowering Cost per Acquisition (CPA): Healthcare businesses often avoid digital marketing due to high costs and low ROI. Traditional advertising methods like print and television are expensive and ineffective, leading to low return on investment. Healthcare digital marketing offers cost-effective solutions, reducing the cost per acquisition and allowing businesses to connect with a wide network of audiences and establish multiple communication channels.

5.5.3 Provides Transparent and Measurable Data and Analytics: Digital marketing offers a measurable and straightforward approach to tracking progress in traditional marketing methods. It provides marketers with valuable insights into which channels yield the highest conversions, enabling them to adapt their strategies for enhanced success rates (Breuer et al., 2021). This approach eliminates uncertainty about the effectiveness of digital marketing, allowing for continuous monitoring and evaluation of analytics to gain a clear understanding of the campaign's effectiveness (webmdignite.com, 2023).

5.5.4 Enhances the Patient Experience: Digital marketing bridges the communication gap between patients and healthcare businesses, enabling proactive communication with offers and updates. Patients can also easily contact healthcare businesses with questions or feedback, fostering improved customer satisfaction and higher retention rates. This approach is crucial in healthcare branding (Gaurav, 2023).

5.6 STRATEGIES FOR HEALTHCARE DIGITAL MARKETING

In the current healthcare landscape, it is essential for providers to establish their unique identity and utilize digital marketing tactics throughout the customer's decision-making process. Healthcare providers should adopt the following digital healthcare marketing strategies (innoservdigital.com, 2023).

5.6.1 Emphasizing the Patient Experience: By showcasing the patient journey and showcasing their expertise and services, healthcare providers can engage with their audience and showcase their expertise. Acknowledging and sharing user-generated content, such as reviews, demonstrates commitment to social listening and making patients feel acknowledged and heard (marq.com, 2023).

5.6.2 Combating Misinformation: Up to 87% of social media users are exposed to health misinformation on platforms they frequent. Healthcare social media marketing offers a platform for trusted medical professionals to provide reassurance and evidence-based medical guidance. An effective public health campaign relies heavily on vaccine advocacy from the American Academy of Pediatrics, a preeminent authority in paediatric medicine (Suarez-Lledo and Alvarez-Galvez, 2021).

5.6.3 Educating the Public: Content in healthcare social media marketing serves as a valuable educational tool, helping the public understand the relevance of research to current healthcare practices. Companies like Cedars-Sinai can use social media platforms to promote articles, increase website traffic, and improve search engine rankings (marq.com, 2023).

5.6.4 Promoting Preventative Care: Advocacy is essential for healthcare organizations to have a substantial influence on social media and market preventive services that can impact medical outcomes. Collaboration with other healthcare organizations can extend the reach of content and broaden the audience (marq.com, 2023).

5.6.5 Establishing Trustworthiness: Healthcare providers should focus on becoming a reliable source of healthcare information and an authoritative voice in the industry. This can be achieved by highlighting the outstanding talent within the company, such as the Mayo Clinic, which prominently features its world-class doctors and researchers on social media (swaay.health, 2020).

5.7 DIGITAL MARKETING CHALLENGES FACED BY THE HEALTHCARE PROVIDERS

Digital marketing is now a vital element for hospitals within today's digital landscape. Nevertheless, healthcare providers encounter a range of obstacles that impede their progress in this domain. The following are the primary issues experienced by healthcare providers in digital marketing:

5.7.1 Data Privacy and Security Concerns: Hospitals face challenges in digital marketing, particularly in protecting patient data. To comply with

HIPAA regulations, they must implement robust security measures, train staff on data protection, and conduct regular audits of digital platforms to ensure data privacy and security (Prabhu, 2023).

5.7.2 Resource and Expertise Limitations: Hospitals often face budget, personnel, and digital marketing limitations. To overcome these, they can invest in staff training, outsource tasks, and use automation tools (weareamnet.com, 2023).

5.7.3 Complex Healthcare Landscape: The healthcare sector is complex, involving multiple stakeholders, regulations, and medical terminology. Effective digital communication can be challenging, but hospitals can simplify concepts, use plain language, and use multimedia content (mds.healthcare, 2023).

5.7.4 Trust and Credibility: Hospitals face challenges in building trust and credibility online due to patients' skepticism about healthcare information. To overcome this, they must establish themselves as reliable sources of truthful information through content marketing, social media engagement, and patient testimonials (Prabhu, 2023).

5.7.5 Targeting the Right Audience: Hospitals offer diverse services to various patient groups, but effective targeting requires understanding their needs, preferences, and behaviors. To improve targeting, hospitals can conduct market research, segment the target audience, and tailor marketing messages to specific patient segments (Prabhu, 2023).

5.7.6 Competition from Other Healthcare Providers: Hospitals must differentiate themselves from competitors like private clinics and online telemedicine platforms by highlighting their unique value propositions, expertise, personalized care, and patient-centered approach, while also highlighting success stories and patient outcomes (weareamnet.com, 2023).

5.7.7 Keeping Pace with Evolving Technology: Hospitals must stay updated with the latest digital marketing trends and technologies to effectively engage their target audience. This involves investing in staff training, participating in industry conferences, and collaborating with digital marketing experts (Prabhu, 2023).

5.8 FUTURE OF HEALTHCARE DIGITAL MARKETING

The global digital transformation in healthcare market is estimated to reach US$ 253.6 billion by 2033, with a CAGR of 14.5% from 2023 to 2033. This growth is driven by the implementation of online health areas such as SMS, telehealth, mail health, mobile health, and other wireless devices across medicinal amenities and tending homes, offering real-time medical treatment. The market has seen a 21.4% CAGR between 2018 and 2022, driven by the implementation of progressive technologies across numerous sectors in the medical industry. Government institutions also introduced health related smartphone appliances and enticement program have played a significant role in the diligence, and online healthcare is considered an promising know-how in superior countries like the United States, Germany, and China (futuremarketinsights.com, 2023).

The increasing implementation of connected health methods, the incorporation of online media, health expertise, and smartphones, are key factors propelling the digital transformation of the healthcare market. As medical technology moves forward, smart gadgets and wearables turn out to be more extensively available; the utilization of associated health clarification grows. The growing requires for distant examination and online communication to vigilant patients to go behind enduring treatment courses are strengthening the demand for associated health and increasing the expansion of the digital conversion in the medical care market (futuremarketinsights.com, 2023).

Increasing per capita healthcare expenditure is stimulating demand for better medical services, with administration and medical organizations investing in IT infrastructure to better satisfy customer needs. Public administration in countries like the United States and Canada are highlighting the accomplishment of digital inventiveness to persuade modernization and digitization in the healthcare field, principally aimed at encouraging hospices and health centers to implement enhanced analytical tools and online medical services (Nikhil Pandey, 2023). Data processing and analysis remain significant challenges in the healthcare sector, with the huge amount of data composed by hospices, health centers, and medical specialists. Virtual or online security is a significant confronts in each sector, counting medical sector, and organizations must be careful against online threats, which can be enormously costly (futuremarketinsights.com, 2023).

5.9 DISCUSSIONS AND CONCLUSION

Digital marketing can significantly grow the business of medical services by drawing in new clients and providing high-quality care. This approach increases patient involvement, contentment, and loyalty, as well as expands the brand/business online. A study conducted in Bangladesh found that people use hospital websites and social media platforms like Facebook groups to gather information about doctors, search for healthcare providers, and post reviews of their experiences. Many also visit hospital or physician websites to read reviews.

However, health services lag behind the industry in digital marketing due to challenges such as patient privacy, security, regulations, lack of guidance on proper use of digital platforms, staff interest in using social media, inadequate infrastructure to handle complaints, and unclear roles in different internet marketing initiatives. To effectively apply digital technology, management commitment and consistency are required. An experimental strategy should be used instead of a planned strategy for electronic communications to prevent improper integration of offline and online marketing communications.

Online marketing has an important brunt on various fronts, such as boosting social media and advertising engagement, playing as a KPI for appraising managerial values, driving up requirement for online products, expanding users' goods searches, and pouring demand for substance policy. The Covid-19 epidemic has tinted the significance of digital marketing during this time, offering benefits such as drawing in new business, growing patient base, boosting client and long-suffering loyalty, building trust, raising brand consciousness, encouraging patients to make use of hospice services, and advertising overhaul to patients' families.

The hospice aims to determine the most suitable online promotion platforms or strategies to utilize. Prior to proceeding, the hospice must establish its objectives, select the suitable online media platforms or strategies, assess the target audience and market share, and decide the budget plan and frequency of marketing efforts. Additionally, choosing the right person to execute the selected marketing plan is essential for its execution.

REFERENCES

airtank.com. (2022, November 16). *The Rise of Digital Marketing in the MedTech and Wellness Industries.* www.airtank.com/blog/the-rise-of-digital-marketing-in-the-medtech-and-wellness-industries

Anand, A., & Bhambri, P. (2018). Rotation, Scale and Translation Invariant Character Recognition System using Neural Network. Punjab Technical University, Jalandhar (M. Tech. thesis).

Bartlett, Richard, Adam Somauroo, and Christian Zerbi. (2021, May 7). *How the Medtech Industry Can Capture Value from Digital Health.* www.mckinsey.com/industries/life-sciences/our-insights/how-the-medtech-industry-can-capture-value-from-digital-health

Bernstein, Corinne. (2021, March 22). *Digital Health.* www.techtarget.com/searchhealthit/definition/digital-health-digital-healthcare

Bhambri, P., & Gupta, O. P. (2018). Implementing Machine Learning Algorithms for Distance based Phylogenetic Trees. I.K. Gujral Punjab Technical University, Jalandhar (Ph.D. thesis).

Bhambri, P., Sinha, V. K., & Jaiswal, M. (2019). Change in Iris Dimensions as a Potential Human Consciousness Level Indicator. In International Conference on Innovations in Communication, Computing and Sciences.

Breuer, Ralph, Elizabeth Guenther, Rukhshana Motiwala, and Christian Zerbi. (2021 September 24). *The Rise of Digital Marketing in Medtech.* www.mckinsey.com/industries/life-sciences/our-insights/the-rise-of-digital-marketing-in-medtech

colorwhistle.com. (2023 July 6). *Why is Digital Marketing Essential for the Healthcare Industry?* https://colorwhistle.com/digital-marketing-for-healthcare-industry/

Digidotes. (2023, June 19). *The 5 Top Benefits of Digital Marketing for Doctors: How to Boost Your Practice Online.* www.linkedin.com/pulse/5-top-benefits-digital-marketing-doctors-how-boost-your-practice/

Frankel, Alexis. (2022, September 20). *10-Step Guide to Effective Healthcare SEO.* www.semrush.com/blog/healthcare-seo/

Furtner, D., Shinde, S. P., Singh, M., Wong, C. H., & Setia, S. (2022). Digital transformation in medical affairs sparked by the pandemic: Insights and learnings from COVID-19 era and beyond. *Pharmaceutical Medicine*, 36(1), 1–10.

futuremarketinsights.com. (2023 April 24). *futuremarketinsights.com.* www.futuremarketinsights.com/reports/digital-healthcare-market

futurionic.com. (2023). *Importance of Digital Marketing for Hospitals, Doctors, and Clinics.* www.futurionic.com/blog/how-is-digital-marketing-important-for-doctors-hospitals-clinics/

Gandolf, Stewart. (2023, September 24). *Healthcare Pay-Per-Click Advertising: Here's What You Should Consider.* https://healthcaresuccess.com/blog/doctor-marketing/healthcare-pay-per-click-advertising.html#:~:text=Nearly%2090%20percent%20of%20the,competitive%20field%20of%20healthcare%20advertising

Gaurav, Dhingra. (2023, July 27). *Top Five Benefits of Digital Marketing for Hospitals.* www.refreshhealthcare.in/blog/healthcare-marketing/benefits-of-digital-marketing

Haleem, A., Javaid, M., Singh, R. P., & Suman, R. (2021). Telemedicine for healthcare: Capabilities, features, barriers, and applications. *Sensors International*, 2, 100117.

Hermes, S., Riasanow, T., Clemons, E. K., Böhm, M., & Krcmar, H. (2020). The digital transformation of the healthcare industry: exploring the rise of emerging platform ecosystems and their influence on the role of patients. *Business Research*, 13, 1033–1069.

Herrmann, M., Boehme, P., Mondritzki, T., Ehlers, J. P., Kavadias, S., & Truebel, H. (2018). Digital transformation and disruption of the health care sector: Internet-based observational study. *Journal of Medical Internet Research*, 20(3), e104.

innoservdigital.com. (2022, February 5). A Healthcare Digital Marketing Guide: 8 Ways To Get More Patients With Digital Marketing in 2022.

innoservdigital.com. (2023, July 21). *Why Digital Marketing is Important For Doctors, Hospitals & Clinics?* www.innoservdigital.com/blog/digital-marketing-benefits-important-for-doctors-hospitals-clinics/

itrobes.com. (2023, June 14). *What is Healthcare Digital Marketing and its Importance?* www.itrobes.com/healthcare-digital-marketing/#:~:text=It%20Improves%20Patient%20Experience,patients%20with%20offers%20and%20updates

Josh. (2021, August 13). *The Importance of Digital Marketing for Doctors and Clinics in 2021.* https://smartclinix.net/importance-of-digital-marketing-for-doctors-and-clinics/

Kaur, J., & Bhambri, P. (2019). Design of Paddy Crop Prediction Technique Based on K-Mean, Naïve Bayes, KNN and SVM Classifiers. I.K. Gujral Punjab Technical University, Jalandhar (M. Tech. thesis).

Kuzhaloli, S., Devaneyan, P., Sitaraman, N., Periyathanbi, P., Gurusamy, M., & Bhambri, P. (2020). IoT based Smart Kitchen Application for Gas Leakage Monitoring. IN Patent App. 202,041,049,866 A.

Lo Presti, L., Testa, M., Marino, V., & Singer, P. (2019). Engagement in healthcare systems: Adopting digital tools for a sustainable approach. *Sustainability*, 11(1), 220.

Lutkevich, Ben. (2022, August 24). *HIPAA (Health Insurance Portability and Accountability Act).* www.techtarget.com/searchhealthit/definition/HIPAA

marq.com. (2023, June 22). *How to Improve Patient Experience.* www.marq.com/blog/how-to-improve-patient-experience?_gl=1*eh9vr6*_gcl_au*MzU3OTI4NzEyLjE2OTg3MzU3NDI.

mds.healthcare. (2023, April 12). *Healthcare Digital Marketing & Its Major Challenges.* https://mds.healthcare/learn/healthcare-digital-marketing-company-and-its-major-challenges/

mymarketing.io. (2023 September 18). *Digital Marketing in the Healthcare Industry.* https://mymarketing.io/blog/digital-marketing-in-the-healthcare-industry/

outlookindia.com. (2023, October 30). *Healthcare SEO For Hospitals-Emerging Search Trends & New Opportunities.* www.outlookindia.com/business-spotlight/healthcare-seo-for-hospitals-news-311447

Pandey, N. (2023, September 27). *Top 10 Digital Transformation Trends and Innovations That Will Reshape Healthcare in 2024.* https://emeritus.org/in/learn/digital-transformation-for-healthcare/

Pandey, N., & Pal, A. (2020). Impact of digital surge during Covid-19 pandemic: A viewpoint on research and practice. *International Journal of Information Management*, 55, 102171.

Perzynska, Kasia. (2023, October 25). *Why Customer Feedback is Important: The Ultimate Guide.* https://survicate.com/customer-feedback/why-customer-feedback-is-important/

Prabhu, Ramnath. (2023, August 21). *Challenges Faced by Hospitals in Digital Marketing: Overcoming the Hurdles.* www.linkedin.com/pulse/challenges-faced-hospitals-digital-marketing-hurdles-ramnath-prabhu/

Prasad, Ajay. (2023, April 25). *Significant Benefits of Digital Marketing for Healthcare Businesses.* www.gmrwebteam.com/blog/significant-benefits-of-digital-marketing-for-healthcare-businesses

Raju, Narasimha. (2023, May 08). *The Role of Digital Marketing in the Healthcare Sector.*

Rayner, Steven. (2023, July 3). *The Role of Digital Marketing in Promoting Medical Devices in the UK*. www.linkedin.com/pulse/role-digital-marketing-promoting-medical-devices-uk-steven-rayner/

River Cartie. (2022, January 25). *Healthcare Email Marketing: Why It Works and How to Get Started*. www.constantcontact.com/blog/email-marketing-for-healthcare/

Seattle New Media. (2023, May 3). *Why is Digital Marketing Important for Healthcare Industry?* www.seattlenewmedia.com/blog/digital-marketing-for-healthcare-industry#:~:text=Make%20data%2Ddriven%20decisions,are%20saying%20about%20their%20services.

sproutsocial.com. (2023, July 24). *Social Media for Healthcare: How to Keep Patients Engaged in the Digital Age*. https://sproutsocial.com/insights/social-media-in-healthcare/

Stoumpos, A. I., Kitsios, F., & Talias, M. A. (2023). Digital Transformation in Healthcare: Technology Acceptance and Its Applications. *International Journal of Environmental Research and Public Health*, 20(4), 3407.

Suarez-Lledo, Victor, & Javier Alvarez-Galvez. (2021). Prevalence of Health Misinformation on Social Media: Systematic Review. *Journal of Medical Internet Research*, 23, 1.

swaay.health. (2020). *Top 10 U.S. Hospitals and Children's Hospitals on Social Media*. https://swaay.health/2020/02/19/top-10-u-s-hospitals-and-childrens-hospitals-on-social-media/

weareamnet.com. (2023, June 20). *7 Healthcare Marketing Challenges (And How to Overcome Them)*. www.weareamnet.com/blog/healthcare-marketing-challenges/

webfx.com. (2023, April 16). *Healthcare PPC: 7 Hospital Advertising Tips for Your Ads*. www.webfx.com/industries/health/hospitals-healthcare/ppc/

webmdignite.com. (2023, February 16). *Importance of Digital Marketing in Healthcare*. https://webmdignite.com/blog/evolving-role-digital-marketing-healthcare

6 Cloud and IoT Integration for Smart Healthcare

Pankaj Bhambri and Suresh Kumar

6.1 INTRODUCTION

Cloud computing offers a flexible and centralized infrastructure for securely storing and managing large quantities of healthcare data. This not only facilitates seamless access to patient records and medical information but also supports real-time analytics and data-driven insights. By leveraging cloud infrastructure, healthcare providers can enhance collaboration, streamline processes, and improve the overall efficiency of healthcare services. Conversely, internet of things (IoT) devices play a role in establishing a linked healthcare ecosystem. Wearable devices, intelligent sensors, and medical IoT devices facilitate the uninterrupted monitoring of sufferers' vital signs as well as wellness metrics. Real-time information can be sent to the cloud, enabling healthcare experts to watch patients from a distance, detect abnormalities, and offer prompt solutions.

The synergy between cloud and IoT in smart healthcare extends beyond data management. The integration enables the development of innovative healthcare applications and services. Telemedicine platforms, remote patient monitoring systems, and personalized healthcare apps become more robust and accessible with the combined power of cloud computing and IoT. Furthermore, the partnership improves the protection and confidentiality of health information by using sophisticated encryption as well as access control protocols within the cloud architecture. The integration of cloud and IoT technologies is crucial in defining the future of smart healthcare systems that are efficient, personalized, accessible, and responsive to the changing demands of patients as well as physicians.

6.1.1 Objectives of Cloud and IoT Integration in Smart Healthcare

The convergence of cloud computing and the internet of things (IoT) in the realm of smart healthcare entails a number of primary goals, with the aim of improving the effectiveness, availability, and calibre of healthcare provisions. Here are some of the primary objectives:

- Real-Time Monitoring and Data Collection: Leverage the cloud's scalability and storage capabilities to handle the vast amount of data generated by

DOI: 10.1201/9781032698519-6

IoT devices in real-time. Enable continuous monitoring of patients' health through wearable devices, sensors, and medical equipment, transmitting data to the cloud instantly.

- Remote Patient Monitoring: Facilitate remote monitoring of patients from anywhere in the world through secure cloud connections. Deploy IoT devices for continuous tracking of vital signs, medication adherence, and other health parameters, allowing healthcare providers to intervene promptly.
- Data Analytics and Predictive Insights: Utilize cloud-based analytics tools to process and analyze the massive datasets collected from IoT devices. Extract meaningful insights from real-time and historical data to identify trends, predict health issues, and personalize treatment plans.
- Enhanced Patient Engagement: Develop interactive and user-friendly applications on cloud platforms to engage patients in their healthcare management. Foster patient participation through wearable devices that provide personalized feedback, reminders, and health education, promoting a proactive approach to wellness.
- Interoperability and Integration: Promote interoperability by adopting cloud standards that facilitate seamless integration of various healthcare systems and IoT devices. Ensure compatibility among different IoT devices and platforms, enabling a cohesive and interconnected healthcare ecosystem.
- Security and Privacy Measures: Implement robust security measures in the cloud infrastructure to protect sensitive healthcare data. Employ encryption, authentication, and secure communication protocols for IoT devices to safeguard patient information and maintain privacy.
- Resource Optimization and Cost Efficiency: Optimize resource utilization by leveraging cloud-based services, reducing the need for extensive on-premise infrastructure. Improve resource allocation and healthcare delivery by utilizing data-driven insights for efficient patient management and treatment plans.
- Scalability and Flexibility: Accommodate varying workloads and data volumes efficiently by leveraging the scalability of cloud resources. Easily scale up the deployment of IoT devices as needed, ensuring flexibility and adaptability to changing healthcare demands.
- Faster Decision-Making: Enable healthcare professionals to access real-time patient data from anywhere, facilitating quicker and more informed decision-making. Process data rapidly in the cloud, providing timely insights for medical practitioners to make critical decisions.
- Telemedicine and Remote Consultations: Utilize cloud infrastructure for hosting telemedicine applications, enabling remote consultations and virtual healthcare services. Ensure seamless connectivity between IoT devices and telemedicine platforms for comprehensive remote patient care.

6.2 FUNDAMENTALS OF CLOUD COMPUTING IN HEALTHCARE

Cloud computing for healthcare is the utilization of distant servers and computing resources, which can be accessed via the internet, for the purpose of storing and processing healthcare information and applications (Bhambri and Gupta, 2005). This innovative method enables healthcare organizations to make use of scalable and cost-efficient solutions without requiring a large on-site infrastructure. Healthcare practitioners can securely store and access patient records, do data analytics to get insights into population wellness and personalized therapy plans, and promote collaboration among medical experts in the cloud. Moreover, the cloud's adaptability facilitates the smooth incorporation of cutting-edge technologies like telemedicine, AI, and machine learning, promoting a more integrated and efficient healthcare system. Healthcare organizations may optimize data accessibility, increase patient care, and optimize administrative procedures by utilizing the core principles of cloud computing.

6.2.1 Cloud Infrastructure Overview

Cloud infrastructure is a versatile and expandable computing environment that can be accessed through the internet. It provides a variety of services including processing power, storage, and networking. These resources, consisting of data centres equipped with servers, are accessible to organizations on a pay-as-you-go basis. This allows organizations to easily expand their operations without the need to maintain large physical infrastructure. Prominent cloud service providers, such as Amazon Web Services (AWS), Microsoft Azure, and Google Cloud Platform, provide a range of services, including Infrastructure as a Service (IaaS), Platform as a Service (PaaS), and Software as a Service (SaaS). Infrastructure as a Service (IaaS) gives virtualized computing resources, Platform as a Service (PaaS) provides a development platform for applications, and Software as a Service (SaaS) delivers software applications via the internet. Cloud infrastructure provides businesses with agility, cost-effectiveness, and the ability to rapidly deploy and scale applications, making it a foundational element for various industries, including healthcare, to optimize operations and innovation. Figure 6.1 shows the various types of cloud infrastructure.

6.2.2 Cloud Services in Healthcare

Cloud services offer healthcare providers the ability to securely store patient records, images, and other critical information in a centralized and easily accessible manner, fostering collaboration and improving overall patient care (Liu et al., 2018). Cloud-based solutions also facilitate seamless integration of various healthcare applications and services, promoting interoperability and enhancing the efficiency of healthcare workflows. Moreover, cloud computing enables advanced analytics, machine learning, and artificial intelligence applications, allowing healthcare professionals to derive valuable insights from the data for personalized medicine, predictive analytics, and improved decision-making. Although there are many advantages, it is crucial to prioritize strong security measures and adherence to healthcare legislation in order to protect patient confidentiality and retain confidence when implementing cloud services in the healthcare industry.

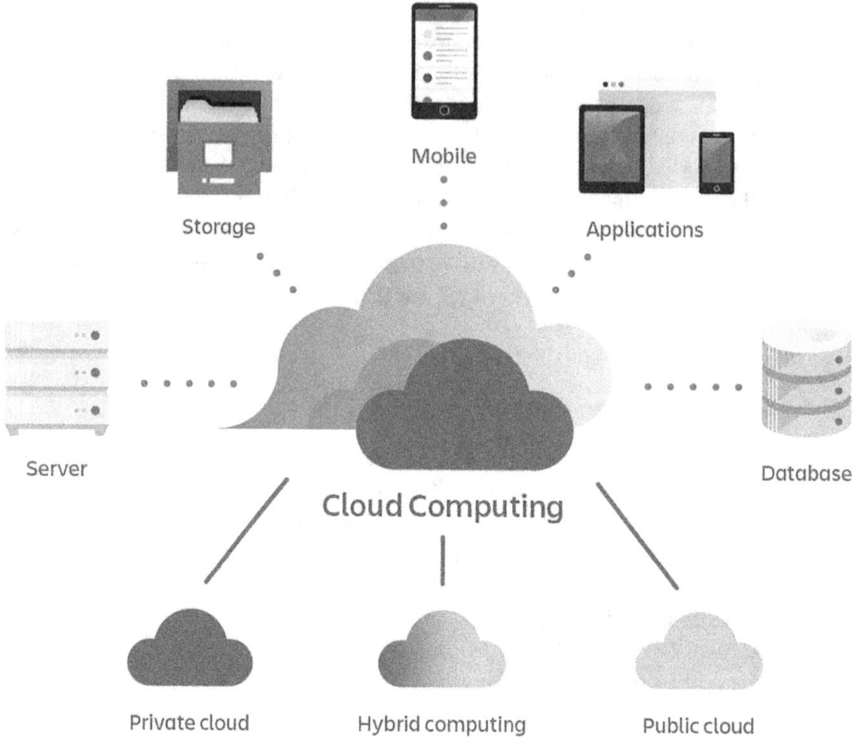

FIGURE 6.1 Types of cloud infrastructure.

6.2.3 Benefits and Challenges

Cloud computing in healthcare brings about several benefits, which are discussed:

- Improved Accessibility and Collaboration: Cloud computing allows healthcare providers to access patient data and collaborate seamlessly across various locations. This accessibility enhances the speed and efficiency of healthcare delivery.
- Scalability: Cloud services provide healthcare organizations with the ability to easily and flexibly adapt their computing resources in response to changes in demand (Singh et al., 2005). This scalability is particularly valuable when dealing with varying workloads, such as during peak times or when implementing new healthcare initiatives.
- Cost Savings: Cloud computing obviates the necessity for substantial on-premises hardware infrastructure and expenses related to maintenance (Al-Masrani and Al-Jumeily, 2016). Healthcare providers have the option to implement a pay-as-you-go model, where they only pay for the specific resources they use. This approach can lead to possible reductions in costs.

- Interoperability: Cloud solutions can integrate diverse healthcare systems and applications, promoting interoperability. Interoperability improves communication among diverse healthcare groups, resulting in a more holistic and integrated approach to patient treatment.
- Advanced Analytics and AI: Cloud computing enables the use of advanced analytics and AI tools. This allows healthcare professionals to derive valuable insights from vast datasets, leading to improved diagnostics, personalized treatment plans, and predictive healthcare analytics.

Along-with these benefits, it also presents its own set of challenges:

- Security and Privacy Concerns: The storage and transmission of sensitive healthcare data on the cloud raises concerns about security and privacy. Healthcare providers need robust security measures and compliance with regulations like HIPAA to ensure the confidentiality of patient information.
- Regulatory Compliance: Strict regulations govern the healthcare industry, making adherence to different regional and worldwide standards essential. Adhering to these regulations while using cloud services can be challenging, requiring careful consideration of data sovereignty and legal requirements.
- Downtime and Reliability: Reliability and uptime are critical in healthcare. If cloud services experience downtime or disruptions, it can impact access to patient records and disrupt healthcare workflows. Ensuring high availability and reliability is essential.
- Data Migration and Integration: Transitioning existing healthcare systems to the cloud can be complex. Data migration and integration challenges may arise, and seamless integration with legacy systems is crucial to maintaining continuity in healthcare operations.
- Dependency on Internet Connectivity: Cloud computing is dependent on internet connectivity. In areas characterized by unstable or restricted internet connectivity, healthcare practitioners may have challenges in accessing crucial patient data and efficiently utilizing cloud-based services.

6.3 ESSENTIALS OF IoT IN SMART HEALTHCARE SYSTEMS

The essentials of IoT in smart healthcare systems lie in their ability to revolutionize patient care, streamline operations, and enhance overall efficiency (Shojafar and Cordeschi, 2017). IoT devices, such as wearable health trackers, remote monitoring sensors, and connected medical equipment, facilitate real-time data collection, enabling healthcare providers to monitor patient health remotely and intervene proactively. This constant stream of data contributes to personalized and data-driven healthcare decisions, leading to more effective treatment plans. Additionally, IoT fosters the integration of medical devices and systems, promoting seamless communication among different components within the healthcare ecosystem. This interconnectedness enhances diagnostic capabilities, optimizes resource utilization, and improves patient outcomes. Despite these advantages, ensuring robust cybersecurity measures is paramount to safeguard patient data and maintain the trust and integrity of smart healthcare systems leveraging IoT technologies.

6.3.1 IoT Architecture in Healthcare

The IoT architecture in healthcare is designed to interconnect a multitude of devices, sensors, and systems to collect, transmit, and analyze data, ultimately enhancing patient care and operational efficiency (Botta et al., 2016). At its core, IoT in healthcare comprises three main layers: The Perception Layer, where devices such as wearables, medical sensors, and monitoring tools collect real-time data; the Network Layer, facilitating the seamless communication and transmission of data securely and efficiently; and the Application Layer, where data is processed, analyzed, and integrated into healthcare systems, supporting functions like remote patient monitoring, predictive analytics, and personalized medicine (Bhambri and Bhandari, 2005). This architecture enables healthcare providers to gain timely insights, improve diagnosis and treatment, and enhance patient outcomes while fostering a more interconnected and data-driven healthcare ecosystem. However, ensuring robust security measures, addressing privacy concerns, and maintaining interoperability remain critical considerations in the implementation of IoT in healthcare.

6.3.2 Applications of IoT in Healthcare

The IoT has a wide range of applications in healthcare, contributing to the development of more efficient and patient-centric healthcare systems. Some notable applications include:

- Remote Patient Monitoring: The use of IoT devices allows for the continuous monitoring of patients in non-traditional healthcare environments. Wearable technologies and sensors have the capability to gather and send crucial physiological indicators, levels of physical activity, and other health measurements to healthcare specialists. This facilitates the ongoing surveillance of chronic illnesses and timely identification of possible problems.
- Smart Medical Devices: Medical gadgets like insulin pumps, cardiac pacemakers, and smart inhalers incorporate IoT technology. These gadgets have the capability to gather and send data, enabling healthcare personnel to track patients and make necessary adjustments to treatment programmes.
- Asset and Inventory Management: The IoT can be utilized for the purpose of monitoring and overseeing medical equipment, drugs, and other valuable resources within a medical centre (Sangwan Singh et al., 2021). This ensures the availability of resources when needed, reduces waste, and improves overall operational efficiency.
- Hospital Management and Workflow Optimization: IoT facilitates the optimization of hospital operations by monitoring and managing various aspects such as patient flow, bed occupancy, and equipment utilization. This helps in reducing waiting times, improving resource allocation, and enhancing overall workflow efficiency.

- Medication Adherence: IoT devices have the capability to send reminders to patients for taking their medications at the scheduled time and also track their compliance with the medication regimen. This is especially advantageous for those with persistent illnesses who necessitate stringent treatment regimens for optimal control.
- Telemedicine and Virtual Consultations: IoT devices support telemedicine by enabling remote consultations and diagnostics. Connected devices can transmit relevant health data to healthcare providers, allowing for virtual monitoring and consultation without the need for in-person visits.
- Fall Detection and Elderly Care: IoT sensors and wearables can be used to detect falls among the elderly or individuals with mobility issues. This helps in providing timely assistance and improving the safety of patients, especially in home or assisted living environments.
- Health and Wellness Wearables: IoT-based wearables, such as fitness trackers and smart watches, are widely used to monitor physical activity, sleep patterns, and overall well-being. This data can be valuable for both individuals and healthcare providers in promoting preventive healthcare measures.
- Supply Chain Monitoring for Pharmaceuticals: IoT can be employed to monitor the transportation and storage conditions of pharmaceuticals and vaccines. This guarantees the authenticity and quality of pharmaceuticals while they are being transported and stored, hence minimizing the chances of deterioration or pollution.
- Infection Control and Environmental Monitoring: IoT sensors can be employed to monitor environmental parameters in healthcare facilities, such as air quality and temperature. This aids in infection control and helps maintain a safe and sterile environment for patients and healthcare workers.

6.3.3 Opportunities and Challenges

The IoT has the capacity to transform the healthcare sector by offering cutting-edge solutions to patient care, surveillance, and management. Nevertheless, in addition to the possibilities, there are several obstacles that require attention. Here are some opportunities and challenges of IoT in healthcare:

- Remote Patient Monitoring: IoT devices provide uninterrupted real-time monitoring of patients, enabling healthcare providers to remotely track vital signs as well as additional health data (Hao et al., 2015). This enables prompt identification of health problems, diminishes the need for hospital readmissions, and enhances overall patient results.
- Data-Driven Insights: IoT produces vast quantities of data which can be examined to extract significant observations regarding patient behavior, the efficacy of treatments, and trends in overall population health. Data analytics can lead to personalized and more effective healthcare interventions, as well as support public health initiatives.
- Improved Patient Engagement: Wearable devices and intelligent healthcare software enable patients to actively engage in the management of their

health. Heightened patient participation can result in increased compliance with treatment regimens, enhanced interaction with healthcare practitioners, and heightened overall patient contentment.

- Efficient Asset Management: IoT can be used for tracking and managing medical equipment, medications, and other healthcare assets. Improved asset utilization and reduced operational costs, leading to better resource management in healthcare facilities.
- Predictive Maintenance: IoT-enabled devices can predict when medical equipment requires maintenance or replacement, reducing downtime and ensuring the availability of critical healthcare infrastructure. Increased reliability of equipment, cost savings, and enhanced patient safety.
- Data Security and Privacy Concerns: The substantial volume of critical health data produced by IoT devices gives rise to issues regarding privacy and security of information (Islam et al., 2015). To tackle these difficulties, it is crucial to implement strong security measures, utilize encryption, and ensure compliance with standards like HIPAA.
- Interoperability Issues: Interoperability issues arise due to the diverse origins of healthcare IoT devices. Standardization efforts, common communication protocols, and industry collaboration are needed to ensure seamless integration of diverse IoT devices.
- Regulatory Compliance: Healthcare regulations and standards may struggle to keep pace with the rapid evolution of IoT technologies. Close collaboration between the healthcare industry and regulatory bodies to establish and update guidelines that address emerging IoT challenges.
- Integration with Existing Systems: Incorporating IoT solutions into current healthcare information technology (IT) systems can be intricate and may necessitate substantial financial commitment. Robust planning, phased implementation, and the use of interoperability standards can help streamline integration processes.
- Reliability and Accuracy: The dependability and precision of data gathered by IoT gadgets are essential for creating well-informed healthcare determinations. Rigorous testing, calibration, and continuous monitoring of IoT devices to ensure data accuracy and reliability.

6.4 CONVERGENCE OF CLOUD AND IoT IN HEALTHCARE

The integration of cloud computing and the IoT in the healthcare industry signifies a significant combination, where cloud-based platforms play a crucial role in handling and examining the extensive data produced by IoT devices. This integration enables seamless storage, processing, and retrieval of healthcare data, fostering real-time monitoring, predictive analytics, and personalized patient care. Cloud platforms offer scalable and secure infrastructure, allowing healthcare organizations to efficiently handle the diverse and evolving IoT ecosystem (Rachna et al., 2022). Through this convergence, healthcare providers can harness the power of cloud computing to centralize data storage, ensure interoperability, and leverage advanced analytics, ultimately improving operational efficiency, enhancing patient outcomes, and facilitating innovative approaches to healthcare delivery and management.

6.4.1 Synergies and Interactions

Cloud platforms provide the scalable infrastructure needed to handle the vast amounts of data generated by IoT devices, enabling seamless storage, processing, and analysis. This collaboration enhances real-time access to patient information, facilitates data-driven decision-making, and supports remote monitoring (Lasierra et al., 2019). By leveraging cloud-based services, healthcare providers can efficiently manage and share critical data, leading to improved collaboration among care teams. Additionally, the cloud-IoT integration enables the deployment of advanced analytics and machine learning algorithms, offering predictive insights for disease prevention and personalized treatment plans. As a result, this convergence not only enhances the efficiency and responsiveness of healthcare systems but also contributes to the delivery of more personalized and effective patient care.

6.4.2 Impact on Patient Care

Through the integration of IoT devices with cloud-based platforms, healthcare professionals gain access to real-time patient data, enabling remote monitoring and timely interventions. This convergence facilitates personalized and proactive healthcare approaches, as health data from wearables, medical devices, and other sensors are securely stored and analyzed in the cloud. Patients can benefit from continuous monitoring, early detection of health issues, and improved treatment plans. Moreover, the cloud infrastructure allows for scalable storage and efficient management of the vast amounts of data generated by IoT devices, fostering data-driven insights that enhance diagnosis and treatment strategies. Overall, the synergy between cloud and IoT in healthcare not only elevates the quality of patient care but also supports healthcare providers in making informed decisions for better health outcomes.

6.4.3 Resource Management Enhancements

Through the seamless integration of cloud and IoT technologies, healthcare providers can remotely monitor and manage patient data, enabling real-time analytics for more informed decision-making. This convergence facilitates improved resource allocation, as cloud-based solutions enhance the efficiency of healthcare processes, streamline data storage and retrieval, and support the deployment of advanced analytics for predictive insights. As a result, healthcare professionals can access critical information swiftly, leading to enhanced patient care, reduced operational costs, and more effective overall resource utilization in healthcare settings.

6.4.4 Overall System Efficiency Improvements

By leveraging the scalability and computational power of cloud infrastructure, healthcare organizations can seamlessly process and analyze vast volumes of data generated by IoT devices (Catarinucci et al., 2015). This integration facilitates real-time monitoring of patient health, predictive analytics, and data-driven decision-making. The cloud's storage capabilities enable secure and accessible archival of patient records and health information. Additionally, the cloud-IoT synergy enhances collaboration among healthcare professionals by providing them with instant access to synchronized and up-to-date patient data. This convergence not only streamlines administrative processes but also contributes to more personalized and proactive patient care, fostering a healthcare ecosystem that is agile, efficient, and capable of delivering improved outcomes.

6.5 TECHNOLOGICAL CONSIDERATIONS AND CHALLENGES

The integration of cloud and IoT in smart healthcare introduces several technological considerations and challenges. Firstly, ensuring seamless interoperability between diverse IoT devices and cloud platforms is critical to enable a cohesive and unified healthcare ecosystem. Standardization efforts and the adoption of common communication protocols become imperative to overcome the complexities arising from the multitude of devices and systems. Data security and privacy concerns also pose significant challenges, as the vast amounts of sensitive health data transmitted between IoT devices and the cloud requires robust encryption, authentication, and compliance with stringent regulatory frameworks. Additionally, addressing issues related to the reliability and low-latency requirements for real-time applications is crucial to maintaining the effectiveness of healthcare services. Balancing the need for scalability with the demand for low-latency responses becomes a delicate technological consideration, requiring sophisticated architecture designs and efficient resource management (Wang and Zhang, 2018). Overall, successful cloud and IoT integration in smart healthcare necessitates a comprehensive approach to technology, encompassing standardization, security, and performance optimization.

6.5.1 Data Security in Cloud and IoT Integration

Data security is a paramount concern in the integration of cloud and IoT for smart healthcare systems. The convergence of these technologies introduces a myriad of interconnected devices and platforms, leading to an increased attack surface and potential vulnerabilities. Ensuring the confidentiality, integrity, and availability of sensitive health data is crucial to prevent unauthorized access and protect patient privacy. Encryption, robust authentication mechanisms, and secure communication protocols are essential components in safeguarding data during its transmission and storage in the cloud. Additionally, compliance with stringent regulatory frameworks, such as HIPAA, is imperative to meet industry standards and address legal requirements. Continuous monitoring, threat detection, and regular updates to security protocols are fundamental in mitigating evolving cyber threats. Establishing a comprehensive and resilient security framework is vital to instill confidence in patients, healthcare providers, and stakeholders, fostering a trustworthy and secure environment for the integration of cloud and IoT in smart healthcare.

6.5.2 Interoperability Challenges and Solutions

The diverse array of IoT devices, each with its own data formats and communication protocols, often leads to difficulties in seamless information exchange and integration within cloud environments. Standardizing data formats and communication protocols is essential to ensure interoperability. Adopting common healthcare interoperability standards, such as HL7 and FHIR, can facilitate data exchange between devices and cloud platforms. Moreover, robust Application Programming Interfaces (APIs) that adhere to these standards can bridge the interoperability gap, enabling smooth communication and data sharing between different devices and cloud-based systems. Collaborative efforts between industry stakeholders, including device manufacturers, cloud service providers, and regulatory bodies, are crucial to establish and adhere to these standards, promoting a cohesive and interoperable ecosystem for smart healthcare solutions.

6.5.3 Scalability Issues and Strategies

As the volume of data generated by IoT devices continues to grow exponentially, ensuring that the cloud infrastructure can scale accordingly becomes crucial (Zhang et al., 2018). In order to address this challenge, healthcare organizations need to implement scalable cloud architectures that can handle the increasing data load efficiently. Cloud services should possess the capability to assign resources dynamically in response to demand, thereby guaranteeing optimal performance during periods of high usage. Furthermore, the utilization of edge computing, which involves processing data in proximity to IoT devices, might mitigate scalability issues by minimizing the volume of data transported to the cloud. Additionally, implementing robust data management and storage strategies, such as data compression and prioritization, can help optimize resource utilization. Continuous monitoring, predictive analytics, and proactive capacity planning are essential strategies to anticipate and address scalability issues, ensuring the seamless integration of cloud and IoT for efficient and responsive smart healthcare systems.

6.6 CASE STUDIES AND REAL-WORLD EXAMPLES

Major set of case studies and real-world examples are:

- Philips Healthcare and Health Suite Digital Platform: Philips has been at the forefront of integrating cloud and IoT technologies into healthcare. Their Health Suite digital platform is specifically engineered to consolidate and scrutinize health data from diverse sources, encompassing IoT devices. The technology developed by Philips allows medical professionals to remotely track patients with chronic illnesses, enabling prompt intervention and minimizing the necessity for hospitalization. The platform incorporates data from wearable devices, sensors, and electronic health records into a centralized cloud infrastructure for comprehensive analysis.

- GE Healthcare and IoT Medical Devices: General Electric (GE) Healthcare has implemented IoT in its medical devices to enhance patient care and streamline healthcare operations. GE's medical devices, such as MRI machines and X-ray equipment, are equipped with IoT sensors. These sensors collect real-time data and transmit it to the cloud for analysis. This allows healthcare providers to monitor equipment performance, predict maintenance needs, and optimize resource utilization.
- Siemens Healthineers and Digital Ecosystems: Siemens Healthineers focuses on creating digital ecosystems that leverage cloud and IoT technologies to improve healthcare outcomes. Siemens Healthineers has integrated cloud solutions to enable the sharing and analysis of medical imaging data. This facilitates collaboration among healthcare professionals, leading to faster and more accurate diagnoses. Additionally, their IoT-enabled devices contribute to the continuous monitoring of patients, supporting preventive and personalized healthcare.
- IBM Watson Health: IBM Watson Health is a cloud-based platform that integrates various health data sources and applies AI for insights. By leveraging IoT devices and cloud computing, IBM Watson Health helps healthcare organizations manage and analyze vast amounts of patient data. The platform supports clinical decision-making, drug discovery, and population health management. The integration of cloud and IoT enables scalable and efficient processing of healthcare information.
- Connected Inhalers for Asthma Management: Several pharmaceutical companies and technology providers have collaborated to develop connected inhalers for asthma patients. IoT-enabled inhalers collect data on medication usage, inhalation patterns, and environmental factors. This information is sent to the cloud, where healthcare professionals can analyze it to personalize treatment plans, provide timely interventions, and improve overall asthma management.

6.7 ANALYTICS AND REAL-TIME MONITORING

The utilization of analytics and real-time monitoring is essential in transforming healthcare by enhancing effectiveness, patient results, and decision-making. The incorporation of these technologies into intelligent healthcare systems has the capacity to revolutionize the manner in which healthcare is provided, rendering it more individualized, forward-thinking, and reliant on data. Let's explore the role of analytics in smart healthcare, real-time monitoring applications, and the generation of data-driven insights for decision-making.

6.7.1 Role of Analytics in Smart Healthcare

- Predictive Analytics for Disease Management: Predictive analytics can utilize past patient data to discern patterns and forecast the development or course of diseases. This enables healthcare providers to implement proactive measures and give individualized treatment strategies.

- Patient Segmentation and Personalization: Analytics helps in segmenting patients based on their health profiles, enabling healthcare providers to offer personalized care plans. This can enhance patient engagement and satisfaction.
- Operational Efficiency and Resource Optimization: Analytics can be applied to optimize hospital operations, streamline resource allocation, and reduce costs. This includes predicting patient admission rates, optimizing staff schedules, and managing medical inventory.
- Fraud Detection and Risk Management: Analytics tools can identify anomalies in healthcare claims and transactions, aiding in fraud detection. It also helps in managing risks associated with patient care, treatment outcomes, and financial aspects.
- Population Health Management: Analytics allows healthcare providers to analyze the health status of entire populations, identify at-risk groups, and implement targeted interventions to improve overall community health.

6.7.2 Real-Time Monitoring Applications

- Remote Patient Monitoring (RPM): RPM entails employing interconnected equipment to continuously monitor patients, capturing data on vital signs, levels of activity, and medication compliance. This facilitates the prompt identification of problems and immediate intervention.
- IoT-enabled Wearables: Wearable devices, which are coupled with sensors, have the capability to consistently monitor the health indicators of patients and transmit data in real-time to healthcare providers. This promotes proactive management of healthcare and minimizes the necessity for regular hospital visits.
- Smart Hospitals and Facilities: Real-time monitoring is applied to hospital infrastructure to optimize energy usage, track equipment performance, and enhance overall operational efficiency.
- Emergency Response Systems: Real-time monitoring aids in emergency situations by providing immediate alerts for critical events. This is crucial for timely response and intervention, especially in cases like cardiac arrests or falls.

6.7.3 Data-Driven Insights for Decision-Making

- Clinical Decision Support Systems (CDSS): Analytics generates insights that can be integrated into CDSS, assisting healthcare professionals in making informed decisions about patient care, treatment options, and medication choices.
- Performance Analytics for Healthcare Providers: Healthcare organizations use data-driven insights to assess and improve the performance of healthcare providers, enhancing the quality of care delivered.

- Continuous Quality Improvement: Data analytics supports ongoing quality improvement initiatives by identifying areas for enhancement, monitoring the effectiveness of implemented changes, and ensuring compliance with best practices.
- Research and Development: Aggregated healthcare data can be used for research purposes, contributing to medical advancements, drug discovery, and the development of innovative treatment approaches.

6.8 BUILDING RESILIENT AND ADAPTIVE HEALTHCARE ECOSYSTEMS

Design principles for resilience are critical in ensuring that healthcare systems can withstand and recover from disruptions effectively. These principles include redundancy in critical systems, interoperability of healthcare technologies, and the ability to scale resources dynamically based on demand. Resilient healthcare systems are designed to not only withstand shocks, such as pandemics or natural disasters, but also to learn from these events, continuously improve, and adapt to future challenges.

Adaptive strategies are essential for healthcare ecosystems to thrive in changing landscapes. The healthcare industry is witnessing rapid technological advancements, shifting patient expectations, and evolving regulatory landscapes. An adaptive healthcare system embraces innovation, leverages data analytics for real-time insights, and fosters a culture of continuous learning and improvement. Strategies should include the integration of telemedicine and digital health solutions, promoting interdisciplinary collaboration among healthcare professionals, and adopting flexible policies that can quickly respond to emerging healthcare trends. Proactive adaptation allows healthcare ecosystems to stay ahead of the curve and provide high-quality, patient-centered care.

Looking towards the future, healthcare ecosystems must consider several factors to maintain resilience and adaptability. These include ongoing investments in digital infrastructure, cybersecurity measures to safeguard patient data, and the development of frameworks for ethical and responsible use of emerging technologies like artificial intelligence. Additionally, fostering a patient-centric approach by prioritizing preventive care, patient education, and personalized treatment plans will contribute to long-term sustainability. Continuous collaboration between public and private sectors, as well as international cooperation, will be crucial in addressing global health challenges. Embracing a future-oriented mindset ensures that healthcare ecosystems remain not only resilient and adaptive but also well-positioned to deliver efficient, equitable, and patient-focused healthcare services.

6.9 CONCLUSION

To summarize, this chapter has explored the profound influence of integrating cloud and IoT technologies on smart healthcare. It has shown the collaborative nature of these technologies in improving patient care, optimizing operations, and fostering innovation within the healthcare industry. Key findings from our exploration include the pivotal role of cloud platforms in securely storing and processing vast healthcare data, the seamless connectivity offered by IoT devices for real-time monitoring and data collection, and the potential for improved decision-making through advanced analytics.

To summarize the key observations, we have observed that the combination of cloud and IoT allows for remote patient monitoring, enables predictive analytics to detect diseases early, and aids in the development of intelligent medical ecosystems. The combination of the flexibility, scalability, and affordability of cloud infrastructure, along with the widespread presence and sensor abilities of IoT devices, leads to a strong synergy that drives the advancement of smart healthcare.

Looking ahead, future directions in cloud and IoT integration for smart healthcare demand a continued commitment to security and privacy measures to protect sensitive patient information. The interoperability of diverse healthcare systems and devices remains a challenge that requires ongoing standardization efforts. Furthermore, the integration of emerging technologies like edge computing and 5G networks will play a crucial role in enhancing the real-time capabilities and responsiveness of smart healthcare solutions.

As the journey towards smart healthcare continues, collaboration among healthcare providers, technology developers, policymakers, and researchers will be paramount. The convergence of cloud and IoT technologies has laid a solid foundation, and future advancements will depend on collective efforts to address challenges, refine existing solutions, and explore novel applications that further empower healthcare professionals and benefit patients. This chapter serves as a snapshot of the current landscape and an invitation to actively contribute to the ongoing narrative of cloud and IoT integration for smart healthcare.

REFERENCES

Al-Masrani, S., & Al-Jumeily, D. (2016). An Integrated Cloud-Based Healthcare Infrastructure. In *Proceedings of the 2016 International Conference on Cloud and Autonomic Computing (ICCAC)* (pp. 179–184). IEEE.

Bhambri, P., & Bhandari, A. (2005, March). Different Protocols for Wireless Security. In *National Conference on Advancements in Modeling and Simulation* (p. 8). LLRIET.

Bhambri, P., & Gupta, S. (2005, March). A Survey & Comparison of Permutation Possibility of Fault Tolerant Multistage Interconnection Networks. In *National Conference on Application of Mathematics in Engineering & Technology* (p. 13). MIMIT.

Botta, A., de Donato, W., Persico, V., & Pescapé, A. (2016). Integration of Cloud Computing and Internet of Things: A Survey. *Future Generation Computer Systems*, 56, 684–700.

Catarinucci, L., de Donno, D., Mainetti, L., Palano, L., Patrono, L., & Stefanizzi, M. L. (2015). An IoT-Aware Architecture for Smart Healthcare Systems. *IEEE Internet of Things Journal*, 2(6), 515–526.

Hao, Q., Jin, Y., Li, Y., & Zomaya, A. Y. (2015). Fog Computing: Fundamentals and Research Challenges. In *2015 IEEE/ACM International Conference on Advances in Social Networks Analysis and Mining (ASONAM)* (pp. 809–814). IEEE.

Islam, S. R., Kwak, D., Kabir, M. H., Hossain, M., & Kwak, K. S. (2015). The Internet of Things for Health Care: A Comprehensive Survey. *IEEE Access*, 3, 678–708.

Lasierra, N., Lozano, J. A., León, C., & Ortega, A. (2019). Integrating the Internet of Things with Cloud Computing in Precision Medicine. *Sensors*, 19(11), 2693.

Liu, Y., Hou, Y. T., Chen, J., Wu, M., & Chen, X. (2018). Smart Healthcare: Making Medical Care More Intelligent. *Global Health Journal*, 2(3), 63–65.

Rachna, R., Bhambri, P., & Chhabra, Y. (2022). Deployment of Distributed Clustering Approach in WSNs and IoTs. In *Cloud and Fog Computing Platforms for Internet of Things* (pp. 85–98). Chapman and Hall/CRC.

Sangwan Singh, Y., Lal, S., Bhambri, P., Kumar, A., & Dhanoa, I. S. (2021). Advancements In Social Data Security And Encryption: A Review. *Natural Volatiles & Essential Oils*, 8(4), 15353–15362.

Shojafar, M., & Cordeschi, N. (2017). An Efficient and Self-tuned Virtual Machine Monitor for Cloud and Fog Computing. *Journal of King Saud University-Computer and Information Sciences*, 3(2).

Singh, P., Singh, M., & Bhambri, P. (2005). Embedded systems. In *U.G.C. Sponsored National Seminar* (pp. 10–15). Presented at the "Embedded Systems" seminar at KMV, Jalandhar held during January 24–25, 2005.

Wang, H., & Zhang, D. (2018). A Cloud-Based Framework for Healthcare Information System. In *2018 IEEE 3rd International Conference on Cloud Computing and Big Data Analysis (ICCCBDA)* (pp. 370–374). IEEE.

Zhang, J., Yu, Y., Zhang, X., Xiong, S., Zhu, J., & Liu, Z. (2018). A Review of the Role of Fog Computing in Healthcare. *Computer Methods and Programs in Biomedicine*, 153, 1–7.

7 IoT-based Effective Wearable Healthcare Monitoring System for Remote Areas

Brij Nandan Singh, Ankit Singh and Kirti Amresh Gautam

7.1 INTRODUCTION

According to research that the World Health Organization (WHO) and UNICEF reported, 585,000 women die each year from complications that are associated with pregnancy and delivery (WHO, 2023). Complications can arise in pregnancy for women everywhere in the world; however, women living in underdeveloped nations have a considerably lower chance of receiving fast and sufficient treatment, and as a result, they have a higher risk of passing away.

Non-communicable diseases (NCDs) refer to medical disorders or diseases that do not arise from transmitting infectious agents. Chronic illnesses of extended duration, often characterized by gradual development, arise from a complex interplay of genetic, physiological, environmental, and behavioral variables (Pawar, 2022). According to the research report titled "India: Health of the Nation's States"—The India State-Level Disease Burden Initiative, which was published in 2017 by the Indian Council of Medical Research (ICMR), it is believed that the percentage of deaths in India that were caused by NCDs occurred to increase from 37.9% in the year 1990 to 61.8% in the year 2016. This represents an increase from 37.9% in the year 1990. Diabetes, cancer, chronic respiratory diseases (also known as CRDs), and cardiovascular illnesses (often known as CVDs) are the four most common types of NCDs. These four illnesses have four behavioral risk factors in common: poor nutrition, inactivity, use of cigarettes and alcohol, and use of harmful substances (Pawar, 2022).

Technology development has allowed this generation to utilize miniature versions of contemporary items. This innovation incorporates a health monitoring system into it (Shivajirao Salunke and Shivleela, 2022). In recent years, remote health monitoring systems have become increasingly popular for personal healthcare, physical fitness, and medical awareness. These devices allow patients or incapacitated individuals to be monitored remotely by their medical providers and authorized personnel.

DOI: 10.1201/9781032698519-7

Integrating the internet of things (IoT) technology has heralded a transformative era in healthcare, revolutionizing how medical data are collected, processed, and utilized. IoT, a network of interconnected devices and sensors capable of exchanging data over the internet, has found prolific applications in various domains, with healthcare at the forefront of innovation (Xu et al., 2023). By amalgamating wearable devices, intelligent sensors, and advanced analytics, IoT in healthcare can enhance patient care, optimize resource allocation, and facilitate real-time monitoring, even in remote or resource-constrained settings.

The healthcare sector is witnessing an unprecedented surge in the utilization of IoT-enabled devices for diverse applications, ranging from patient monitoring and chronic disease management to drug adherence and telemedicine (Al-Fuqaha et al., 2015). These devices, equipped with an array of sensors, collect a wealth of physiological data and ensure a continuous and comprehensive stream of information regarding an individual's health status. According to Hussain et al. (2018), when such data are analyzed intelligently, they aid in early diagnosis and intervention, not to mention that they assist in the development of individualized treatment regimens, which ultimately results in improved patient outcomes.

Furthermore, IoT plays a pivotal role in creating a seamless healthcare ecosystem, facilitating communication between various stakeholders, including patients, healthcare providers, and medical facilities. It fosters the establishment of interconnected healthcare systems that promote real-time data sharing, enabling timely clinical decision-making and reducing administrative overhead (Islam et al., 2015). Moreover, adopting IoT technologies in healthcare aligns with the paradigm shift towards patient-centric care, empowering individuals to actively manage their health through access to real-time data and personalized health insights (Pramanik et al., 2017).

As the IoT landscape in healthcare continues to evolve, it is crucial to address the challenges of data security, privacy, and interoperability, ensuring that the benefits derived from this technological revolution are maximized while minimizing potential risks (Pramanik et al., 2017). Moreover, IoT solutions must be scalable and cost-effective to provide equal access to modern healthcare services, especially in underserved and distant locations.

Cloud-based health monitoring can detect medical emergencies and deliver biofeedback via early warning. The method lets geriatric patients stay in touch with a family member who knows their health. Remote health monitoring devices may transfer all data to the cloud for medical practitioners and authorized staff to view. These gadgets may help people survive unknown illnesses (Hamim et al., 2019).

7.1.1 Role of IoT in Healthcare Transformation

The web-enabled IoT collects, transfers, and processes data from sensors, processors, and communications devices by utilizing the capabilities provided by wireless cloud technology; this fundamental aspect of the internet of things enable its operators to get remote access to the many linked devices. The devices must have the option of connecting to communicate with other intelligent devices located at great distances from them without needing any outside mediation (Hamim et al., 2019)

Creating an IoT may be divided into four distinct stages. Various phases are responsible for carrying out specific procedures (Bhambri et al., 2005). Stage 1 involves identifying and collecting several interconnected elements that are primary data sources for further analysis. Typically, it comprises many sensors that may be categorized as either wired or wireless. During Stage 2, relevant data is gathered to establish an internet connection. In this stage, an analog-to-digital conversion is also performed. During Stage 3 of the data processing pipeline, data undergoes preprocessing procedures facilitated by information technology (IT) systems before advancing to the final step (Stage 4). In Stage 4, the filtered, analyzed, and processed data is then saved in a cloud-based storage system, a traditional back-end data system (Fuller, 2016).

7.1.2 Significance of Wearable Devices in Remote Areas

Wearable devices have the potential to be significant in rural areas for a variety of reasons, and one of those reasons is that they are more convenient. In more rural areas, where there are typically fewer medical facilities and resources accessible, individuals can struggle to maintain track of their health and seek quick medical attention when needed. The use of wearable technology has the potential to assist in the reduction of this gap by enabling medical professionals to monitor the health of their patients remotely by giving individuals rapid feedback on their health (Huhn et al., 2022).

One of the most significant advantages that may be obtained via the utilization of wearable technology in remote areas is the capability to keep track of one's health. Through the use of wearable technology, it is possible to monitor the health of people who live in distant areas by providing real-time feedback on their vital signs. These vital indicators include the individual's heart rate, breathing rate, and body temperature. In the event that this is carried out, it will be feasible to watch over the health of those who reside in isolated areas.

Because of this, individuals can monitor their health and seek medical help when required, which may be especially beneficial in regions where access to healthcare institutions is restricted. For instance, research that was carried out in Burkina Faso, which is situated in Africa, made use of wearable devices in order to generate data at the individual level in the real world. Rural locations, where there were fewer resources available, were the ones where this was handled.

In addition to this function, wearable technology may monitor environmental, behavioral, physiological, and psychological data. Wearable technology has the potential to be significant in rural areas for a variety of reasons, and one of those reasons is that it is more convenient. In more rural areas, where there are typically fewer medical facilities and resources accessible, individuals can struggle to maintain track of their health and seek quick medical attention when needed. Wearable technology has the potential to help reduce this gap by providing individuals with instant feedback on their health and by enabling medical professionals to monitor the health of their patients remotely (Haghi et al., 2021).

Wearable technology has the potential to be useful in various domains, one of which is monitoring physical activity in remote places. Wearable technology, which can detect the amount of physical activity individuals participate in even in different locations, enables individuals to receive feedback on their activity levels and be encouraged to remain active. This technology also enables individuals to be encouraged to remain active (Bhambri and Singh, 2006). A research study on older people who lived in rural locations revealed that an intervention based on wearable devices significantly impacted the participants' physical performance levels. It may be of particular use in areas where access to recreational facilities is limited since it enables individuals to monitor their physical activity levels and adapt to their lifestyle as necessary. It may be especially advantageous in places with restricted access to recreational facilities. It can be especially helpful in areas where people do not have easy access to recreational amenities (Jang et al., 2018).

Wearable electronic devices also have the potential to make a difference in terms of access to medical treatment in rural regions. People who reside in more rural areas of the country, where they may have to travel considerable distances to receive specialized care, may benefit from having clinicians send them wearable devices to monitor their health. Not only does this make it feasible to collect data, but it can also make it possible to exchange crucial data with physicians in other areas, making access to high-quality treatment easier. Wearable technology may also monitor patients remotely, allowing medical professionals to track their patients' conditions and take appropriate action as necessary (Ellis, 2023).

Another field that might benefit from the usage of wearable technology in distant regions is data collecting for research purposes. The most recent wearable medical gadgets are revolutionizing the methods and results of clinical research by allowing physicians to remotely collect a plethora of data from a distance. It gives the researchers a larger sample size that is more typical of the whole, enabling them to obtain a greater variety of data. Wearable devices may also gather data on environmental elements such as air quality and temperature. This data, which can help understand the influence of ecological factors in health, can be collected using wearable devices (Jang et al., 2018).

Wearable technology has the potential to be beneficial in several different areas, including emergency response. In an emergency, it may be possible to track the whereabouts of persons in more remote places using gadgets. For instance, wearable devices equipped with global positioning system (GPS) capabilities can collect exact information on the locations of the participants' time spent. It enables first responders to rapidly discover persons who may need assistance, which can be of particular use in regions prone to experiencing a high frequency of natural catastrophes (Bhat et al., 2019).

7.2 LIVE HEALTH MONITORING USING WEARABLE IoT

Wearable IoT devices have the potential to transform healthcare by allowing real-time health monitoring. These devices have the potential to gather crucial data that could potentially save lives and offer valuable insights into the symptoms and patterns of various physiological or psychological disorders. The internet of things allows for the implementation of remote care, a concept once only found in fiction. Wearable devices enable the continuous monitoring of patients, offering valuable information for assessing health status and even making preliminary medical diagnoses. Doctors no longer need to speculate when patients will return for their next appointment. Wearable gadgets offer remote patient monitoring, providing healthcare personnel with real-time access to vital indicators such as heart rate and blood pressure regardless of the patient's location (Wan et al., 2018).

Numerous studies have been conducted to investigate the potential of real-time health monitoring devices that are enabled by IoT and can be worn (Bhambri and Mangat, 2005). These devices have been the subject of a significant deal of research. Recent research has led to the creation of a new cloud-based health monitoring system (WISE) that is based on IoT and wearable technology. This system enables real-time monitoring of an individual's health as it occurs. Through the deployment of the BASN architecture, WISE is able to make it feasible to provide health monitoring in real-time. A number of wearable sensors have been added to the collection. Some examples of these sensors are those that detect blood pressure, temperature, and heart rate (Wan et al., 2018). This work presents the design, methodology, and experimental findings of the WISE system that might be implemented in the future.

Wearable IoT devices have the potential to improve clinical treatment and provide continuous health monitoring, as indicated by the findings of another study published in the same field. Mobile health applications can process sensor data locally or at a gateway to facilitate remote diagnostics. Wearable devices are perfect for health monitoring as they allow users to be monitored in their homes. This capability enables health professionals to assess how symptoms progress over time. Monitoring vital signs is a crucial use for wearables. Monitoring vital signs, including body temperature, pulse rate, respiration rate, blood pressure, blood sugar, and sweat rate, can be instrumental in detecting and tracking medical conditions. Wearables are portable, convenient, and non-invasive, making vital signs measurements easy in hospitals and at home. Additionally, wearable gadgets can continually check vital indicators (Bhat et al., 2019).

IoT-enabled wearables hold immense potential to revolutionize the healthcare industry. Wearable technologies enable healthcare professionals to monitor vital signs remotely, eliminating the need for in-person visits. They also empower patients to actively track and manage their health conditions daily. They also provide the ability for consumers to track and monitor their physical activity. IoT-enabled hygiene devices can be activated whenever there is a concern for compromised health and sanitation conditions. Wearable respiratory monitoring sensors, placed as a patch on the chest, can alert patients to variations in their heart rate, temperature, and breathing patterns via their cellphones. These signals can be used to spot early indicators of a deterioration in lung function. Exacerbations that necessitate immediate medical treatment can be sent via the gadget (Islam et al., 2015).

7.2.1 WISE Framework and Architecture

The WISE framework offers a holistic approach to real-time health monitoring through wearable IoT devices. It provides a well-organized framework for gathering, analyzing, and interpreting data from wearable devices to monitor and manage personal health conditions. The framework emphasizes utilizing IoT technology to facilitate ongoing monitoring and immediate analysis of health data (Downey et al., 2019).

Several significant elements go into the design of the WISE system for accurate health monitoring utilizing wearable IoT devices.

Choosing the appropriate hardware: The system must accurately detect and choose suitable wearable IoT devices according to the precise health metrics that need to be monitored. It is crucial to take into account elements such as the accuracy of the sensor, the longevity of the battery, the level of comfort, and the networking options that are accessible (Chong et al., 2020).

Collecting and Transmitting Data: Establishing dependable communication channels between the wearable devices and the IoT infrastructure is crucial. Uploading information to the cloud via wireless protocols, including Bluetooth Low Energy (BLE), Wi-Fi, and cellular networks, is possible.

IoT Infrastructure: An infrastructure comprising sensors, gateways, communication protocols, and cloud-based platforms is necessary for the system to function. The careful selection and configuration of these components guarantees smooth data collection, storage, and processing (Kumar et al., 2019).

Storage and processing: The health data obtained is securely kept in a cloud-based storage system. The system should employ encryption and access limits to protect data. It should also include scalable data processing algorithms for dealing with enormous amounts of real-time data (Wan et al., 2018; Bhambri et al., 2020).

Real-time Monitoring and Analysis: The system uses powerful algorithms and machine learning techniques to monitor and analyze real-time health data. These algorithms can detect patterns, abnormalities, and trends in data, allowing for the early diagnosis of health concerns or hazards. Developers ought to furnish users and healthcare providers with precise and prompt notifications (Wan et al., 2018).

7.3 REMOTE HEALTHCARE CHALLENGES AND SOLUTIONS

Medical technological advancements have made it possible to create wearables that have a substantial impact on health outcomes. However, the lack of reliable internet access is a key obstacle in implementing IoT because most IoT devices rely on advanced technologies that require strong internet connections. Additionally, the cost of wearables, medical devices, and the internet is unavailable globally or are costly for many people, especially in remote and rural areas of developing countries.

Data security and privacy are most important to achieve the maximum benefit of IoMT to resolve communication gaps because no platform is 100% secure from hackers and data breaches (Gajarawala and Pelkowski, 2021). Therefore, the healthcare system must administer robust cybersecurity measures and regulation mechanisms to protect patient data. Wearables have meager encryption and protection; because of that, most patients refuse to wear the devices in rural and urban populations

(Tran et al., 2019). Telehealth providers can simultaneously provide medical help and clinical expertise to patients across geographical barriers. Patients with smartphones, laptops, computers, online meetings, and the internet can easily use telehealth via telephone, email, video calls, or conferences (Singh et al., 2005). The lack of multi-state licensure for the implementation of telehealth presents barriers, including medical education and financial obligations. Therefore, governments and administrations must develop systematic, regulated interstate medical licensure for healthcare workers practicing telemedicine from state to state (Gajarawala and Pelkowski, 2021).

Data accuracy and misdiagnosis are also possible due to internet bandwidth, which may affect the validity and reliability of motor task measurements, resulting in inaccurate data-based decisions by the healthcare worker. Besides these issues, some severe cases like medical liability (informed consent, standards, and protocols), fraud and abuse, etc., do not violate government policies and regulations in the IoT sector.

7.3.1 Accessibility Issues in Remote and Rural Areas

Access to healthcare is defined as an individual's approach to obtaining the medical facilities for early and timely prevention, diagnosis, treatment, and disease management to achieve the best health outcomes (Millman, 1993). According to the Rural Policy Research Institute (RUPRI), various countries have implemented the concept of universal health coverage concerning quality of care, availability, affordability, accessibility, and acceptability as a strategic background for their national policies. The assessment and quality assurance of healthcare comprises three major components: overage (pooled funds—solidarity principle), healthcare services (healthcare funds), and healthcare infrastructure with the workforce (Healthy People, 2020; WHO, 2012).

As proposed in the *Declaration of Alma-Ata*, the accessibility of quality healthcare services is a complex and multi-dimensional challenge in remote or rural areas, leading to health disparities between urban and rural populations, particularly in developing countries (Franco et al., 2021). In most countries, rural and remote areas encounter difficulties such as geographical approach, transportation, communication gap, shortage of efficient healthcare workers and facilities, limited public health education, fund constraints, etc., (Figure 7.1) (Jon Ander Mendia, 2022). The premises of Alma-ata in "*Health for All By 2000*" professed health as a right and primary healthcare (PHC) is obligatory for maintaining population health (Franco et al., 2021). PHC is inexpensive, most influential in disease prevention, and can be delivered quickly in inpatient care. Inequity in the PHC delivery system in urban and rural populations leads to significant discrepancies in overall statistics of a country's healthcare system because the rural inhabitants encompass approximately half of the world's population and have less accessibility to healthcare.

These accessibility issues should be addressed using implementable government strategies, healthcare infrastructure development, community engagement programs, telehealth initiatives, and recent advanced technology. Healthcare services delivery and management are revolutionizing using IoMT, in which interconnected medical equipment and regulated devices collect and send real-time patient data to

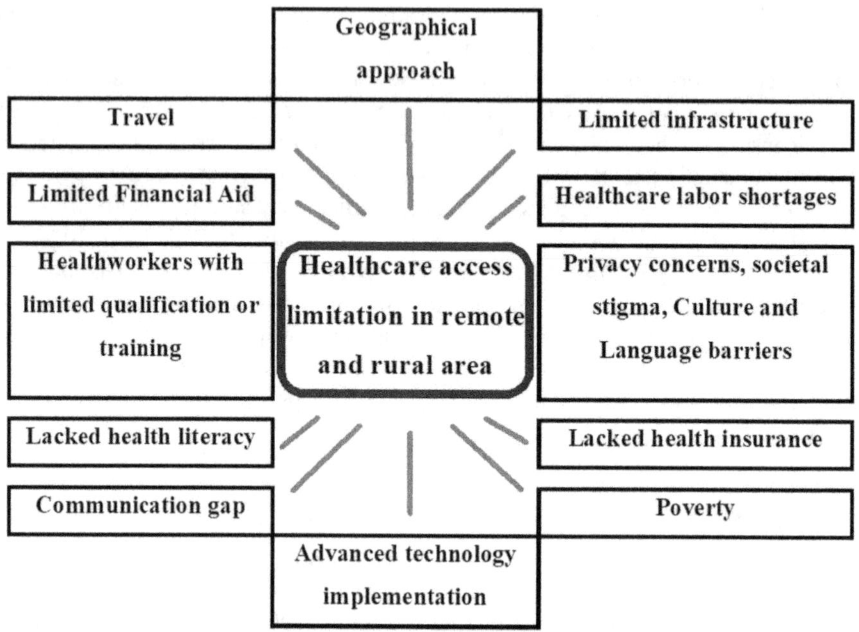

FIGURE 7.1 Factors affecting healthcare accessibility in remote or rural areas.

healthcare practitioners. IoMT can significantly increase health outcomes in addition to lowering health costs.

7.3.2 Resource Constraints and Infrastructure Limitations

Resource constraints and limited infrastructure are the most persistent challenges in providing healthcare services among remote and rural populations, impacting the quality and availability of healthcare services. Researchers, governments, and policymakers are investigating and addressing critical issues like financial limitations, shortages of skilled personnel, insufficient medical equipment, and lack of advanced technology, including artificial intelligence, IoT, cloud systems, high-speed internet facilities, and outreach efforts to gain maximum health benefits.

According to research looking at patterns in out-of-pocket expenses (OOPEs) for healthcare across all socioeconomic categories, OOP payments have been rising over time, particularly in rural regions. In rural and urban regions, the percentage of households on OOPEs increased from 64%, 65% to 81%, and 78%, respectively (Karan et al., 2014). Based on the findings of a recent study by Fu et al., 2021, families in rural areas with patients suffering from non-communicable diseases are more likely than urban households to face catastrophic medical costs and financial hardship. Additionally, researchers found that the disparities in catastrophic health spending between urban and rural areas could be predicted by family income, literacy, and knowledge of the health state of household heads. This was due to the fact that these factors were shown to be significantly different. This was accomplished with great success because of the utilization of the Fairlie nonlinear decomposition as well as the Blinder-Oaxaca decomposition (Fu et al., 2021). By acclimatizing IoMT, the complications mentioned above can be addressed and answered significantly.

Inadequate funding and **a shortage of healthcare experts** make investing in procuring new medical equipment, hiring skilled healthcare professionals, and managing existing infrastructure challenging. Many remote and rural healthcare facilities lack access to modern medical equipment, diagnostic tools, and technology, leading to imprecision and delayed treatment. Attributable to these limitations, doctors, nurses, and other medical staff are the most interested in delivering healthcare services in remote areas.

Limited access to technology in many parts of the world, development in technology is cumulative exponentially. However, only the urban population is acquainting themselves with this advancement, and only a limited fraction of the rural population is profited, especially regarding access to high-speed internet. Due to infrastructural issues, telemedicine, and other sophisticated healthcare services may be inefficient.

Patient education and awareness are the most critical factors for preventing preventable diseases and achieving good health outcomes. Community engagement and education, whether online or offline, can manage awareness regarding the prevention of conditions.

Limited electricity, water supply, and lack of transportation facilities hamper medical supplies and maintenance, disrupting hygienic conditions and operating medical equipment.

7.3.3 Addressing Communication Gaps Through IoT

The Sustainable Development Goals (SDGs) include a number of major objectives, one of which is to achieve universal health care, as stated by Hogan et al. (2018). This indicates that by the year 2030, every single person will have unfettered access to primary health care (PHC), which is also known as primary medical care. The World Health Organization (WHO) and the World Bank announced that "poverty caused by illness" is a result of the fact that 122 million people are considered to be "poor" (living on less than \$3.10 per day) and 100 million people are recorded as "extremely poor" (living on less than \$1.90 per day) due to the costs associated with healthcare (World Health Organization-World Bank, 2017). This "poverty caused by illness" is a result of medical expenses. Addressing the challenges mentioned above, employing government strategies, and including advanced and robust technology like IoMT, achieving SDGs in speculated time is possible.

By leveraging IoMT, healthcare workers and patients can address communication gaps and streamline processes that have long been challenging. IoMT can facilitate real-time monitoring, remote consultations, data-sharing and collaboration, medication management, personalized healthcare plans, data analytics, emergency response chronic disease management, efficient resource allocation, and cost-effective solutions. The healthcare system faced several issues treating patients with and without COVID-19, so many practice models have been introduced, including telehealth. Other models are used in inpatient and outpatient settings.

Remote patient monitoring systems (RPMS) for home-based care are used for chronic conditions, infectious disorders during isolation, post-surgery, neonates, the elderly, and mobility problems. In RPMS, data is collected wirelessly, transmitted to the cloud system, and then analyzed and interpreted by artificial intelligence machine learning or healthcare providers (Boikanyo et al., 2023).

Telemedicine or telehealth tremendously increases healthcare solutions in remote and rural areas, where long-distance travel is critical. Healthcare professionals, by virtual visits and using information and communication technologies, have been delivering services efficiently since the COVID-19 pandemic. Telehealth was initially developed with the intention of providing primary medical care to those who are located in rural areas or who were underserved. However, widespread adoption is difficult due to regulatory, legal, and reimbursement barriers. Successful telehealth implementation can result in efficient, quality care, and minimizing costs (Gajarawala and Pelkowski, 2021).

Consumer health wearables encompass devices for personal fitness and are highly in trend in urban areas. Nevertheless, it is typically not regulated by health authorities. Fitness experts or trainers highly endorse these consumer-grade devices for some specific health applications. The diagnosis and treatment of cardiovascular illnesses, neurological diseases, and liver diseases in COVID-19 can be accomplished through the utilization of wearable devices that are equipped with high-speed internet facilities and are supported by machine learning and algorithms (Chakrabarti et al., 2022).

Clinical-grade (medical grade) wearables include patient-worn regulated wearable devices generally approved by health authorities, such as electronic skin patches, schizophrenia, metabolic disorders, ECG monitors, blood pressure monitors, and others. These devices are well-appointed with actuators, sensors, and software connected to the cloud that direct real-time data collection, analysis, and interpretations for early detection and improved diagnosis. Wearables provide long-term monitoring in some sectors, which is tedious or impossible using conventional medical approaches (Xu et al., 2020).

7.3.4 Case Studies of Successful Implementations

Implementing IoMT has numerous successful stories that have changed healthcare services by improving remote monitoring and patient outcomes. IoMT enhances clinical trials, optimizes medical device performance, and reshapes the healthcare landscape by making it more patient-centric, cost-effective, and efficient.

Merchant et al., investigated the influence of digital health intervention on the number of visited and hospitalized events of asthma patients. As per the findings of Merchant et al., (2018), it was discovered that the number of visits per 100 patient-years experienced a substantial drop from 11.6 to 5.4 visits ($p < 0.05$) and 13.4 to 5.8 events ($p < 0.05$) in the 365 days prior to enrollment and 365 days immediately after enrollment, respectively. Nelson and colleagues assessed the accuracy of collected data from wearables, including Apple Watch and Fitbit. An echocardiogram (ECG) of the same subjects was used, and an agreement was observed with both methods, 91% and 5%, respectively (Nelson and Allen, 2019).

Throughout the COVID-19 pandemic, the Food and Drug Administration (FDA) of the United States has sped up the process of approving a wide range of medical devices for the treatment of COVID-19-related illnesses for use in emergency scenarios. These devices are intended to be used in the event of an emergency. Examples include the Whoop Strap, which is used to measure respiratory rate; disposable patches and biosensors developed by Philips for the purpose of diagnosing COVID-19; the "DETECT" technology developed by Scripps, which is capable of collecting data from smart wearable devices; Taiwan's testing and tracing architecture; Eko's electrocardiogram low ejection fraction tool for assessing cardiac complications associated with COVID-19; "Lumify" and other hand-held portable ultrasound solutions; and AI-CT algorithms for COVID-19 detection developed by Aidoc Medical, an Israeli technology company (Dwivedi et al., 2022).

Through the utilization of Zigbee or Wi-Fi, Fu et al. (2021) developed a non-invasive oximeter that utilizes the parameters of blood oxygen saturation level, heart rate, and pulse in order to evaluate the effectiveness of medical intervention (Fu et al., 2021). The findings of another study (Agustine et al., 2018) describe the development of an alarm system that, when coupled with a pulse oximeter and a wireless local area network (WLAN) router, notifies patients when their oxygen saturation drops below a prescribed threshold.

IoMT application-based devices coined for non-invasive monitoring of blood glucose trends. Paul et al., utilizing the near-infrared sensors, determined the glucose level from the figure tip without pricking it, and they succeeded in taking the readings non-invasively.

7.4 WEARABLE HEALTH MONITORING ALGORITHMS

The use of wearable health monitoring technologies has revolutionized the field of medical epidemiology. Millions of people are generating massive amounts of data from their smartwatches, fitness trackers, and other wearables relevant to their health. Wearable technology has the potential to totally transform the healthcare system by its ability to provide continuous monitoring and early identification of health conditions. Algorithms for wearable health monitoring are necessary to transform sensor data into useful information. These algorithms include preprocessing data, extracting features, machine learning, and fusing data. They allow for early warning system detection, predictive analysis, and immediate health advice.

7.4.1 Uses of Wearable Health Monitoring Algorithms

Various domains in healthcare benefit from wearable health monitoring algorithms, which are as follows:

a. *Chronic Disease Management:* The care of a wide variety of chronic illnesses, such as diabetes, cardiovascular disease, and respiratory illness, has the potential to be considerably strengthened by the implementation of wearable technology. Algorithms that analyze the data obtained from continuous glucose monitors, ECG sensors, and pulse oximeters can provide real-time feedback and early warnings.
b. *Fitness and Wellness*: Many individuals nowadays use wearable technologies to monitor their fitness routines, track their sleeping patterns, and evaluate their overall state of health. After algorithms evaluate sensor data, sleep quality, physical activity, and calories burnt may be determined.
c. *Remote Patient Monitoring:* The application of wearable medical sensors extends the reach of healthcare outside of conventional clinic settings. Using algorithms to detect early deterioration signs in patients with chronic conditions is possible. It paves the door for prompt interventions and decreases hospital readmission rates.
d. *Early Disease Detection:* Wearable sensors and sophisticated algorithms may one day allow for early detection and treatment of diseases, including atrial fibrillation, hypertension, and possibly COVID-19. Better outcomes might be possible with earlier diagnosis.

7.4.2 Challenges and Ethical Considerations

The algorithms used in wearable health monitoring devices have their fair share of challenges and ethical considerations. Some of these include:

a. *Data Security and Confidentiality:* Wearable technology allows for collecting personally identifiable health information. Because of the possibility of data breaches, keeping sensitive information secure is even more essential.
b. *Accuracy and Dependability:* The data obtained through wearable technology should not be relied upon. Validating algorithms is necessary to ensure the accuracy of health evaluations and recommendations.
c. *Informed Consent:* The use of wearable health monitoring technologies necessitates the development of protocols for obtaining informed consent. Individuals need to have a solid understanding of data collection and exploitation implications.

7.4.3 Data Preprocessing and Filtering Techniques

Data preprocessing and filtering techniques are fundamental to accurately analyzing wearable health monitoring data. Raw data collected from sensors can be noisy, contain artifacts, and require cleaning, enhancement, and filtering for meaningful interpretation. This section explores the significance of data preprocessing and filtering techniques, their applications, and their impact on the quality of wearable health data—the various steps involved in this process, which are mentioned below.

Raw Data Collection: Data preprocessing starts with collecting raw data from various sources. The quality of the raw data significantly affects the success of subsequent data preprocessing steps. A variety of forms, such as organized, semi-structured, and unstructured data, are frequently used to describe raw data. It may be noisy, incomplete, or contain missing values.

Data Filtering: Data filtering is an essential step to reduce noise in data. Noise refers to random or irrelevant variations in data that can hinder the extraction of meaningful information. Filtering techniques are crucial in various fields, including image processing, signal processing, and time-series analysis.

Mean Filtering: The mean filtering approach is a straightforward method that is highly successful in eliminating noise in data. The process involves replacing the value of each pixel with the average value of the pixels in its immediate vicinity. Image processing and signal denoising are two fields that make extensive use of this technology.

Median Filtering: Median filtering is a nonlinear approach that is particularly successful at removing im-pulse noise, often known as salt-and-pepper noise. The value of each pixel is changed to reflect the median value of the pixels in its immediate vicinity.

Gaussian Filtering: Gaussian filtering is a smoothing technique that uses a weighted average of pixel values in the neighborhood. It effectively reduces Gaussian noise and is commonly used in image smoothing.

Frequency Domain Filtering: Frequency domain filtering involves transforming data into the frequency domain, where filtering is performed, and then converting it back into the time or spatial domain. This technique is commonly used in signal processing to remove specific frequency components.

Adaptive Filtering: Adaptive filtering is a specialized filtering technique used in applications where the characteristics of the noise or interference are constantly changing. It adjusts the filter coefficients in real-time to effectively cancel noise.

Data Cleaning: Data cleaning identifies and rectifies errors, inconsistencies, and inaccuracies in the raw data. Addressing outliers, dealing with duplication, and resolving missing data are all part of the process. The processes of data cleansing guarantee that the data that is utilized for analysis is correct and dependable.

Data Transformation: The term "data transformation" refers to the process of converting data into a format that is suitable for analysis or modeling. This format can be used for either of these purposes. It may include normalization, standardization, and encoding of categorical variables. The accurate translation of data signifies that data coming from various sources and having a range of scales may be utilized productively together.

Feature Engineering: By utilizing previously collected data, feature engineering generates new features or variables. These engineered features can capture additional information, improve model performance, and help discover hidden patterns in the data. Feature engineering requires domain expertise and creativity.

7.4.4 Real-Time Monitoring and Alerting Systems

Real-time monitoring and alerting systems are essential components of contemporary healthcare. These systems make use of technology to enable continuous surveillance, early detection of health risks, and fast response. It is essential to have these systems in place in order to improve patient outcomes and lower the costs of healthcare. This section delves into the significance of real-time monitoring and alerting systems, their applications, and the technologies that enable them. Real-time monitoring in healthcare allows for the immediate tracking of patient vital signs, disease markers, and other health-related data. It provides timely alerts for healthcare professionals to intervene and initiate necessary treatments promptly, leading to better patient outcomes.

7.4.4.1 Applications of Real-Time Monitoring

Real-time monitoring and alerting systems applied in various healthcare contexts, including:

- *Patient monitoring:* Continuous tracking of vital signs, such as heart rate, blood pressure, and oxygen saturation.
- *Disease management:* Monitoring chronic diseases like diabetes and asthma to adjust treatment as needed.
- *Clinical decision support:* Providing real-time information to assist healthcare professionals in making critical decisions.
- *Early warning systems:* Alerting medical staff to abnormal events, such as sudden cardiac arrest or sepsis.

7.4.4.2 Technologies Empowering Real-Time Monitoring

Real-time monitoring and alerting systems rely on a suite of technologies, including:

- *Wearable devices:* For instance, fitness trackers and smartwatches, which are designed for constant monitoring.
- *Internet of Things (IoT):* Connecting medical devices and sensors for data collection.
- *Cloud computing:* Storing and analyzing vast amounts of real-time data.
- *Artificial intelligence:* Powering predictive algorithms for early detection and decision support.

7.4.4.3 Challenges and Considerations

While real-time monitoring and alerting systems offer significant benefits, they come with challenges, including:

- *Data security and privacy:* Safeguarding sensitive patient data.
- *Integration with existing systems:* Ensuring seamless integration with electronic health records and other healthcare IT infrastructure.
- *Scalability and reliability:* Managing large volumes of real-time data while ensuring system uptime.

7.4.5 Performance Metrics and Validation

As part of the process of determining whether or not healthcare interventions, diagnostic tools, and predictive models are effective, performance metrics and validation are essential components. They provide a systematic way to measure healthcare-related outcomes' accuracy, reliability, and generalizability. This section explores the importance of performance metrics and validation in healthcare, various evaluation methods, and the role of evidence-based medicine.

In healthcare, decisions and interventions can have life-altering consequences. Determining the effectiveness and safety of healthcare practices, technologies, and treatments is crucial. Performance metrics and validation provide a structured approach to making informed decisions and ensuring the highest quality of care.

7.4.5.1 Types of Performance Metrics

Performance metrics in healthcare encompass a wide range of measures, including:

- *Sensitivity and specificity:* Assessing the accuracy of diagnostic tests.
- *Positive predictive value (PPV) and negative predictive value (NPV):* Predictive power of tests.
- *Area under the receiver operating characteristic curve (AUC-ROC):* Discriminatory power of models.
- *Concordance statistics:* Agreement between observed and predicted outcomes.
- *Validation in Healthcare:* Validation in healthcare encompasses the rigorous process of confirming the effectiveness, safety, and accuracy of healthcare interventions, tools, and models. Validation may involve clinical trials, laboratory testing, and real-world data analysis to ensure that healthcare practices are evidence-based.

7.5 FUTURE DIRECTIONS AND RECOMMENDATIONS

The healthcare field is dynamic, continually evolving with emerging technologies and new trends. As healthcare providers and researchers embrace innovation, it's essential to anticipate the future landscape of healthcare and make recommendations for its growth and improvement. This section explores the upcoming technologies and trends in healthcare, offers guidance for implementation, and discusses potential extensions and enhancements. It is driven by technological advancements and evolving patient needs in the coming years. Through the implementation of artificial intelligence, telemedicine, and customized medicine, the delivery of healthcare will undergo a transformation that will make it more effective, accessible, and patient-centered.

7.5.1 Emerging Technologies and Trends

IoT is accelerating health monitoring system development to improve patient outcomes and healthcare quality. The evolution mixes new technology. IoT-based health monitoring systems use the following sophisticated technologies and trends:

Wearable Devices: There has been a significant increase in the number of people using wearable gadgets in recent years. Some examples of these devices are smartwatches, fitness trackers, and biosensors. These devices are used to monitor vital signs, physical activity, and sleep patterns. These devices have the power to wirelessly relay data to healthcare practitioners, which allows for the remote monitoring of a patient's health and early detection of prospective health concerns (Dang et al., 2023).

Artificial Intelligence (AI) and Machine Learning (ML): AI and ML algorithms are currently used for IoT health monitoring systems to interpret the vast data generated from various sensors. These algorithms can recognize trends, forecast health issues, and offer patients and medical professionals individualized insights and suggestions (Greco et al., 2020).

Edge Computing: Real-time data processing and analysis can be done at the network's edge, closer to data production. Edge computing technology makes this possible. Edge computing minimizes latency, increases reaction times, and promotes data security and privacy in health monitoring systems. It's accomplished by processing data locally on IoT devices or gateways (Abdulmalek et al., 2022).

Sensor Technology: The creation of small, low-power sensors for monitoring various health factors, such as heart rate, blood pressure, glucose levels, and oxygen saturation, has been made possible by advancements in sensor technology. Continuous monitoring can be accomplished by implanting these sensors into the human body or seamlessly integrating them into wearable devices (Dang et al., 2023).

Blockchain Technology: In IoT-based health monitoring systems, blockchain technology allows for storing safe and decentralized health data. It protects both the data's integrity and privacy. It enables consumers to have greater control over their health data. It allows healthcare providers to share patient information seamlessly while protecting patients' privacy and maintaining high security (Kumar et al., 2023).

5G Connectivity: The development of 5G networks provides a link that is both high-speed and low latency, which is necessary in order to support the transfer of data in real-time via health monitoring systems that are based on the internet of things. The fifth-generation wireless network, or 5G, enables faster and more reliable data exchange, as well as remote monitoring and telemedicine. It contributes to the scalability and efficiency of healthcare services (Rejeb et al., 2023).

These are just a few examples of the emerging technologies and trends in IoT-based health monitoring systems in this field as technology advances, leading to more effective and personalized healthcare solutions.

7.5.2 Challenges and Future Directions

Advancements in medical technology allowed the generation of wearables for significant health outcomes; however, limited internet connectivity is a major issue for implementing the IoT because approximately every IoT is associated with advanced technologies that rely on robust internet facilities. Additionally, the cost of wearables, medical devices, and the internet is unavailable globally or costly for many people, especially in remote and rural areas of developing countries.

Data security and privacy are most important to achieve the maximum benefit of IoMT and resolve communication gaps because no platform is 100% secure from hackers and data breaches (Smith, 2018). Therefore, the healthcare system must administer robust cybersecurity measures and regulation mechanisms to protect patient data. Wearables have meager encryption and protection, and because of that, most patients in rural and urban populations refuse to wear the device (Tran et al., 2019). Mittlesteadt et al., reported that Fitbit data did not outperform the continuous electroencephalographic (EEG) monitoring data to detect epileptic seizures (Mittlesteadt et al., 2020). The accuracy of wearable devices must be comparable to conventional diagnostics procedures.

Telehealth providers can simultaneously provide medical help across geographical barriers and clinical expertise with patients. Patients with smartphones, laptops, computers, online meetings, and the internet can easily use telehealth via telephone, email, video calls, or conferences. The lack of multistate licensure for telehealth implementation presents barriers, including medical education and financial obligations. Therefore, governments and administrations must develop systematic, regulated interstate medical licensure for healthcare workers practicing telemedicine from state to state (Smith, 2018).

Data accuracy and misdiagnosis are also possible due to internet bandwidth that may affect the validity and reliability of motor task measurements, resulting in inaccurate data-based decisions by healthcare workers. Besides these issues, some severe cases like medical liability (informed consent, standards, and protocols), fraud, and abuse, etc., do not violate government policies and regulations in the IoMT sector.

REFERENCES

Abdulmalek, S., Nasir, A., Jabbar, W. A., Almuhaya, M. A. M., Bairagi, A. K., Khan, M. A.-M., & Kee, S.-H. (2022). IoT-Based Healthcare-Monitoring System towards Improving Quality of Life: A Review. *Healthcare*, *10*(10), 1993. https://doi.org/10.3390/healthcare 10101993

Agustine, L., Muljono, I., Angka, P. R., Gunadhi, A., Lestariningsih, D., & Weliamto, W. A. (2018). Heart Rate Monitoring Device for Arrhythmia Using Pulse Oximeter Sensor Based on Android. *2018 International Conference on Computer Engineering, Network and Intelligent Multimedia (CENIM)*, 106–111. https://doi.org/10.1109/CENIM.2018.8711120

Al-Fuqaha, A., Guizani, M., Mohammadi, M., Aledhari, M., & Ayyash, M. (2015). Internet of Things: A Survey on Enabling Technologies, Protocols, and Applications. *IEEE Communications Surveys & Tutorials*, *17*(4), 2347–2376. https://doi.org/10.1109/COMST.2015.2444095

Bhambri, P., & Mangat, A. S. (2005, March). Wireless Security. In *National Conference on Emerging Computing Technologies* (pp. 155–161). HRMMV.

Bhambri, P., & Singh, I. (2005, March). Electrical Actuation Systems. In *National Conference on Application of Mathematics in Engineering & Technology* (pp. 58–60). MIMIT.

Bhambri, P., Singh, I., & Gupta, S. (2005, March). Robotics Systems. In *National Conference on Emerging Computing Technologies* (p. 2). HRMMV.

Bhambri, P., Sinha, V. K., & Dhanoa, I. S. (2020). Development of Cost Effective PMS with Efficient Utilization of Resources. *Journal of Critical Reviews*, 7(19), 781–786.

Bhat, G., Tuncel, Y., An, S., & Ogras, U. Y. (2019). Wearable IoT Devices for Health Monitoring. *TechConnect Briefs*, *2019*, 357–360. https://eecs.wsu.edu/~gbhat/data/techconnect_paper.pdf

Boikanyo, K., Zungeru, A. M., Sigweni, B., Yahya, A., & Lebekwe, C. (2023). Remote Patient Monitoring Systems: Applications, Architecture, and Challenges. *Scientific African*, *20*, e01638. https://doi.org/10.1016/j.sciaf.2023.e01638

Chakrabarti, S., Biswas, N., Jones, L. D., Kesari, S., & Ashili, S. (2022). Smart Consumer Wearables as Digital Diagnostic Tools: A Review. *Diagnostics*, *12*(9), 2110. https://doi.org/10.3390/diagnostics12092110

Chong, K. P. L., Guo, J. Z., Deng, X., & Woo, B. K. P. (2020). Consumer Perceptions of Wearable Technology Devices: Retrospective Review and Analysis. *JMIR mHealth and uHealth*, *8*(4). https://doi.org/10.2196/17544

Dang, V. A., Vu Khanh, Q., Nguyen, V.-H., Nguyen, T., & Nguyen, D. C. (2023). Intelligent Healthcare: Integration of Emerging Technologies and Internet of Things for Humanity. *Sensors*, *23*(9), 4200. https://doi.org/10.3390/s23094200

Downey, C., Ng, S., Jayne, D., & Wong, D. (2019). Reliability of a Wearable Wireless Patch for Continuous Remote Monitoring of Vital Signs in Patients Recovering from Major Surgery: A Clinical Validation Study from the TRaCINg Trial. *BMJ Open*, *9*(8). https://doi.org/10.1136/bmjopen-2019-031150

Dwivedi, R., Mehrotra, D., & Chandra, S. (2022). Potential of Internet of Medical Things (IoMT) Applications in Building a Smart Healthcare System: A Systematic Review. *Journal of Oral Biology and Craniofacial Research*, *12*(2), 302–318. https://doi.org/10.1016/j.jobcr.2021.11.010

Ellis, L. D. (2023, May 19). *Exploring the Promise of Wearable Devices to Further Medical Research.* Https://Postgraduateeducation.Hms.Harvard.Edu/Trends-Medicine/Exploring-Promise-Wearable-Devices-Further-Medical-Research

Franco, C. M., Lima, J. G., & Giovanella, L. (2021). Atençãoprimária à saúdeemáreasrurais: acesso, organização e força de trabalhoemsaúdeemrevisãointegrativa de literatura. *Cadernos de SaúdePública*, *37*(7). https://doi.org/10.1590/0102-311x00310520

Fu, X., Sun, Q., Sun, C., Xu, F., & He, J. (2021). Urban-Rural Differences in Catastrophic Health Expenditure Among Households with Chronic Non-Communicable Disease Patients: Evidence from China Family Panel Studies. *BMC Public Health*, *21*(1), 874. https://doi.org/10.1186/s12889-021-10887-6

Fuller, J. R. (2016, May 26). *The 4 Stages of an IoT Architecture*. Https://Techbeacon.Com/Enterprise-It/4-Stages-Iot-Architecture.

Gajarawala, S. N., & Pelkowski, J. N. (2021). Telehealth Benefits and Barriers. *The Journal for Nurse Practitioners*, *17*(2), 218–221. https://doi.org/10.1016/j.nurpra.2020.09.013

Greco, L., Percannella, G., Ritrovato, P., Tortorella, F., & Vento, M. (2020). Trends in IoT based Solutions for Health Care: Moving AI to the Edge. *Pattern Recognition Letters*, *135*, 346–353. https://doi.org/10.1016/j.patrec.2020.05.016

Haghi, M., Danyali, S., Ayasseh, S., Wang, J., Aazami, R., & Deserno, T. M. (2021). Wearable Devices in Health Monitoring from the Environmental towards Multiple Domains: A Survey. *Sensors*, *21*(6), 2130. https://doi.org/10.3390/s21062130

Hamim, M., Paul, S., Hoque, S. I., Rahman, M. N., & Baqee, I.-A. (2019). IoT Based Remote Health Monitoring System for Patients and Elderly People. *2019 International Conference on Robotics, Electrical and Signal Processing Techniques (ICREST)*, 533–538. https://doi.org/10.1109/ICREST.2019.8644514

Healthy People 2020. (2020). Washington, DC: U.S. Department of Health and Human Services, Office of Disease Prevention and Health Promotion. www.healthypeople.gov/2020/topics-objectives/topic/Access-to-Health-Services.

Hogan, D. R., Stevens, G. A., Hosseinpoor, A. R., & Boerma, T. (2018). Monitoring Universal Health Coverage within the Sustainable Development Goals: Development and Baseline Data for An Index of Essential Health Services. *The Lancet Global Health*, *6*(2), e152–e168. https://doi.org/10.1016/S2214-109X(17)30472-2

Huhn, S., Matzke, I., Koch, M., Gunga, H.-C., Maggioni, M. A., Sié, A., Boudo, V., Ouedraogo, W. A., Compaoré, G., Bunker, A., Sauerborn, R., Bärnighausen, T., & Barteit, S. (2022). Using Wearable Devices to Generate Real-World, Individual-Level Data in Rural, Low-Resource Contexts in Burkina Faso, Africa: A Case Study. *Frontiers in Public Health*, *10*. https://doi.org/10.3389/fpubh.2022.972177

Hussain, M., Al-Haiqi, A., Zaidan, A. A., Zaidan, B. B., Kiah, M., Iqbal, S., Iqbal, S., & Abdulnabi, M. (2018). A Security Framework for mHealth Apps on Android Platform. *Computers and Security*, *75*, 191–217. https://doi.org/10.1016/j.cose.2018.02.003

Islam, S. M. R., Kwak, D., Kabir, M. H., Hossain, M., & Kwak, K. S. (2015). The Internet of Things for Health Care: A Comprehensive Survey. *IEEE Access*, *3*, 678–708. https://doi.org/10.1109/ACCESS.2015.2437951

Jang, I.-Y., Kim, H. R., Lee, E., Jung, H.-W., Park, H., Cheon, S.-H., Lee, Y. S., & Park, Y. R. (2018). Impact of a Wearable Device-Based Walking Programs in Rural Older Adults on Physical Activity and Health Outcomes: Cohort Study. *JMIR MHealth and UHealth*, *6*(11), e11335. https://doi.org/10.2196/11335

Karan, A., Selvaraj, S., & Mahal, A. (2014). Moving to Universal Coverage? Trends in the Burden of Out-of-Pocket Payments for Health Care across Social Groups in India, 1999–2000 to 2011–12. *PLoS ONE*, *9*(8), e105162. https://doi.org/10.1371/journal.pone.0105162

Kumar, M., Kumar, A., Verma, S., Bhattacharya, P., Ghimire, D., Kim, S., & Hosen, A. S. M. S. (2023). Healthcare Internet of Things (H-IoT): Current Trends, Future Prospects, Applications, Challenges, and Security Issues. *Electronics*, *12*(9), 2050. https://doi.org/10.3390/electronics12092050

Kumar, S., Tiwari, P., & Zymbler, M. (2019). Internet of Things is a Revolutionary Approach for Future Technology Enhancement: A Review. *Journal of Big Data*, *6*(1). https://doi.org/10.1186/s40537-019-0268-2

Mendia, J. A. (2022). Limitations of Healthcare Access in Rural Areas. *Family Medicine & Medical Science Research*, *11*(1). https://doi.org/10.37532/2327-4972.22.11.116

Merchant, R., Szefler, S. J., Bender, B. G., Tuffli, M., Barrett, M. A., Gondalia, R., Kaye, L., Van Sickle, D., & Stempel, D. A. (2018). Impact of a Digital Health Intervention on Asthma Resource Utilization. *World Allergy Organization Journal*, *11*, 28. https://doi.org/10.1186/s40413-018-0209-0

Millman, M. (1993). *Access to Health Care in America*. National Academies Press. https://doi.org/10.17226/2009

Mittlesteadt, J., Bambach, S., Dawes, A., Wentzel, E., Debs, A., Sezgin, E., Digby, D., Huang, Y., Ganger, A., Bhatnagar, S., Ehrenberg, L., Nunley, S., Glynn, P., Lin, S., Rust, S., & Patel, A. D. (2020). Evaluation of an Activity Tracker to Detect Seizures Using Machine Learning. *Journal of Child Neurology*, *35*(13), 873–878. https://doi.org/10.1177/0883073820937515

Nelson, B. W., & Allen, N. B. (2019). Accuracy of Consumer Wearable Heart Rate Measurement During an Ecologically Valid 24-Hour Period: Intraindividual Validation Study. *JMIR MHealth and UHealth*, *7*(3), e10828. https://doi.org/10.2196/10828

Pawar, Bharati Pravin. (2022, February 18). *Health & Family Welfare Department National Health Mission, India*. https://pib.gov.in/PressReleaseIframePage.aspx?PRID=1796435.

Pramanik, M. I., Lau, R. Y. K., Demirkan, H., & Azad, M. A. K. (2017). Smart Health: Big Data Enabled Health Paradigm within Smart Cities. *Expert Systems with Applications*, *87*, 370–383. https://doi.org/10.1016/j.eswa.2017.06.027

Rejeb, A., Rejeb, K., Treiblmaier, H., Appolloni, A., Alghamdi, S., Alhasawi, Y., & Iranmanesh, M. (2023). The Internet of Things (IoT) in Healthcare: Taking Stock and Moving Forward. *Internet of Things*, *22*, 100721. https://doi.org/10.1016/j.iot.2023.100721

Shivajirao Salunke, A., & Shivleela, M. (2022). *Real Time Healthcare Monitoring and Analysis System Using Iot* (Vol. 9). www.jetir.org

Singh, M., Singh, P., Kaur, K., & Bhambri, P. (2005, March). Database Security. In *National Conference on Future Trends in Information Technology* (pp. 57–62). SJPMLIET.

Smith, E. (2018, September 20). *American Telemedicine Association Applauds Landmark Expansion of Medicare Telehealth Coverage*. American Telemedicine Association. www.americantelemed.org/press-releases/american-telemedicine-association-applauds-landmark-expansion-of-medicare-telehealth-coverage/

Tran, V.-T., Riveros, C., & Ravaud, P. (2019). Patients' Views of Wearable Devices and AI in Healthcare: Findings from the ComPaRe e-Cohort. *npj Digital Medicine*, *2*(1), 53. https://doi.org/10.1038/s41746-019-0132-y

Wan, J., AAH Al-awlaqi, M., Li, M., O'Grady, M., Gu, X., Wang, J., & Cao, N. (2018). Wearable IoT Enabled Real-Time Health Monitoring System. *EURASIP Journal on Wireless Communications and Networking*, *11*(1). https://doi.org/10.1186/s13638-018-1308-x

WHO. (2012). *The World Health Report 2010, Health Systems Financing: The Path to Universal Coverage*. www.who.int/publications/i/item/9789241564021

WHO. (2023, February). *Trends in Maternal Mortality 2000 to 2020: Estimates by WHO, UNICEF, UNFPA, World Bank Group and UNDESA/Population Division*. WHO.

World Health Organization-World Bank. (2017). *Tracking Universal Health Coverage: 2017 Global Monitoring Report*. www.worldbank.org/en/topic/universalhealthcoverage/publication/tracking-universal-health-coverage-2017-global-monitoring-report

Xu, G., Qi, C., Dong, W., Gong, L., Liu, S., Chen, S., Liu, J., & Zheng, X. (2023). A Privacy-Preserving Medical Data Sharing Scheme Based on Blockchain. *IEEE Journal of Biomedical and Health Informatics*, *27*(2), 698–709. https://doi.org/10.1109/JBHI.2022.3203577

Xu, H., Li, P., Yang, Z., Liu, X., Wang, Z., Yan, W., He, M., Chu, W., She, Y., Li, Y., Cao, D., Yan, M., & Zhang, Z. (2020). Construction and Application of a Medical-Grade Wireless Monitoring System for Physiological Signals at General Wards. *Journal of Medical Systems*, *44*(10), 182. https://doi.org/10.1007/s10916-020-01653-z

8 Voice Signal-Based Disease Diagnosis using IoT and Learning Algorithms for Healthcare

Pulkit Kumar and Harpreet Kaur Channi

8.1 INTRODUCTION

In an era defined by rapid technological advancements and an ever-growing emphasis on patient-centred healthcare, innovative solutions have become imperative in the medical field. The convergence of emerging technologies like the internet of things (IoT) and advanced machine learning algorithms has paved the way for a transformative approach to healthcare, with the potential to redefine the landscape of disease diagnosis and patient care. The traditional paradigm of healthcare diagnosis often involves invasive, time-consuming, and costly procedures. Furthermore, access to specialized medical facilities can be limited, particularly in remote or underserved regions. These limitations have underscored the need for novel, non-invasive, and widely accessible diagnostic methods that can provide timely and accurate results. Voice, as a diagnostic tool, offers an intriguing prospect. The human voice is a rich source of information, carrying subtle cues related to a person's health and well-being. The patterns, frequencies, and characteristics of one's voice can reveal a wealth of information, ranging from respiratory conditions to neurodegenerative disorders and mental health conditions. Leveraging voice signals for healthcare diagnostics not only offers a non-invasive and patient-friendly approach but also the potential to extend the reach of healthcare services to a global audience (Rattan et al. 2005). IoT provides a critical infrastructure for collecting and transmitting voice data efficiently and securely. IoT devices equipped with specialized sensors can capture voice signals and transmit them to a central platform for analysis. Machine learning algorithms, particularly natural language processing (NLP) and pattern recognition techniques, can then decipher these signals, discerning valuable insights related to a patient's health.

The objectives of this research are multifaceted. First and foremost, it aims to develop a robust voice-based diagnostic system that can accurately detect various diseases. This system will be underpinned by state-of-the-art IoT sensors and

DOI: 10.1201/9781032698519-8

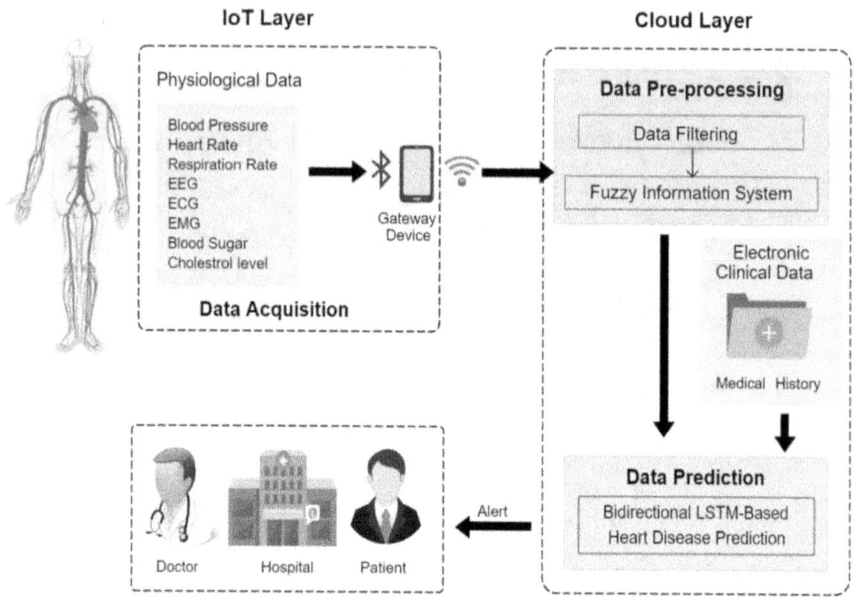

FIGURE 8.1 IoT based smart healthcare monitoring system (Nancy et al. 2022).

devices, ensuring the seamless collection and transmission of voice data. Machine learning algorithms will then play a pivotal role in pattern recognition and classification, leading to timely and precise disease diagnoses. Figure 8.1 shows the IoT based smart healthcare monitoring system.

8.1.1 Literature Review

The patient data stored in such PHR systems constitute big data whose analysis with the use of appropriate machine learning algorithms is expected to improve diagnosis and treatment accuracy, to cut healthcare costs and, hence, to improve the overall quality and efficiency of healthcare provided. Poulymenopoulou et al., (2014) describe a health data analytics engine which uses machine learning algorithms for analyzing cloud based PHR big health data towards knowledge extraction to support better healthcare delivery as regards disease diagnosis and prognosis (Poulymenopoulou et al., 2014). An intelligent optimization model is proposed for monitoring patients with Parkinson's disease (PD) based on UPDRS assessment (Unified Parkinson's Disease Rating Scale) from voice records in a smart home. ALO-DEELM model is compared with different machine learning (ML) prediction algorithms and showed the superiority based on different measures. In these studies, various speech signal processing algorithms have been used to extract clinically useful information for PD assessment, and the calculated features were fed to learning algorithms to construct reliable decision support systems (Anter and Zhang 2020). (Sakar et al., 2019) apply, to the best of the knowledge for the first time, the tunable Q-factor wavelet transform

(TQWT) to the voice signals of PD patients for feature extraction, which has higher frequency resolution than the classical discrete wavelet transform (Sakar et al., 2019). The healthcare system also predicts the disease for a particular patient base on current reading using various supervised learning algorithms (Yadav and Jadhav 2019).

8.2 IoT AND HEALTHCARE

The integration of IoT in the healthcare industry represents a groundbreaking shift in how healthcare services are delivered and experienced (Sharma et al., 2020). IoT, which involves connecting everyday objects and devices to the internet, plays a pivotal role in collecting, transmitting, and analyzing healthcare data in real-time. This section explores the profound implications of IoT in healthcare, ranging from the digital transformation of medical devices to the personalization of patient care (Kashani et al., 2021).

8.2.1 IoT in the Healthcare Industry

IoT has revolutionized healthcare by extending its reach beyond the traditional boundaries of hospitals and clinics. In essence, it transforms healthcare by connecting medical devices, wearables, and healthcare infrastructure to the internet. This interconnectivity results in the continuous collection and transmission of health data, which can be leveraged to enhance patient care and streamline healthcare processes. For instance, medical devices equipped with IoT capabilities, such as ECG monitors and blood glucose meters, can transmit real-time data to healthcare providers and offer patients greater insight into their health conditions (Kodali et al., 2015). The transformative power of IoT is evident in its ability to facilitate seamless data exchange among devices, healthcare professionals, and patients. This digital transformation enhances the efficiency of healthcare services.

8.2.2 The Role of IoT in Remote Monitoring

Remote monitoring, as empowered by IoT, redefines the healthcare paradigm by enabling the continuous monitoring of patients' health and symptoms without the need for in-person visits. This approach is particularly crucial for individuals with chronic diseases, the elderly, and those residing in geographically remote or underserved areas. Remote monitoring effectively bridges the gap between patients and healthcare providers, ensuring that healthcare services are accessible to a broader demographic, regardless of their physical location. The core strength of IoT in remote monitoring lies in its ability to facilitate real-time data acquisition. Devices such as blood pressure monitors, pulse oximeters, and wearable sensors continuously collect health-related data. This data is then transmitted to healthcare providers' systems, enabling close surveillance of patients' conditions (Tekeste Habte et al., 2019). Figure 8.2 shows the benefits of IoT in healthcare.

In the context of IoT-enabled healthcare devices, interoperability and data sharing are fundamental considerations. These devices must seamlessly communicate with each other and with electronic health record (EHR) systems. Interoperability

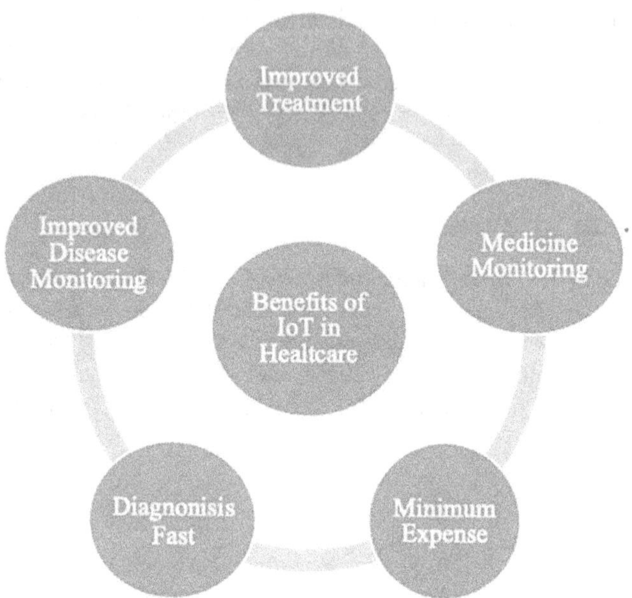

FIGURE 8.2 Benefits of IoT in healthcare (Upadhyay et al., 2023).

ensures that healthcare providers have access to a unified patient profile, simplifying decision-making, and treatment coordination (Javaid and Khan 2021). For example, ingestible sensors, sometimes referred to as "smart pills," are designed to monitor medication adherence and collect data from within the body. These sensors transmit data about the patient's medication intake and physiological responses. Healthcare providers can remotely assess treatment efficacy and adherence, further enhancing patient care and medication management (Said and Tolba 2021).

8.3 VOICE SIGNAL ANALYSIS IN HEALTHCARE

Voice signal analysis in healthcare refers to the process of using advanced techniques and technology to extract valuable medical information from a person's voice (Bhambri and Gupta 2005). This field has gained significant attention due to its non-invasive, cost-effective, and patient-friendly approach to healthcare diagnostics (Sirisha and Reddy 2018). By analyzing the characteristics of a person's voice, such as pitch, tone, speed, and even subtle changes imperceptible to the human ear, healthcare professionals and researchers can gather insights about various health conditions. Here are some key aspects of voice signal analysis in healthcare:

8.3.1 Voice as a Diagnostic Tool

The human voice serves as a unique and continuous reflection of an individual's physiological and psychological state. Voice signal analysis recognizes that subtle changes in one's voice, often imperceptible to the human ear, can serve as critical indicators of various medical conditions. By focusing on aspects like pitch, tone, speech rate, articulation, and the presence of anomalies (such as tremors or hesitations), healthcare professionals and researchers can identify patterns associated with specific diseases (Bhambri and Bhandari 2005). For instance, variations in voice characteristics can be linked to respiratory disorders like asthma, neurological ailments such as Parkinson's disease, mental health conditions like depression, and even early signs of neurodegenerative disorders such as Alzheimer's disease. As a diagnostic tool, voice signal analysis leverages the distinctive features of an individual's vocal characteristics to detect and monitor health-related changes over time (Singhal and Sharma 2023).

8.3.2 Advantages and Challenges of Voice-Based Diagnosis

The utilization of voice for healthcare diagnosis offers a multitude of advantages. It stands out as a non-invasive technique, eliminating the need for uncomfortable or potentially risky procedures that may be associated with traditional diagnostic methods. This is especially advantageous in the context of chronic diseases that require frequent monitoring (Singh et al., 2005). Voice analysis can also be a cost-effective solution, as it doesn't demand high expenditures on specialized equipment or consumables, which can make healthcare more affordable. Furthermore, voice-based diagnostics are inherently patient-friendly and accessible. Voice data can be collected remotely, without the necessity for in-person visits, enhancing convenience for patients, especially in situations where mobility or access to healthcare facilities is limited (Almada and Maranhão 2021).

8.4 IoT INFRASTRUCTURE FOR VOICE DATA COLLECTION

The "IoT Infrastructure for Voice Data Collection" section elucidates the foundational components and technologies essential for acquiring and securely managing voice data in healthcare applications. This infrastructure encompasses IoT sensors and devices, data transmission and connectivity, as well as data security and privacy measures (Hossain et al., 2016).

8.4.1 IoT Sensors and Devices

Wearable devices with integrated microphones have gained prominence for voice data collection. These devices offer continuous voice signal capture, rendering them suitable for applications requiring remote patient monitoring and real-time data acquisition (Mikusz et al., 2018). They excel in the context of chronic diseases and mental health conditions, as they allow for unobtrusive, prolonged voice data collection, enabling healthcare providers to gain insights into patient well-being over time. Dedicated remote monitoring devices equipped with specialized microphones play a pivotal role in healthcare applications of voice data collection. These devices are meticulously designed for gathering voice data from patients, ensuring high-quality recordings that can be subjected to machine learning algorithms for analysis. They are indispensable in diagnosing and monitoring respiratory conditions, neurodegenerative disorders, and mental health conditions, among others (Ilyas et al., 2020).

8.4.2 Data Transmission and Connectivity

Efficient data transmission protocols are a linchpin of IoT infrastructure. These protocols enable the secure and reliable transfer of voice data from sensors to centralized systems for analysis. Common IoT communication protocols like MQTT and CoAP are frequently employed for voice data transmission, guaranteeing the delivery of data, even in real-time scenarios. IoT infrastructure for voice data collection harnesses wireless networks for data transmission, which can include Wi-Fi, cellular networks, or dedicated IoT networks such as LoRaWAN. The choice of connectivity hinges on application-specific considerations, including the desired range, data volume, and power consumption. Stable and low-latency connections are critical for real-time applications.

8.5 MACHINE LEARNING FOR VOICE-BASED DISEASE DIAGNOSIS

The integration of machine learning into healthcare has opened up new avenues for diagnostic and monitoring techniques. In the realm of voice-based disease diagnosis, machine learning serves as a powerful tool to analyze and interpret voice data, providing valuable insights into various medical conditions. This section explores the application of machine learning in healthcare, focusing on natural language processing (NLP) in healthcare, pattern recognition and classification, and real-world case studies featuring algorithms (Ouhmida et al., 2021).

8.5.1 Natural Language Processing (NLP) in Healthcare

8.5.1.1 NLP Fundamentals

Natural Language Processing (NLP) is a subfield of artificial intelligence that concentrates on the interaction between computers and human language. It equips machines with the capability to comprehend, analyze, and generate human language. In healthcare, NLP is a game-changer, as a vast amount of medical information is present in unstructured text, including electronic health records, medical literature, and patient narratives. NLP empowers healthcare professionals and researchers to harness this data for improved diagnostic and decision-making processes (Iroju and Olaleke 2015). The initial step involves cleaning and preparing textual data. It includes tasks like tokenization (breaking text into words or phrases), stop-word removal (eliminating common words with little meaning), and stemming (reducing words to their base form). NLP techniques can extract structured information from unstructured text, making it easier to integrate textual data into healthcare databases and decision support systems (Hudaa et al., 2019).

8.5.2 Pattern Recognition and Classification

8.5.2.1 Pattern Recognition Basics

Pattern recognition is a fundamental concept in machine learning and artificial intelligence. It involves the identification of regularities or patterns in data, which can be used to make data-driven decisions, including categorizing data into predefined classes. In the context of voice-based disease diagnosis, pattern recognition algorithms are employed to identify unique voice characteristics associated with specific medical conditions. These algorithms leverage the principles of supervised learning, where they are trained on labelled datasets to recognize patterns and make predictions (Dougherty 2012).

8.5.2.2 Classification Algorithms

Machine learning models, particularly classification algorithms, play a central role in voice-based disease diagnosis. These algorithms are responsible for categorizing voice data into different disease or health status groups. Support Vector Machines (SVM) is a powerful classification algorithm that finds the optimal hyperplane to separate data points into different classes. It is effective in distinguishing between healthy and disease-affected voice patterns (Weiss and Kapouleas 1989).

8.5.3 Case Studies and Algorithms

8.5.3.1 Real-World Case Studies

The practical application of machine learning in voice-based disease diagnosis is exemplified through real-world case studies. These case studies illustrate how machine learning algorithms are implemented in clinical and research settings, showcasing their potential in diagnosing and monitoring medical conditions using voice data. Here are a few examples:

- Respiratory Conditions: Machine learning algorithms have been applied to voice data to diagnose and monitor respiratory conditions like asthma and chronic obstructive pulmonary disease (COPD). These algorithms can detect changes in voice characteristics, such as wheezing or breathlessness, and use these patterns for early diagnosis and monitoring of these conditions (Cukic et al., 2012).
- Neurodegenerative Disorders: Voice data analysis has proven effective in the early diagnosis and monitoring of neurodegenerative disorders like Parkinson's disease and Alzheimer's disease. Machine learning models can identify specific vocal markers associated with these conditions, aiding in early intervention and treatment planning (Brandebura et al., 2023).

8.6 VOICE SIGNAL-BASED DISEASE DIAGNOSIS APPLICATIONS

Voice signal analysis has emerged as a promising tool for disease diagnosis and monitoring across a range of medical conditions. Its applications extend from diagnosing respiratory conditions to monitoring neurodegenerative disorders, assessing mental health conditions, and exploring emerging applications in healthcare. Here, we delve into the details of these applications:

8.6.1 Respiratory Conditions

8.6.1.1 Asthma and COPD Diagnosis

Voice signal analysis offers a unique approach to diagnose and monitor respiratory conditions, notably asthma and chronic obstructive pulmonary disease (COPD) (Singhal and Sharma 2023). Voice signal analysis can be particularly useful in the following ways:

- Early Detection: By monitoring subtle changes in voice patterns, such as increased wheezing or variations in pitch, healthcare providers can detect early signs of exacerbations or worsening symptoms in asthma and COPD patients.
- Remote Monitoring: Voice signal analysis is a valuable tool for remote monitoring of respiratory conditions. Patients can use wearable devices equipped with specialized microphones to record their voice regularly from the comfort of their homes. Remote monitoring minimizes the need for frequent in-person visits and allows for continuous disease tracking (Islam et al. 2020).

8.6.2 Neurodegenerative Disorders

8.6.2.1 Early Detection of Parkinson's Disease

Voice analysis has proven to be a valuable tool in the early detection of neurodegenerative disorders, particularly Parkinson's disease. This debilitating condition is characterized by specific voice changes, including reduced pitch variability and altered speech rhythm. Voice recordings can be analyzed using machine learning algorithms to detect these vocal characteristics. The application of voice signal analysis in Parkinson's disease diagnosis is beneficial in the following ways:

- Non-Invasive Screening: Voice-based diagnosis provides a non-invasive and cost-effective screening method for Parkinson's disease. By analyzing voice recordings, clinicians can identify potential early indicators of the disease, facilitating timely referrals for further neurological evaluation.
- Longitudinal Monitoring: Voice signal analysis can be used for longitudinal monitoring of Parkinson's disease progression. Changes in voice characteristics over time can offer insights into the severity and trajectory of the condition (Gallagher and Montgomery 2007).

8.6.2.2 Alzheimer's Disease Monitoring

Voice signal analysis is also being explored for monitoring Alzheimer's disease, a progressive neurodegenerative disorder characterized by cognitive decline. Voice data collected over time can aid in tracking the progression of Alzheimer's disease, allowing for timely interventions and treatment adjustments. The applications in Alzheimer's disease monitoring include:

- Progress Tracking: Voice-based disease monitoring offers a non-invasive and patient-friendly approach to track the progression of Alzheimer's disease. Changes in language complexity, fluency, and coherence can be detected through voice analysis, enabling clinicians to assess the cognitive status of patients over time.
- Therapeutic Feedback: In therapeutic settings, voice signal analysis can provide feedback to speech therapists and caregivers. Therapeutic exercises that involve controlled speech patterns and language exercises can be monitored and adjusted based on the analysis of voice data, thereby facilitating more effective therapy (de la Fuente Garcia et al., 2020).

8.6.4 Other Emerging Applications

8.6.4.1 Heart Disease Detection

Emerging applications of voice signal analysis include the detection of heart disease. Research suggests that certain voice characteristics may be associated with underlying heart conditions. Changes in voice patterns, such as the presence of murmurs or anomalies, could provide clues to cardiac issues. The applications in heart disease detection include:

- Non-Invasive Screening: Voice-based screening for heart disease offers a non-invasive and accessible method for early detection. This can be particularly beneficial in primary care settings and for patients at risk of cardiovascular issues.
- Cost-Effective Assessment: Voice signal analysis is a cost-effective means of screening for heart disease, especially when compared to traditional diagnostic tests like echocardiography or cardiac catheterization (Das et al., 2023).

8.6.4.2 Vocal Cord Disorders

Voice signal analysis is valuable in diagnosing vocal cord disorders. Conditions like vocal cord nodules or polyps can affect voice quality. By analyzing voice data, healthcare professionals can identify anomalies and voice irregularities that may be indicative of these disorders. The applications in vocal cord disorder diagnosis include:

- Non-Invasive Evaluation: Voice-based diagnosis provides a non-invasive means of evaluating vocal cord health. It can be used in the assessment of conditions that affect vocal quality, allowing for early intervention and treatment planning.
- Post-Surgical Assessment: Voice signal analysis can also be used to assess vocal cord function post-surgery. This aids in determining the effectiveness

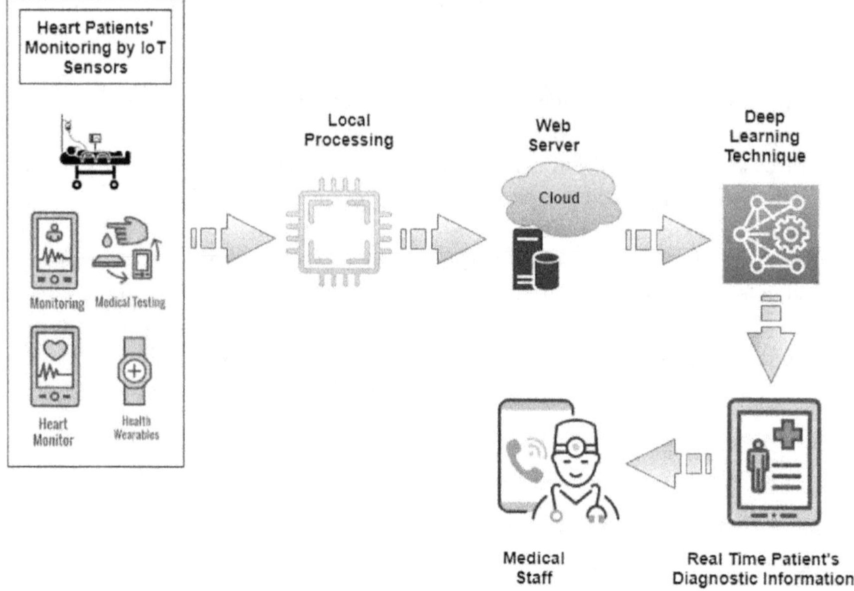

FIGURE 8.3 Heart patient monitoring using the IoT (Umer et al., 2022).

of surgical interventions and the need for additional therapies or follow-up procedures (Compton et al., 2023). Figure 8.3 shows the heart patient monitoring using the IoT.

8.7 ETHICAL AND PRIVACY CONSIDERATIONS

The integration of voice signal-based disease diagnosis in healthcare raises important ethical and privacy concerns that must be carefully addressed. This section delves into these considerations, encompassing informed consent and patient rights, data security and encryption, and regulatory compliance and standards.

8.7.1 Informed Consent and Patient Rights

8.7.1.1 Informed Consent Basics

Informed consent is a cornerstone of ethical healthcare practice. It is the process through which healthcare providers ensure that patients fully understand the nature of a medical procedure or data collection and willingly agree to participate. In the context of voice signal-based disease diagnosis, informed consent plays a vital role. Patients must be informed about the purpose and scope of voice data collection, how the data will be used, who will have access to it, and the potential benefits and risks. This understanding enables patients to make informed decisions regarding their participation. Patients have the right to voluntarily agree to participate in voice signal data collection. They should not be coerced, and their participation should be based on their free will. Patients can choose to withdraw their consent at any time without facing negative consequences.

8.7.1.2 Patient Rights

Respecting patient rights is integral to the ethical use of voice signal data in healthcare, patients have the right to assert ownership of their voice data. They should be informed that their data remains their property, and they may choose to access, amend, or delete their records at any time. Patients have the right to access their own voice data. They should be able to review the information collected and how it has been utilized. Patients have the right to transparency regarding how their voice data is processed and shared. Transparency includes the disclosure of data-sharing practices and the involvement of third parties. Patients have the right to expect robust data security and privacy measures. Their data should be protected from unauthorized access, breaches, and misuse. Patients have the right to ensure that their participation in voice signal data collection does not result in discrimination or stigmatization.

8.7.2 Data Security and Encryption

8.7.2.1 Encryption Measures

Data security is a paramount consideration in voice signal-based disease diagnosis. Robust encryption measures should be employed to safeguard voice data. Voice data should be encrypted from the point of collection to storage and transmission. End-to-end encryption ensures that data is accessible only to authorized individuals or entities, preventing unauthorized access or data breaches. Only authorized personnel, such as healthcare providers, should have access to patient data. Implementing audit trails allows for the monitoring of data access and usage. Clear data retention policies should be in place, once voice data is no longer needed for diagnosis or treatment, it should be de-identified to remove personally identifiable information. This minimizes privacy risks. Data that is no longer needed should be securely destroyed to prevent unintended access (Chadha et al., 2023).

8.8 CHALLENGES AND FUTURE DIRECTIONS

The field of voice signal-based disease diagnosis using IoT and learning algorithms in healthcare is rapidly evolving, but it faces several challenges. This section outlines these challenges and discusses future directions, including addressing technological limitations, expanding diagnostic capabilities, enhancing user acceptance and adoption, and promoting research and innovation.

8.8.1 Addressing Technological Limitations

One of the primary technological challenges in voice signal-based disease diagnosis is the variability in data quality. Voice data collected from different sources, such as various types of microphones or recording conditions, can vary significantly in terms of background noise, signal quality, and acoustic characteristics. Addressing this limitation requires the development of robust pre-processing techniques to standardize and enhance data quality, making it suitable for machine learning analysis. Another significant challenge is the limited availability of labelled voice data for training machine learning algorithms. Many medical conditions have specific voice markers, but acquiring and curating large and diverse datasets to train and validate models can be a resource-intensive process (Singhal and Sharma 2023).

8.8.2 Expanding Diagnostic Capabilities

While voice data provides valuable insights, combining it with other healthcare modalities, such as physiological sensor data or imaging, can enhance diagnostic capabilities. Future directions should explore multi-modal data integration to offer a more comprehensive and accurate assessment of patients' health conditions. This requires the development of sophisticated fusion techniques and machine learning models that can effectively utilize and integrate data from diverse sources. Expanding diagnostic capabilities also involves the implementation of longitudinal monitoring (Shah et al., 2021). Tracking changes in voice patterns and health markers over time can provide a more dynamic and personalized approach to disease diagnosis. It enables the early detection of disease progression, optimizing treatment plans, and interventions. Future developments may focus on continuous monitoring using wearable devices and real-time data analysis. (Vaidya et al., 2018).

8.9 CONCLUSION

In conclusion, the integration of voice signal-based disease diagnosis using IoT and learning algorithms in healthcare represents a significant stride towards more accessible, personalized, and efficient medical diagnostics. Despite facing technological challenges, such as data variability and interoperability, the field shows great promise in expanding diagnostic capabilities through multi-modal integration and personalized medicine. User acceptance and adoption hinge on trust, privacy assurance, and regulatory compliance, highlighting the importance of transparent communication and healthcare provider training. Continuous research and innovation, coupled with rigorous validation through clinical trials, will be instrumental in realizing the full potential of this transformative approach. With ethical considerations and bias mitigation at the forefront, the future of voice-based diagnosis holds tremendous potential to revolutionize healthcare, ultimately leading to improved patient outcomes and a more inclusive, equitable healthcare system.

REFERENCES

Almada, M. and J. Maranhão (2021). "Voice-based diagnosis of covid-19: ethical and legal challenges." *International Data Privacy Law* 11(1): 63–75.

Anter, A. M. and Z. Zhang (2020). "E-health Parkinson disease diagnosis in smart home based on hybrid intelligence optimization model." In *Proceedings of the International Conference on Advanced Intelligent Systems and Informatics 2019*, Springer.

Bhambri, P. and A. Bhandari (2005, March). "Different protocols for wireless security." In *National Conference on Advancements in Modeling and Simulation* (p. 8). LLRIET.

Bhambri, P. and S. Gupta (2005, March). "A survey & comparison of permutation possibility of fault tolerant multistage interconnection networks." In *National Conference on Application of Mathematics in Engineering & Technology* (p. 13). MIMIT.

Brandebura, A. N., A. Paumier, T. S. Onur and N. J. Allen (2023). "Astrocyte contribution to dysfunction, risk and progression in neurodegenerative disorders." *Nature Reviews Neuroscience* 24(1): 23–39.

Chadha, H., S. Gupta, A. Khanna and N. Kumar (2023). "AI-based security protocols for IoT applications: a critical review." *Recent Advances in Computer Science and Communications (Formerly: Recent Patents on Computer Science)* 16(5): 2–18.

Compton, E. C., T. Cruz, M. Andreassen, S. Beveridge, D. Bosch, D. R. Randall and D. Livingstone (2023). "Developing an artificial intelligence tool to predict vocal cord pathology in primary care settings." *The Laryngoscope* 133(8): 1952–1960.

Cukic, V., V. Lovre, D. Dragisic and A. Ustamujic (2012). "Asthma and chronic obstructive pulmonary disease (COPD)–differences and similarities." *Materia Socio-Medica* 24(2): 100.

Das, R. C., M. C. Das, M. A. Hossain, M. A. Rahman, M. H. Hossen and R. Hasan (2023). Heart disease detection using ML. In *2023 IEEE 13th Annual Computing and Communication Workshop and Conference (CCWC)*, IEEE.

de la Fuente Garcia, S., C. W. Ritchie and S. Luz (2020). "Artificial intelligence, speech, and language processing approaches to monitoring Alzheimer's disease: a systematic review." *Journal of Alzheimer's Disease* 78(4): 1547–1574.

Dougherty, G. (2012). *Pattern Recognition and Classification: An Introduction*, Springer Science & Business Media.

Gallagher, C. and E. B. Montgomery Jr (2007). "Early detection of Parkinson's disease." *Handbook of Clinical Neurology* 83: 457–477.

Hossain, M. S., G. Muhammad, S. M. M. Rahman, W. Abdul, A. Alelaiwi and A. Alamri (2016). "Toward end-to-end biomet rics-based security for IoT infrastructure." *IEEE Wireless Communications* 23(5): 44–51.

Hudaa, S., D. B. P. Setiyadi, E. L. Lydia, K. Shankar, P. T. Nguyen, W. Hashim and A. Maseleno (2019). "Natural language processing utilization in healthcare." *International Journal of Engineering and Advanced Technology* 8(6): 1117–1120.

Ilyas, M. U., M. Ahmad and S. Saleem (2020). "Internet-of-things-infrastructure-as-a-service: the democratization of access to public internet-of-things infrastructure." *International Journal of Communication Systems* 33(16): e4562.

Iroju, O. G. and J. O. Olaleke (2015). "A systematic review of natural language processing in healthcare." *International Journal of Information Technology and Computer Science* 8: 44–50.

Islam, R., M. Tarique and E. Abdel-Raheem (2020). "A survey on signal processing based pathological voice detection techniques." *IEEE Access* 8: 66749–66776.

Javaid, M. and I. H. Khan (2021). "Internet of things (IoT) enabled healthcare helps to take the challenges of COVID-19 Pandemic." *Journal of Oral Biology and Craniofacial Research* 11(2): 209–214.

Kashani, M. H., M. Madanipour, M. Nikravan, P. Asghari and E. Mahdipour (2021). "A systematic review of IoT in healthcare: applications, techniques, and trends." *Journal of Network and Computer Applications* 192: 103164.

Kodali, R. K., G. Swamy and B. Lakshmi (2015). An implementation of IoT for healthcare. In *2015 IEEE Recent Advances in Intelligent Computational Systems (RAICS)*, IEEE.

Mikusz, M., Houben, S., Davies, N., Moessner, K., & Langheinrich, M. (2018). Raising awareness of IoT sensor deployments. In *Living in the Internet of Things: Cybersecurity of the IoT – 2018*, London (pp. 1–8). doi: 10.1049/cp.2018.0009

Nancy, A. A., D. Ravindran, P. M. D. Raj Vincent, K. Srinivasan and D. Gutierrez Reina (2022). "IoT-cloud-based smart healthcare monitoring system for heart disease prediction via deep learning." *Electronics* 11(15): 2292.

Ouhmida, A., O. Terrada, A. Raihani, B. Cherradi and S. Hamida (2021). "Voice-based deep learning medical diagnosis system for parkinson's disease prediction." In *2021 International Congress of Advanced Technology and Engineering (ICOTEN)*, IEEE.

Poulymenopoulou, M., F. Malamateniou and G. Vassilacopoulos (2014). "Machine learning for knowledge extraction from PHR big data." In *Integrating Information Technology and Management for Quality of Care* (pp. 36–39), IOS Press.

Rattan, M., P. Bhambri and Shaifali (2005, February). "Institution for a sustainable civilization: negotiating change in a technological culture." In *National Conference on Technical Education in Globalized Environment-Knowledge, Technology & The Teacher* (p. 45). SBBSIET.

Said, O. and A. Tolba (2021). "Design and evaluation of large-scale IoT-enabled healthcare architecture." *Applied Sciences* 11(8): 3623.

Sakar, C. O., G. Serbes, A. Gunduz, H. C. Tunc, H. Nizam, B. E. Sakar, M. Tutuncu, T. Aydin, M. E. Isenkul and H. Apaydin (2019). "A comparative analysis of speech signal processing algorithms for Parkinson's disease classification and the use of the tunable Q-factor wavelet transform." *Applied Soft Computing* 74: 255–263.

Shah, P., J. Sands and N. Normanno (2021). "The expanding capability and clinical relevance of molecular diagnostic technology to identify and evaluate EGFR mutations in advanced/metastatic NSCLC." *Lung Cancer* 160: 118–126.

Sharma, R., P. Bhambri and A. K. Sohal, (2020). "Energy bio-inspired for MANET." *International Journal of Recent Technology and Engineering* 8(6): 5580–5585.

Singh, M., P. Singh, K. Kaur and P. Bhambri (2005, March). "Database security." In *National Conference on Future Trends in Information Technology* (pp. 35–41). SJPMLIET.

Singhal, A. and D. K. Sharma (2023). "Voice signal-based disease diagnosis using IoT and learning algorithms for healthcare." In *Implementation of Smart Healthcare Systems Using AI, IoT, and Blockchain* (pp. 59–81), Elsevier.

Sirisha, G. and A. M. Reddy (2018). "Smart healthcare analysis and therapy for voice disorder using cloud and edge computing." In *2018 4th International Conference on Applied and Theoretical Computing and Communication Technology (iCATccT)*, IEEE.

Tekeste Habte, T., H. Saleh, B. Mohammad, M. Ismail, T. Tekeste Habte, H. Saleh, B. Mohammad and M. Ismail (2019). "IoT for healthcare." In *Ultra Low Power ECG Processing System for IoT Devices* (pp. 7–12). Springer. ttps://www.springerprofessional.de/en/ultra-low-power-ecg-processing-system-for-iot-devices/16104002

Umer, M., S. Sadiq, H. Karamti, W. Karamti, R. Majeed and M. NAPPI (2022). "IoT based smart monitoring of patients' with acute heart failure." *Sensors* 22(7): 2431.

Upadhyay, S., M. Kumar, A. Upadhyay, S. Verma, Kavita, M. Kaur, R. A. Khurma and P. A. Castillo (2023). "Challenges and limitation analysis of an IoT-dependent system for deployment in smart healthcare using communication standards features." *Sensors* 23(11): 5155.

Vaidya, A., P. Mulatero, R. Baudrand and G. K. Adler (2018). "The expanding spectrum of primary aldosteronism: implications for diagnosis, pathogenesis, and treatment." *Endocrine Reviews* 39(6): 1057–1088.

Weiss, S. M. and I. Kapouleas (1989). An empirical comparison of pattern recognition, neural nets, and machine learning classification methods. In *International Joint Conferences on Artificial Intelligence (IJCAI)*. https://www.ijcai.org/Proceedings/89-1/Papers/125.pdf

Yadav, S. S. and S. M. Jadhav (2019). "Machine learning algorithms for disease prediction using Iot environment." *International Journal of Engineering and Advanced Technology* 8(6): 4303–4307.

9 Artificial Intelligence-Enabled Internet of Medical Things for Enhanced Healthcare Systems

Wasswa Shafik

9.1 INTRODUCTION

As technology has improved, smart healthcare has changed a lot. It now includes microelectronics, big data, IoT, cloud computing, mobile internet, and mobile health (Nair and Sahoo, 2023). The incorporation of modern medical sensors and different hardware in the health sector has led to the development of a new concept called "IoMT," sometimes called "the Internet of Health Things," which, along with the technologies, has transformed traditional healthcare into a more efficient, all-round, and personalized experience. The global market for smart health is projected to increase by a mean growth rate of 16.2% (Kok, 2023). This creates a dire need for fast, comprehensive, accurate, and intelligent eHealthcare systems, as highlighted by the emergency of global pandemics. Through different medical electronic devices, these systems will be able to collect, analyze, and make sense of a large amount of information about the health and well-being of the patient (Bhattarai and Peng, 2023; Deshmukh et al., 2023).

The convergence of IoMT, AI, and big data has added new dimensions to such systems, which are now capable of analyzing the collected data to provide better insights, thereby ushering in a new era in healthcare, such as early-stage chronic disease prediction and personalized and physiological health monitoring systems, among others (Fahim et al., 2024). Through the IoMT environment, monitoring health can be attained with the aid of numerous wearable medical sensors that record and keep track of patient medical conditions in real-time (Shafik et al., 2020; Shafik, 2023). The data produced by such sensors enables medical physicians to reliably and efficiently recognize and respond to critical situations regarding patients to enable them to become more informed regarding their health conditions for future diagnosis and treatment (Mathur et al., 2023).

The large amount of patient information collected by several devices in the IoMT environment has ushered in new opportunities that leverage the power of AI

DOI: 10.1201/9781032698519-9

(Bhambri et al., 2020). Currently known as AI-enabled health, opportunities such as the ability to quickly analyze and interpret patient information diagnose, and predict future diseases have been reported (Kalinaki et al., 2024). Advanced AI techniques have made it possible for medical physicians to remotely track habits and reveal patient medical status from the captured data emanating from several sensors, along with sensor usage patterns. Through the IoMT environment, AI techniques, for example, support vector machines, random forest, logistic regression, decision trees, k-nearest neighbour, naïve Bayes, and several neural networks have been used for various health-related applications (Irfana Parveen et al., 2023).

The IoMT architecture in Figure 9.1 depicts the comprehensive growth of exploiting smart sensors to accumulate data and regulate smart healthcare structures. However, there are notable challenges that face smart healthcare, as discussed (Narasimharao et al., 2023). Furthermore, medical institutions rely on internet-based technologies, from connected infusion pumps to telemetry patient monitors, to provide best-in-class patient care. According to Kok and Setyadi (2023), they predicted that by 2022, the number of connected medical devices "Things" will reach up to 30 billion. During their study, they considered four main health factors that soar with the smart healthcare system, including in homes (like mobile help, vitality, and intelligent clinic, among others), communities (for instance, Xerafy, American Well, and Skytron, among others), clinics, hospitals, and on the body (Pandey and Pandey, 2023).

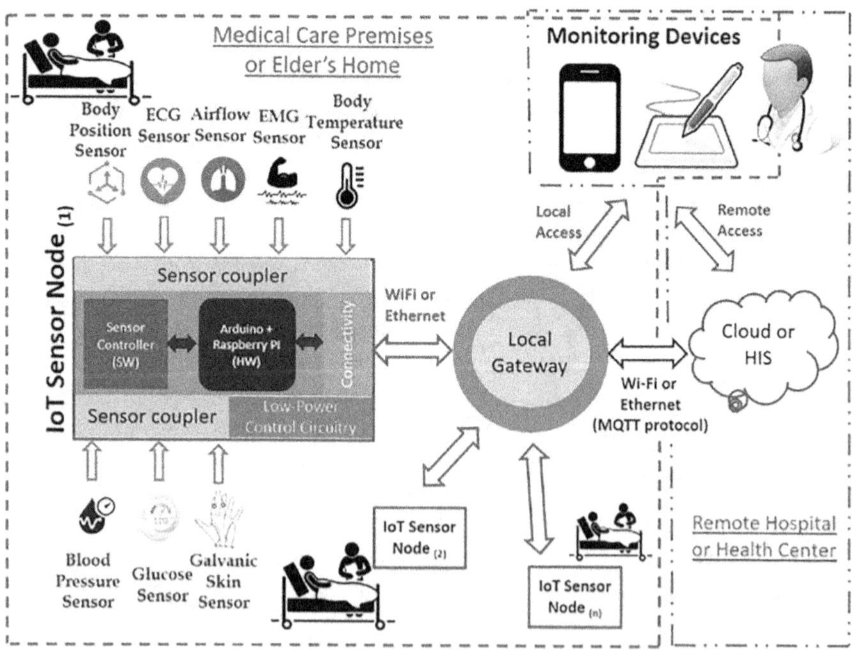

FIGURE 9.1 IoMT architecture with comprehensive growth (Petrellis et al., 2019).

Healthcare providers and officials in the healthcare domain need to keep track of viral infections to ensure the necessary isolation of patients along with real-time measures to contain infections (Bhambri and Singh, 2006). In light of current developments, the medical devices that comprise the IoMT and their convergence with AI described above have demonstrated tremendous potential in improving the overall health of billions of people worldwide, resulting in improved quality of life (Banday and Bhat, 2023). With the paradigm of artificial intelligence-enabled internet of medical things (AIoMT) being new, few studies have been dedicated to detailing the different electronic devices deployed.

9.1.1 Key Contributions of the Chapter

The significant contributions of this chapter are listed:

- The chapter provides a detailed description of the diverse electronic sensors used in AIoMT in the wider medical industry.
- The different electronic signals transmitted by the different AIoMT sensors are presented.
- The significant challenges and prospects faced in using the identified electronic devices in healthcare have been discussed.
- Finally, some benefits and challenges for the AIoMT are reviewed, limitations of AIoMT are presented as well, and the future research direction of AIoMT in the healthcare industry and its future scope are depicted.

9.1.2 Chapter Organization

Section 9.2 presents electronic sensors in IoMT and electronic sensor traits, disposable health sensors, ingestible sensors, patch sensors, connected health sensors, wearables, smart clothing, and implantable sensors. Section 9.3 presents the electronic signals in sensors. Section 9.4 discusses the identified challenges of electronic devices in the AIoMT, including data security threats. Section 9.5 explains the benefits of the AIoMT evaluated. Section 9.6 demonstrates the challenges of evaluated AIoMTs. Section 9.7 entails the limitation of AIoMT. Section 9.8 demonstrates the future research direction of IoMT in the healthcare industry. Finally, Section 9.9 entails the concluding chapter of AIoMT's future scope.

9.2 MEDICAL WEARABLE ELECTRONICS

When used in the smart healthcare industry, IoMT combines various processing units with communication technologies, for instance, electronic wireless sensors that remotely monitor patient health status, to enable the prompt transmission of clinical information to healthcare medics (Gupta et al., 2023; Sharma et al., 2020). IoMT makes it possible for caregivers to continuously monitor their patient's health, which enhances clinical judgment, lowers patients' medical costs, and ultimately improves patient outcomes. This section presents notable electronic sensor traits related to

IoMT applications and presents a brief discussion of the four main commonly used electronic sensor signals.

9.2.1 Electronic Sensor Traits

As the IoMTs are applied in the medical facility, these electronic sensors show different characteristics, and their contrast causes an impact on the patient (Bhambri et al., 2019). To support its many uses, a plethora of electronic biosensors have been invented and incorporated into the healthcare domain enabled by IoT (Dwivedi et al., 2022). Smart home care, clinical diagnostics, preventive medicine, fitness tracking, and a few monitoring services are some of these.

9.2.2 Disposable Health Sensors

Diagnostics, patient monitoring, and treatment support are the three main uses for disposable health sensors. The sensors are frequently strip-type, implementable, and ingestible. All these are focused on depending on the patient body nature (Guan et al., n.d.).

9.2.3 Ingestible Sensors

The microfabricated integrated circuit for this tiny electronic sensor is made of thin layers of magnesium, copper, and gold (Singh et al., 2005). As the taken pill enters the stomach, a reaction between the circuit layers and gastric juice occurs. The sensor experiences an electrochemical reaction as a result (Gupta et al., 2023). The patches of sensors then receive a digital code that denotes the drug type and appropriate dosage along with the time of dosage administration since this reaction energizes the sensor.

9.2.4 Patch Sensors

The patient may monitor their daily activities and medication schedules in appreciation of the transmission of all this data to a smartphone application, which then sends it to the discover portal. Medics and other healthcare professionals can find important data on their patients' daily health reports within the portals to help them choose the most appropriate treatments. By enhancing drug adherence, for instance, authors (Dwivedi et al., 2022) have reported the Proteus Digital Medicine model, which has transformed the healthcare industry by lowering treatment failure rates and the demand for patient retreatment.

9.2.5 Connected Health Sensors

The end-use market, electronic sensors, and platform sensors are additional subcategories of connected e-health sensors (Idrees and Khlief, 2023). Wearables, embedded technology, and intrusive sensors are examples of end-use market sensors for IoMT.

9.2.6 Wearables

Wearable sensors are continuously worn or put near the human skin to closely keep track of the patient's actions without restricting their usual range of mobility (Gezimati and Singh, 2023). Mobility trackers are an especially well-liked kind of wearable health technology that has several practical uses in other domains such as sports, determining the risk of falling, and keeping an eye on the senior population, where some devices are demonstrated in Figure 9.2.

9.2.7 Smart Clothing

Numerous wearable gadgets have been deployed to measure important aspects of human health in addition to being helpful in encouraging individuals to keep track

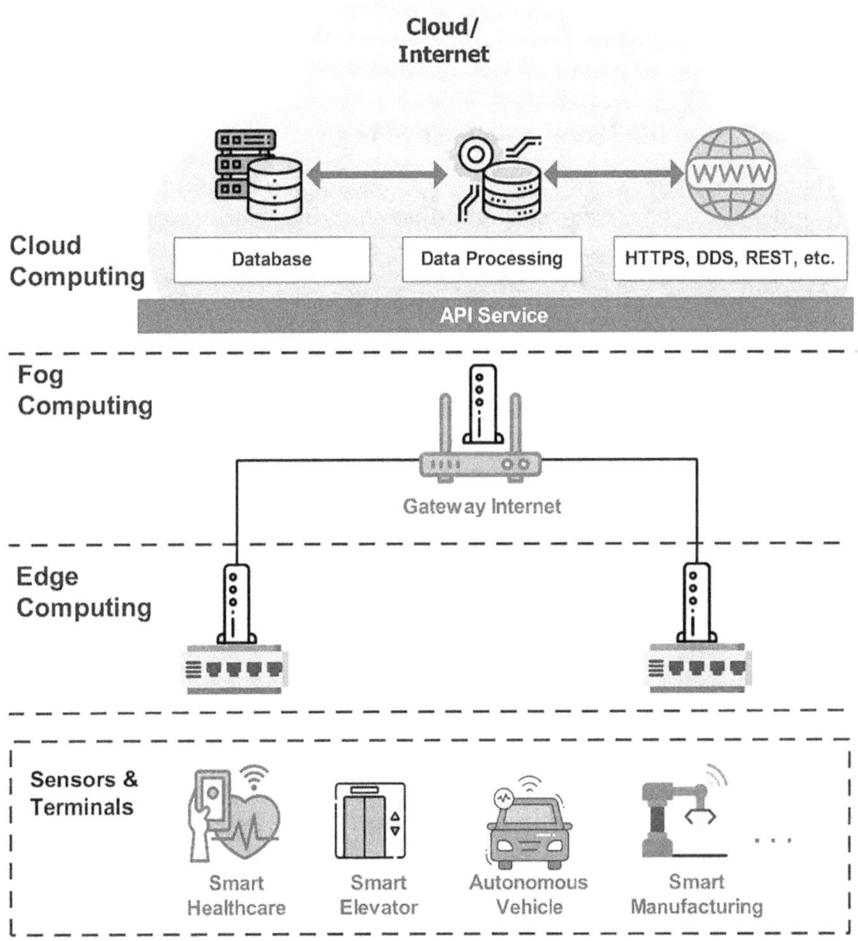

FIGURE 9.2 Current state of computation entailing digital healthcare (Quy et al., 2022).

of daily workouts and sustain a more active and healthier lifestyle. The most typical of these measurements include electrocardiogram (ECG) and electroencephalogram (EEG) measurements. Body-worn smart gear is one innovative innovation intended to combine wearable sensors with essential health monitoring capabilities (Bhutnal and Moparthi, 2023). Compared to current technologies, which frequently only record a small number of physiological data, smart clothing enables people with intermittent illnesses to benefit from several health monitoring systems. Smart clothes substantially decrease the cost of sensors as well, but the efficiency in terms of wireless communication and packet transfer is still not that efficient.

9.2.8 Implantable Sensors

Implantable sensors are becoming increasingly popular these days due to low-power technology. A major challenge of these implantable sensors is the sizing, efficient communication, and low power consumption. The efficient transfer of data from these sensors is important in terms of proper working.

9.3 ELECTRONIC SIGNALS IN SENSORS

The human body generates different signals, which can be classified based on IoMT. Within this subsection, we majorly classified them into four in terms of their frequency range obtained from the IoMT.

9.3.1 Gait Analysis

Human movements are widely studied, and over the past years, numerous people died due to physical inactivity. Almost 100,000 deaths can be prevented annually if US citizens increase their physical activity by ten minutes each day. That is, gait analysis can play an important role. To keep track of physical activity, proper tracking, monitoring, and measurement are important. It is important to assess human locomotion quantitatively. The most commonly used human locomotion sensing is seen in the step tracker application. Sensors used in this application need to be highly precise, small in weight, user-friendly, and easy to use in all environments (Gupta et al., 2023).

9.3.2 Photoplethysmography

Photoplethysmography (PPG) is used for both making biomedical and non-biomedical wearables. This signal is at the center of measuring heart rate variability. In the traditional method, heart rate variability is measured using HRV by means of an electrocardiogram (ECG) signal. HRV data was used to measure the peak-to-peak time interval between cardiac cycles. HRV analytics can provide a wide range of information to the autonomous nervous system (Dwivedi et al., 2022). However, there are several limitations to acquiring ECG data regarding collecting them at home as it requires proper positioning and operation.

Trained medical staff are needed to properly position the electrodes in the right position to get proper results, which is sometimes quite unlikely and time-consuming.

Moreover, some patients complain about other complications, like irritation and itching, while going through this process. On the contrary, in the reactance method, the photodiode is placed on the same side as the light source. It measures the intensity of the travelling light. This method is very commonly used in wristband watches. Some of the common devices that use this technique are the pulse oximeter, which is put on the fingertip, and Fitbit watches, respectively (Gupta et al., 2023).

9.3.3 Electromyography

Through the electromyography (EMG) method, the response of the nerves is measured at the moment electrical stimulation is applied to the nervous system. This stimulation is often referred to as an action potential, and the cumulative addition of the action potential of the motor unit denotes the electromyography signal at the skin surface. Conventionally, there are two techniques to gather the EMG data. One method uses a needle to collect blood samples, and another method uses an electrode on top of the skin's surface (Gupta et al., 2023). EMG signals acquired from the same muscle but from different sensor locations will result in different results.

9.3.4 Auscultation

Cardiac patients have to go through cardiac auscultation, in which a physician uses a stethoscope in the first place to diagnose the initial cardiac problems. There is a dire need for a noninvasive and fast technique to identify the primary cardiac condition. Stethoscope auscultation plays an important role in this. The main heart sounds used in medical applications are S1 and S2. S1 signals occur during ventricular contraction, which relates to a QRS complex in ECG. While the cardiovascular system is being analyzed, it is also important to analyze the functions of the lungs. This way, respiratory disorders can easily be identified through lung auscultation. In the case of a physically fit person, lung auscultation does not give much information in terms of audible sounds. Wheezing sounds often indicate a lung disease called chronic obstructive pulmonary disease (Nair and Sahoo, 2023).

People with this disease often encounter breathing problems. Capturing and detecting these sounds is another important thing. Apart from the anatomy of the heart and lungs, it is vital to understand the anatomy of surface anatomy. People have a misconception that the best sound of auscultation is captured just slightly above the heart, but this is not the case (Kok, 2023). It depends on the direction of the blood flow, and some of the smart wearable devices are demonstrated in Figure 9.3.

Besides the identified electronic sensors, recent medical wearables development showed great potential in accurately and precisely measuring different health-related parameters without the need for a consultation from a doctor using the sampled sensors. Although research is ongoing and there is a need to further look into this issue, some IoMTs include epileptic seizure detection, myocardial ischemia monitoring, fatigue detection, physical therapy, wearables, monitoring of sleep apnea, and stress monitoring, among others (Bhattarai and Peng, 2023; Kok, 2023). Both commercial and research items are being investigated in recent studies. However, most supercomputing personal medical applications are still in the improvement phase.

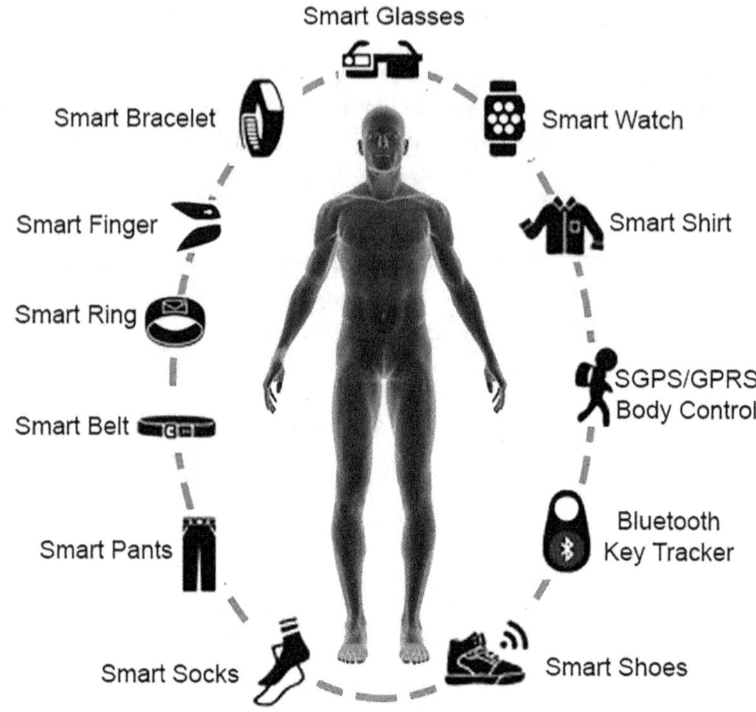

FIGURE 9.3 Sampled wearable medical electronics in IoMTs (Rodrigues et al., 2018).

9.4 CHALLENGES OF ELECTRONIC DEVICES IN THE AIoMT

In contrast to other sectors (IoT applications) where IoT adoption is equally widespread, network managers in the healthcare setup or sector confront difficulties when adopting this IoMT technology. Strict privacy laws, connectivity restrictions brought on by erratic physical settings, and the growing danger of security breaches are just a few of the issues (Mathur et al., 2023). Information health technology departments are responsible for ensuring that IoMT equipment is secure, available all the time, and dependable throughout the entire year. Here is a closer look at the top challenges encountered in IoMT applications, and some suggestions have been made (Mathur et al., 2023; Narasimharao et al., 2023). The challenges can be categorized into seven for instance: data management, interoperability, power consumption, privacy and security of data, cost, efficiency, and environmental impact, among others, amidst a few challenges that are not entailed within these categories, which are also discussed.

9.4.1 Data Security Threats

Cyber-attacks and medical cyber threats are likely to compromise Medicare data in medical facilities that have not fully encompassed security-based measures in handling patients' data. The danger of exposure is greatly increased when the IoMT data are merged with the existing pool of patient medical data, and the exposure to danger is greatly excavated (Irfana Parveen et al., 2023). A data breach investigation report conducted by Ponemon Institute and Verizon revealed that the compromised data primarily consisted of sensitive health information. The likelihood of data breaches are higher when devices are connected to external systems and one another. US government data of breaches to healthcare in the first five months of 2022 have approximately doubled compared to last year (Pandey and Pandey, 2023).

9.4.2 Data Interoperability

Without a doubt, the more we get data digital, the more chances there are to have the data altered, mainly in the medical industry. Nevertheless, the majority of data in the medical sector is kept in siloed databases, and incompatible computer systems and proprietary software are not interoperable. Consequently, it is complex to exchange, analyze, and realize these kinds of data. This hinders the evolution of medicine since technologies that depend on this data, like big data, AI, and mobile applications, might not be utilized to their full capacity (Banday and Bhat, 2023).

9.4.3 Regulatory Challenges

Clinical-grade IoMT must have permission and require clearance from national regulators before they may be introduced to the national and international markets. These devices require new regulations from legislators and regulatory agencies that are not familiar enough with how these IoMTs are used (Ding et al., 2023). Those kinds of limitations also delay the IoMT's being used in medical care due to the limited technological acceptance from those in authority.

9.4.4 High Infrastructure Costs

A significant initial outlay is required due to the price of the hardware, specialized IoMT infrastructure, developing consumer-facing applications, and cloud computing. The high infrastructure expenses for IoMT pose a barrier, even though the eventual return on investment is certain. Back in 2015, there were 4.5 billion IoMT devices in operation, and in fact, a Frost and Sullivan report shows that there will be close to 30 billion in less than two years. Deloitte's analysis predicts that by 2022, the IoMT market will be worth $158.1 billion, up from its $41 billion value in 2017 (Chunka et al., n.d.). Furthermore, the IoMT sector is expected to expand to a value of $29 billion by 2026, resulting in an increased number of wearable devices.

9.4.5 Cybersecurity

Cybersecurity is a difficult matter that requires knowledge and experience from a variety of professions for comprehension, which the majority of medical persons are not widely informed of. It is comfortable for policy experts and others to become lost in the technical details of cybersecurity, despite the fact that technology measures are an essential component of cybersecurity in the medical sector (Patra et al., 2023). In addition, cybersecurity knowledge is usually arranged in silos based on disciplinary boundaries, which lowers the number of insights that can be gained through cross-fertilization (Gupta et al., 2023). This introduction may give connection insight. Importantly, it attempts to leave the reader with two major issues to consider.

9.5 AIoMT BENEFITS

Within this subsection, we present AIoMT with two benefits and the challenges as detailed subsequently:

9.5.1 Medical Diagnosis

AIoMT aids in a quick and precise medical diagnosis because it is the first step undertaken to treat patient ailments, thereby reducing patient mortality rates. This ultimately leads to improved health and quality of life for individuals. Robots such as the Husky and Veebot have shown great potential in spotting skin tumours accurately and drawing blood, respectively (Wang and Li, 2023). A hundred percent accuracy in the robotic diagnosis of 340 brains using magnetic resonance imaging. Compatibly, AIoMTs are equipped with the ability to alert medical workers when patients' health deteriorates, as has been shown in this study, where doctors were alerted by Google's DeepMind AI system when patients had acute kidney injury.

9.5.2 Medical Treatment

Because treatment plays an important role in a patient's life, AIoMT has the potential to provide prompt treatment to various patient ailments due to its accuracy, thereby saving lives. In what is now referred to as precision medicine, AIoMT is accelerating the transition from traditional medicine to personalized medicine, targeted treatment, and uniquely composed drugs (Patra et al., 2023). Different AI models have shown great potential in the treatment of COVID-19 as indicated in the studies highlighted. Moreover, with the help of smartphones, AI can aid in prescribing medication to different patients who are unable to move to hospital settings physically.

9.5.3 Patient Empowerment

AIoMT has the potential to empower individuals to help them make better and more informed health decisions. The large amount of patient data collected by wearable medical devices discussed in the previous section, along with the embedded AI, helps in analyzing this data, which could alert people with a higher risk of becoming ill long before such ailments become serious (Wang and Li, 2023). Doing so allows individuals affected by certain chronic illnesses to curb their disease better, thereby enabling them to live healthier lives through mobile apps.

9.5.4 Reduction in Medical Costs

Artificial intelligence is capable of speeding up the creation of life-saving medicines, thereby saving money in medical costs incurred on healthcare delivery systems (Narasimharao et al., 2023). AIoMT can optimize medication development in clinical trials, leading to minimization of the time taken to certify developed drugs fully.

9.5.5 Reduction in Human Error

The use of AI in the IoMT has shown great benefits in minimizing human errors by medical workers, which saves lives. AIoMT has shown the potential to diagnose patients with a reported 72% more accurate diagnosis compared to the high error rate of medical workers. Without the use of technology in surgical procedures done by medical practitioners, the operation can lead to life-threatening consequences (Mahalakshmi and Lalithamani, 2023).

9.6 CHALLENGES OF AIoMTs

Although AI and its convergence with the IoMT have shown tremendous potential to revolutionize healthcare, several technological challenges in their deployment have to be addressed to realize their adaptability and monetization in hospitals/clinics and society in general.

9.6.1 Privacy Concerns

Patients have serious concerns about the large amount of data collected by the different IoMTs. Leakage of such sensitive data through hackers and other means has consequences such as patient blackmail, tarnishing the reputation of health service providers, and the likelihood of loss of lives (Pandey et al., 2023). Studies have shown the possibility of AI compromising privacy by predicting the personal information of patients regardless of whether the algorithm has ever been presented with such records. This modus operandi for AI in healthcare may result in lawsuits, especially if the AI's conclusions are made available for public consumption.

9.6.2 Missteps and Errors

AIoMT systems are not flawless, as a patient could be hurt if the wrong treatment is prescribed or if the system fails to detect tumors on a radiological exam, among others. Moreover, if AIoMT systems become popular, a slight error in one has the potential to hurt several (Lee et al., 2023). Furthermore, because AI systems work with consumer-facing smart wearable devices and use the data they generate, those systems may produce invalid results, as indicated in this study using Fitbit trackers.

9.6.3 Data Management and Power Issues

The heterogeneity of medical devices running different applications in the AIoMT system creates a data management problem, such as storage and incompatible dataset formats created by various legacy third-party systems. Moreover, the large volume of data (big data) generated needs to be stored and analyzed. Hence, the need for scalable and intelligent machine learning algorithms for processing such a large amount of patient data becomes vital. Finally, most devices in the AIoMT have low power capacities, which affect the operational time (Riya et al., 2023).

9.6.4 Bias

AI-enabled health suffers from the dangers of prejudice and inequality because such systems, by design, learn from the information fed into them, leading to the absorption of biases from supplied datasets (Alabdan et al., 2023). Regardless of whether the AIoMT systems are trained on accurate, reliable, and representative datasets, bias will still be reflected, as noted in a study where an AI system trained on healthcare datasets learns to recommend lower painkiller doses to patients of African American race. Such a decision is purely based on systemic bias instead of biological traits.

9.7 LIMITATION OF AIoMT

Regardless of the benefits of AIoMTs, some limitations are identified and discussed subsequently. As a result of the ongoing development of technology, business processes in every industry, including medicine, are undergoing continuous change. One of these industries experiencing this problem is the healthcare industry. In the coming years, the IoTs, IoMTs, and generally AIoMT will bring countless fabulous opportunities for the healthcare industry. Using IoMT, we are able to derive additional value from the data we acquire. The IoMT improves the effectiveness and quality of the results delivered by various devices. However, there are a few limitations that are encountered in every technological progress, including data privacy concerns, security issues due to the use of wireless medical devices, the cost of these AIoMTs, and inaccuracy while handling real-time medical data and operation.

9.8 FUTURE RESEARCH DIRECTION

The adoption of AI in the health sector through its convergence with the IoMT is transforming healthcare delivery in aspects such as patient experience, how medical workers practice medicine, and how drugs are being manufactured. Soon, AIoMT is expected to improve the precision of wearable medical devices and their ability to collect, store, and interpret data about patients' health conditions. Consequently, this will allow medical workers to engage with their patients with the help of telemedicine to achieve improved healthcare service delivery. Overall, the new means of getting healthcare services will drastically reduce the healthcare costs incurred for all groups of patients. Because much of how AI operates is unknown to any layman, the policies and legal frameworks that govern its use, especially in the healthcare sector, will have to be instituted to promote public confidence in its use and protect citizens from any fallout from its irresponsible deployment. The European Union has made initiatives in that direction through its quest to come up with the AI Act, which is aimed at promoting uniformity in the governance of AI technologies in different sectors, among which include the health sector. The other initiative is the Pan-Canadian AI strategy, which, along with the European one, will help the medical community and regulators monitor the adoption and explainability of various AI technologies and how their use impacts different contexts in the healthcare industry. Through a combination of standards and regulations, the accuracy, security, reliability, and health use of AI technologies will need to be instituted. This is because AI technologies are capable of learning patterns and modifying their recommendations in ways not envisioned by their creators. This poses regulatory issues, which will need to be addressed as the technology evolves. Adopting a community-led approach by medical workers, technologists, researchers, and other stakeholders is one way that can be adopted to develop standards for data collection and testing of AI-enabled health technologies. AIoMT trends such as chatbot technologies (voice assistants) are seen to revolutionize the healthcare sector with their increased adoption by different healthcare providers. As evidenced by their extensive usage during the COVID-19 global pandemic and other health emergencies, voice assistants like Google Assistant, Apple Siri, and Amazon Alexa proved very useful in responding to COVID-19-related public questions.

9.9 CONCLUSIONS AND FUTURE SCOPE

Due to its potential to transform the delivery of medical care, the IoMT has rapidly gained the interest of researchers since its inception. They are able to monitor and manage a number of health-related disorders and issues. The IoMT devices allow us to monitor our medical records and take the necessary safety precautions. IoMT plays a significant role in boosting the effectiveness and precision of electronic devices in the medical industry. In this chapter, a comprehensive examination of a range of electronic equipment discovered in the AIoMT has been conducted. For convenience, the identified and extensively used medical equipment, including electrical signals for AIoMT sensors, are highlighted subsequently. In addition, AIoMT's architecture demonstrates significant development by utilizing intelligent sensors to collect, aggregate, and manage data for intelligent healthcare buildings. Thanks to AIoMT, the patient experience is improved, and workflows are optimized. Patients stand to benefit from increased participation and fewer in-person physician appointments. Providers can better assist patients now that they have access to more accurate data, improved diagnostics, and more effective time management. AIoMT will very certainly be supplemented in the future by more innovations that will further streamline the medical profession for practitioners and patients. This chapter is limited in that it cannot cover the many issues related to electronic devices and AIoMT that have been raised.

REFERENCES

Alabdan, R., Alruban, A., Hilal, A. M., & Motwakel, A. (2023). Artificial-Intelligence-Based Decision Making for Oral Potentially Malignant Disorder Diagnosis in Internet of Medical Things Environment. *Healthcare*, *11*(1), 113.

Banday, M. T., & Bhat, L. (2023). Towards Building Internet-of-Things-Inclusive Healthcare for Neglected Tropical Diseases. In *The Internet of Medical Things (IoMT) and Telemedicine Frameworks and Applications* (pp. 39–75). IGI Global.

Bhambri, P., & Singh, M. (2005). Artificial Intelligence. In *Seminar on E-Governance—Pathway to Progress* (p. 14). SSIET.

Bhambri, P., Sinha, V. K., & Dhanoa, I. S. (2020). Development of Cost Effective PMS with Efficient Utilization of Resources. *Journal of Critical Reviews*, *7*(19), 781–786.

Bhambri, P., Sinha, V. K., Dhanoa, I. S., & Kaur, J. (2019). Genome DNA Sequence Matching using HBM Algorithm. *International Journal of Control and Automation*, *12*(5), 531–539.

Bhattarai, A., & Peng, D. (2023). An Integrated Secure Efficient Computing Architecture for Embedded and Remote ECG Diagnosis. *SN Computer Science*, *4*(1), 1–15.

Bhutnal, V., & Moparthi, N. R. (2023). Internet of Things-Enabled Diabetic Retinopathy Classification from Fundus Images. In *IOT with Smart Systems* (pp. 757–764). Springer.

Chunka, C., Banerjee, S., & Sachin Kumar, G. (n.d.). A Secure Communication Using Multi-factor Authentication and Key Agreement Techniques in Internet of Medical things for COVID-19 Patients. *Concurrency and Computation: Practice and Experience*, e7602.

Deshmukh, A., Tyagi, A. K., Hansora, H., & Menon, S. C. (2023). Applications of Distributed Ledger (Blockchain) Technology in E-Healthcare. In *The Internet of Medical Things (IoMT) and Telemedicine Frameworks and Applications* (pp. 248–261). IGI Global.

Ding, X., Zhang, Y., Li, J., Mao, B., Guo, Y., & Li, G. (2023). A Feasibility Study of Multi-mode Intelligent Fusion Medical Data Transmission Technology of Industrial Internet of Things Combined with Medical Internet of Things. *Internet of Things*, 100689.

Dwivedi, R., Mehrotra, D., & Chandra, S. (2022). Potential of Internet of Medical Things (IoMT) Applications in Building a Smart Healthcare System: A Systematic Review. *Journal of Oral Biology and Craniofacial Research*, *12*(2), 302–318.

Fahim, K. E., Kalinaki, K., & Shafik, W. (2024). Electronic Devices in the Artificial Intelligence of the Internet of Medical Things (AIoMT). In *Handbook of Security and Privacy of AI-Enabled Healthcare Systems and Internet of Medical Things* (pp. 41–62). CRC Press.

Gezimati, M., & Singh, G. (2023). Internet of Things Enabled Framework for Terahertz and Infrared Cancer Imaging. *Optical and Quantum Electronics*, *55*(1), 1–17.

Guan, Z., Li, Y., Yu, S., & Yang, Z. (n.d.). Deep Reinforcement Learning-Based Full-Duplex Link Scheduling in Federated Learning-based Computing for IoMT. *Transactions on Emerging Telecommunications Technologies*, e4724.

Gupta, S., Sharma, H. K., & Kapoor, M. (2023). Application and Challenges of Blockchain in IoMT in Smart Healthcare System. In *Blockchain for Secure Healthcare Using Internet of Medical Things (IoMT)* (pp. 39–53). Springer.

Idrees, A. K., & Khlief, M. S. (2023). Efficient Compression Technique for Reducing Transmitted EEG Data without Loss in IoMT Networks Based on Fog Computing. *The Journal of Supercomputing*, 1–26.

Irfana Parveen, C. A., Anjali, O., & Sunder, R. (2023). Internet of Things: A Review on Its Applications. In *Information and Communication Technology for Competitive Strategies (ICTCS 2021)* (Vol. 400, pp. 123–134). Springer. https://doi.org/10.1007/978-981-19-0095-2_13

Kalinaki, K., Fahadi, M., Alli, A. A., Shafik, W., Yasin, M., & Mutwalibi, N. (2024). Artificial Intelligence of Internet of Medical Things (AIoMT) in Smart Cities: A Review of Cybersecurity for Smart Healthcare. In *Handbook of Security and Privacy of AI-Enabled*

Healthcare Systems and Internet of Medical Things (pp. 271–292). CRC Press, Taylor and Francis Group.

Kok, C. L. (2023). A Low Cost, Power Efficient, Social Distancing Notification Embedded System Based on Intelligent Wireless Sensor Network. In *The Internet of Medical Things (IoMT) and Telemedicine Frameworks and Applications* (pp. 262–275). IGI Global.

Kok, C. L., & Setyadi, Y. (2023). Li-Ion-Based DC UPS for Remote Application. In *The Internet of Medical Things (IoMT) and Telemedicine Frameworks and Applications* (pp. 276–289). IGI Global.

Lee, H. Y., Lee, K. H., Lee, K. H., Erdenbayar, U., Hwang, S., Lee, E. Y., Lee, J. H., Kim, H. J., Park, S. B., & Park, J. W. (2023). Internet of Medical Things-Based Real-Time Digital Health Service for Precision Medicine: Empirical Studies Using MEDBIZ Platform. *Digital Health*, *9*, 20552076221149660.

Mahalakshmi, R., & Lalithamani, N. (2023). Preventing COVID-19 Using Edge Intelligence in Internet of Medical Things. In Gupta, D., Khanna, A., Bhattacharyya, S., Hassanien, A.E., Anand, S., & Jaiswal, A. (eds) *International Conference on Innovative Computing and Communications. Lecture Notes in Networks and Systems* (vol. 473, pp. 213–227). Springer. https://doi.org/10.1007/978-981-19-2821-5_18

Mathur, G., Pandey, A., & Goyal, S. (2023). Applications of Machine Learning in Healthcare. In *The Internet of Medical Things (IoMT) and Telemedicine Frameworks and Applications* (pp. 177–195). IGI Global.

Nair, A. K., & Sahoo, J. (2023). Internet of Things in Smart and Intelligent Healthcare Systems. In *Intelligent Internet of Things for Smart Healthcare Systems* (1st ed.). CRC Press. eBook ISBN9781003326182.

Narasimharao, M., Swain, B., Nayak, P. P., & Bhuyan, S. (2023). Development of Real-Time Cloud Based Smart Remote Healthcare Monitoring System. In *Ambient Intelligence in Health Care* (pp. 217–224). Springer.

Pandey, R., Pandey, A., Maurya, P., & Singh, G. D. (2023). Prenatal Healthcare Framework Using IoMT Data Analytics. In *The Internet of Medical Things (IoMT) and Telemedicine Frameworks and Applications* (pp. 76–104). IGI Global.

Pandey, S. K., & Pandey, S. (2023). IoT and Healthcare: Study of Conceptual Framework and Applications. In *The Internet of Medical Things (IoMT) and Telemedicine Frameworks and Applications* (pp. 1–16). IGI Global.

Patra, M. K., Kumari, A., Sahoo, B., &Turuk, A. K. (2023). Smart Healthcare System Using Cloud-Integrated Internet of Medical Things. In *Exploring the Convergence of Computer and Medical Science Through Cloud Healthcare* (pp. 60–83). IGI Global.

Petrellis, N., Birbas, M., & Gioulekas, F. (2019). On the Design of Low-Cost IoT Sensor Node for e-Health Environments. *Electronics*, *8*(2), 178.

Quy, V. K., Hau, N. V., Anh, D. V., & Ngoc, L. A. (2022). Smart Healthcare IoT Applications Based on Fog Computing: Architecture, Applications and Challenges. *Complex & Intelligent Systems*, *8*(5), 3805–3815.

Riya, K. S., Surendran, R., Tavera Romero, C. A., & Sendil, M. S. (2023). Encryption with User Authentication Model for Internet of Medical Things Environment. *Intelligent Automation & Soft Computing*, *35*(1).

Rodrigues, J. J., Segundo, D. B. D. R., Junqueira, H. A., Sabino, M. H., Prince, R. M., Al-Muhtadi, J., & De Albuquerque, V. H. C. (2018). Enabling Technologies for the Internet of Health Things. *IEEE Access*, *6*, 13129–13141.

Shafik, W. (2023). A Comprehensive Cybersecurity Framework for Present and Future Global Information Technology Organizations. In *Effective Cybersecurity Operations for Enterprise-Wide Systems* (pp. 56–79). IGI Global.

Shafik, W., Matinkhah, S. M., & Ghasemzadeh, M. (2020). Theoretical Understanding of Deep Learning in UAV Biomedical Engineering Technologies Analysis. *SN Computer Science*, *1*(6), 1–13.

Sharma, R., Bhambri, P., & Sohal, A. K. (2020). Energy Bio-Inspired for MANET. International *Journal of Recent Technology and Engineering*, *8*(6), 5580–5585.

Singh, P., Singh, M., & Bhambri, P. (2005). Security in Virtual Private Networks. In *Seminar on Network Security and Its Implementations* (p. 11). Doaba College.

Wang, J., & Li, X. (2023). Secure Medical Data Collection in the Internet of Medical Things Based on Local Differential Privacy. *Electronics*, *12*(2), 307.

10 Role of AI and IoT Based Medical Diagnostics Smart Health Care System for Post-Covid-19 World

Ritu, Pankaj Bhambri and Bebesh Tripathy

10.1 INTRODUCTION

The COVID-19 pandemic has had a profound impact on economies and societies across the globe, changing the face of healthcare as we know it. Our approach to providing medical services has undergone a paradigm shift as a result of the challenges presented by the pandemic. This chapter tries to investigate how artificial intelligence (AI) and the internet of things (IoT) are crucial in creating a smart and adaptable healthcare ecosystem that is suited for the post-COVID-19 era.

Traditional healthcare systems have been under unprecedented pressure since the pandemic—they are dealing with a shortage of resources, overcrowded hospitals, and a rise in the demand for remote medical care. The demands of this new era call for creative solutions that push healthcare toward greater accuracy, efficiency, and patient-centered care in addition to addressing these issues. The convergence of AI and IoT is the subject of this chapter. These two technological giants have the capacity to completely transform healthcare delivery and medical diagnostics. We specifically look at how cooperatively they can improve diagnostics, remotely monitor patient health, and support the development of a robust and flexible IT system.

The main objective as we delve into the nuances of AI and IoT applications in the healthcare space is to comprehend how these technologies, when seamlessly integrated, can not only mitigate the challenges brought about by the pandemic but also lay the foundation for an infrastructure for healthcare that is ready for the future. The investigation includes wearable device integration for ongoing patient monitoring, the application of machine learning algorithms for precise diagnosis, and the moral issues guiding the uptake of these revolutionary technologies. We hope to shed light on the promising path of healthcare evolution in the post-COVID-19 era, where AI and IoT emerge as positive change agents and provide a glimpse into a future of healthcare that is patient-centered, anticipatory, and adaptive.

DOI: 10.1201/9781032698519-10

10.1.1 Post-Covid Healthcare Challenges

The post-COVID-19 environment brings with it a plethora of complex issues that highlight the pressing need for global healthcare systems to change and advance. The aftermath of the virus itself is a major concern, since survivors frequently struggle with chronic health problems known as "long COVID." These side effects require specialized and prolonged care, ranging from neurological symptoms to cardiovascular issues and respiratory distress. Medical personnel are under additional pressure to comprehend, diagnose, and effectively treat these varied and ever-evolving health challenges, which adds to the already burdensome healthcare system.

Furthermore, during the height of the crisis, hospitals and other healthcare facilities were overcrowded due to the pandemic's considerable increase in the demand on their resources. The backlog of neglected non-COVID medical procedures and treatments has made the resumption of regular healthcare services increasingly necessary. The accumulation of cases combined with an increase in the need for mental health services presents a significant obstacle for medical professionals in terms of staffing levels, resource allocation, and system resilience.

There has also been a noticeable shift in healthcare preferences, as evidenced by the rise in demand for remote healthcare solutions. Once a supplemental service, telemedicine is now essential for ongoing care, monitoring chronic conditions, and consultations. This shift to remote healthcare calls for a reassessment of conventional healthcare delivery models in addition to a strong technology infrastructure. Furthermore, the pandemic's economic effects have made already-existing health disparities worse by depriving a large number of people of access to necessary healthcare services and adequate health insurance. A comprehensive and equitable approach is necessary to address the socioeconomic aspect of the post-COVID healthcare challenges and maintain universal access to healthcare, regardless of one's financial situation.

Healthcare systems must adopt creative solutions in order to navigate these difficulties. It is now essential to integrate technologies like artificial intelligence and the internet of things in order to anticipate future healthcare needs and provide effective diagnosis and treatment. A paradigm change is necessary in the post-COVID healthcare environment to promote inclusivity, resilience, and adaptability in the face of extraordinary obstacles.

10.1.2 Significance of healthcare

During the COVID-19 pandemic, healthcare has never been more important because it is the backbone of the multipronged attack against the virus. Its vital role in the management and treatment of diseases comes first. When it comes to delivering medical care, healthcare providers—from diagnosing and treating COVID-19 cases to implementing life-saving interventions—are at the forefront of their field. Furthermore, the healthcare industry is essential to the implementation and management of preventive care. To stop the virus from spreading, this involves conducting extensive testing, tracking down contacts, and disseminating public health information.

Emergency response and readiness are now critical since healthcare facilities must quickly adjust to the changing needs of the pandemic. In order to lessen the effects of the virus, it is essential to have the capacity to manage spikes in the number of patients, obtain the resources required, and guarantee the availability of qualified staff. In addition, current research endeavors focused on comprehending the virus, creating efficacious treatments, and expanding medical comprehension are fundamentally dependent on the healthcare sector. The pandemic's effect on mental health highlights another aspect of the importance of healthcare. Psychologists and counselors are among the healthcare professionals who are essential in helping people who are struggling with the psychological effects of the pandemic. Additionally, healthcare facilities play a significant role in community education and communication by clearing up misconceptions and promoting a clear knowledge of preventive measures.

Healthcare promotes cooperation and information exchange on a global basis. Because of the interconnectedness of the world, cooperation among healthcare systems is necessary to meet the challenges presented by the pandemic. Lastly, immunization programs demonstrate the critical role that healthcare plays in halting the virus's spread and establishing herd immunity. To put it simply, the importance of healthcare in the context of COVID-19 goes beyond treatment alone; it includes an all-encompassing and proactive response to a global health emergency. Protecting public health, helping communities navigate the complexity of the pandemic, and building the kind of collective resilience needed for a post-COVID-19 world are all critical tasks performed by the healthcare sector.

10.2 AI IN MEDICAL DIAGNOSTICS

10.2.1 Machine Learning Algorithms

In the field of medical diagnostics, artificial intelligence (AI) has become a disruptive force that is changing how medical professionals approach the identification and interpretation of diseases. AI is revolutionizing the field of diagnostics by using sophisticated algorithms and machine learning techniques to decipher complicated medical images, analyze large datasets, and offer previously unheard of insights. The numerous uses of AI in medical diagnostics are covered in detail in this section.

Machine learning algorithms, which have the ability to learn from and adapt to data inputs, are the foundation of artificial intelligence in medical diagnostics. To find patterns, correlations, and anomalies, these algorithms examine a variety of medical data, such as patient records, imaging results, and laboratory results. Rapid processing of large volumes of data by machine learning makes diagnostics more precise and timely. AI systems are particularly good at early illness diagnosis, risk assessment, and differentiating minute differences that might be invisible to the human eye.

10.2.2 Predictive Analysis

Predictive analytics is another area in which AI excels, helping to identify high-risk individuals or groups and forecasting possible health outcomes. AI models are able to forecast the probability of a disease by examining past patient data and pertinent risk factors. This allows healthcare providers to take preventative and early intervention measures with certainty. This predictive capability is extremely helpful in effectively managing long-term health issues and allocating resources, particularly in light of the post-COVID-19 healthcare landscape.

Predicting possible health outcomes is one of the noteworthy uses of predictive analytics, which essentially gives medical professionals a proactive window into the occurrence of disease. AI models can forecast the probability that a person will experience a particular condition by spotting minute correlations and risk factors. This insight is extremely valuable in light of the COVID-19 healthcare challenges, as the pandemic's aftermath has increased the demand for early detection and preventative measures. Predictive analytics becomes revolutionary in the treatment of chronic conditions. Healthcare professionals can customize interventions to each patient's needs and optimize treatment plans for greater efficacy when they can predict how a disease will progress (LeCun et al., 2015). Predictive analytics, for example, can provide information about possible exacerbations of conditions like diabetes or cardiovascular diseases, allowing for prompt modifications to medication, lifestyle advice, or other preventive measures.

In the post-COVID-19 era, when healthcare systems are juggling rising demands and possible resource constraints, the efficiency benefits of predictive analytics extend to resource allocation, making this an important factor to take into account. Healthcare practitioners can target interventions at the most benefiting individuals or populations by identifying high-risk individuals or populations and allocating resources accordingly (O'Donoghue et al., 2020). This focused strategy helps healthcare systems be more resilient and sustainable overall in the face of changing challenges, in addition to optimizing the delivery of healthcare. Moreover, the incorporation of predictive analytics in the healthcare sector expedites the transition towards a preventive and patient-focused care paradigm. Healthcare professionals can take a proactive approach that is in line with the larger objectives of public health and personal well-being by anticipating and addressing health concerns prior to their manifestation, as opposed to merely responding to symptomatic presentations. The combination of AI and predictive analytics in healthcare is a shining example of innovation, providing proactive healthcare strategies, resource optimization, and a revolutionary approach to disease management. These predictive capabilities promise to improve patient outcomes and strengthen healthcare systems against future uncertainties as we navigate the complexity of the post-COVID-19 world.

10.2.3 Personalized Medicine

Artificial Intelligence is a key component in the personalized medicine era when it comes to creating treatment plans that are specific to each patient (Rajkomar et al., 2019). AI algorithms can help optimize therapeutic strategies by combining genetic data, lifestyle factors, and responses to prior treatments. This represents a major step towards more patient-centric healthcare as it not only maximizes the effectiveness of medical interventions but also reduces their side effects.

Personalized medicine relies heavily on genetic data, which AI makes exceptionally precise use of when planning a patient's course of treatment. AI algorithms can identify specific genetic markers linked to particular diseases or conditions by analyzing an individual's genetic makeup (Miotto et al., 2017). With this knowledge, medical practitioners can anticipate a patient's susceptibility, evaluate the likelihood that a disease will manifest, and recommend focused treatments that target the underlying molecular causes of the condition (Islam et al., 2015). This newfound understanding of genomics represents a dramatic shift from conventional methods, opening the door to more effective treatments that are also customized to address the underlying genetic factors affecting a patient's health.

In addition to genetics, AI takes lifestyle into account when creating individualized treatment programs. A comprehensive understanding of a person's health can be obtained through the analysis of data pertaining to nutrition, exercise, stress levels, and environmental exposures. With the use of AI algorithms, patterns and correlations between these lifestyle factors and health outcomes can be found, allowing for the creation of recommendations that are tailored to each patient's particular needs and situation (Panda et al., 2019). This holistic approach emphasizes the value of comprehensive, individualized care by acknowledging that lifestyle choices and genetic predispositions interact intricately to determine health.

Furthermore, by continuously learning from and adjusting to patient responses, AI supports personalized medicine. AI algorithms improve their predictive abilities by analyzing real-time data on treatment outcomes and patient feedback. Treatment plans can be dynamically adjusted through this iterative learning process, guaranteeing that interventions stay in line with each person's changing preferences and health status. This flexibility reduces side effects and increases the effectiveness of medical interventions, which is a big step in the direction of more patient-centered healthcare. A paradigm shift in healthcare is being brought about by the combination of AI and personalized medicine, wherein treatments are now proactive rather than reactive and customized to the individual characteristics of each patient (Tuli et al., 2020). AI-powered personalized medicine is a shining example of innovation in the modern healthcare landscape, offering a truly personalized, cost-effective, and patient-centered healthcare experience in the future.

10.3 IoT-ENABLED HEALTHCARE

The integration of internet of things (IoT) technology into healthcare has revolutionized the industry by creating a dynamic ecosystem that fosters continuous monitoring, real-time data collection, and advanced connectivity. In this era of IoT-enabled healthcare, a multitude of smart devices, ranging from wearable gadgets to sophisticated medical equipment, collaborates to create a comprehensive network that transcends traditional healthcare boundaries.

The ability to monitor patients in real-time is at the forefront of this transformation. Sensor-equipped wearables, like fitness trackers and smartwatches, allow users to monitor their sleep patterns, physical activity, and vital signs (Potluri et al., 2019). These gadgets provide a thorough picture of a patient's health by continuously sending this data to medical professionals. IoT enables remote monitoring for people with chronic conditions, enabling medical professionals to track the course of the disease and take immediate action when abnormalities arise. This capability is especially important in the post-COVID-19 environment, as there is a greater need than ever for remote healthcare solutions, and continuous monitoring is essential to both proactive and reactive healthcare approaches.

Moreover, IoT's networked nature in healthcare goes beyond patient tracking to maximize the effectiveness of healthcare provision. When smart medical devices are combined with IoT, data sharing and communication between different parts of the healthcare system can be done easily. The care coordination, administrative efficiency, and general responsiveness of healthcare facilities are all improved by this interconnectedness. Consequently, this enables healthcare providers to better allocate resources, shorten response times, and provide patients with a higher caliber of care.

IoT adoption in the healthcare industry is not without its difficulties, including worries about interoperability, data security, and privacy. Nonetheless, there are a lot of potential advantages as long as healthcare systems and technology keep up. In addition to providing a response to the immediate problems faced by the post-COVID-19 world, IoT-enabled healthcare establishes the foundation for a future in healthcare that is more connected, data-driven, and patient-focused.

10.3.1 Remote Patient Monitoring

Remote Patient Monitoring (RPM) stands as a transformative approach to healthcare, leveraging technological advancements, particularly in the realm of IoT, to enable continuous and remote monitoring of patients outside traditional healthcare settings. This paradigm shift has become especially crucial in the post-COVID-19 world, where the demand for effective remote healthcare solutions has surged. RPM utilizes a variety of devices, ranging from wearable sensors to smart home devices, to collect and transmit real-time health data to healthcare professionals.

The importance of RPM resides in its capacity to provide healthcare outside of hospital and clinic walls. It is now possible to monitor patients in the comfort of their own homes who are recovering from acute illnesses or chronic conditions. Sensor-equipped wearables record vital signs, medication compliance, and other pertinent health data. After that, the information is safely sent to healthcare professionals, providing a constant flow of data that permits proactive intervention, early identification of possible problems, and individualized modifications to treatment regimens.

In addition, RPM helps patients feel empowered because they take an active role in their own care. IoT-enabled devices ongoing monitoring not only improves patient engagement but also makes it possible to understand health trends over time with greater depth (Topol, 2019). In addition to addressing the pandemic's challenges, this move toward remote patient monitoring also advances the larger objectives of enhancing patient outcomes, accessibility, and efficiency in healthcare. RPM is essential to creating a future in which healthcare is not limited to hospital walls but is instead seamlessly integrated into patients' daily lives as technology advances and healthcare delivery models change.

10.3.2 Smart Medical Devices

Smart medical devices herald a new era in which technology and medical instrumentation combine to improve patient care and expedite healthcare procedures. They represent a substantial advancement in healthcare. With their built-in intelligence and connectivity, these gadgets are essential in changing conventional medical procedures into ones that are more effective, patient-focused, and data-driven. These gadgets, which range from connected glucose monitors to smart infusion pumps, are prime examples of how cutting-edge technology and medical knowledge can work together.

The potential for improving patient outcomes, treatment, and diagnosis is present when smart medical devices are integrated into healthcare systems. In order to facilitate real-time data collection and transmission, these devices frequently include sensors and IoT connectivity. Smart thermometers have the capability to transmit temperature data instantaneously to healthcare providers, thereby facilitating the early detection of fever-related conditions. Continuous glucose monitoring devices empower people with diabetes and improve healthcare providers' ability to manage the condition proactively by providing a real-time view of blood glucose levels.

Smart medical devices support patient engagement and treatment adherence in addition to diagnostics (Rana et al., 2019). For example, connected inhalers can monitor drug use trends, giving doctors insight into how well patients are adhering to their treatment regimens and complying with them. This feature guarantees better care while also allowing medical professionals to tailor interventions according to specific patient information. The potential for streamlining healthcare workflows exists with the integration of these devices. For example, smart infusion pumps can be configured to deliver exact medication doses and send usage information to healthcare providers at the same time. This improves patient safety by lowering the possibility of errors and increasing treatment accuracy.

While the use of smart medical devices expands the scope of healthcare, it also raises issues with data security, interoperability, and the moral use of patient data. As these issues are resolved, smart medical devices have the potential to completely transform the way that healthcare is provided. They will play a part in a future in which technology will enhance the skills of healthcare providers, enhance patient outcomes, and create a more responsive and integrated healthcare system.

10.4 INTEGRATION OF AI AND IoT

The integration of AI and IoT represents a powerful synergy that holds the potential to revolutionize numerous industries, with healthcare being a particularly promising domain (Wynants et al., 2020). This amalgamation leverages the strengths of both technologies to create a seamless and intelligent ecosystem capable of transforming how healthcare is delivered and experienced. At the core of this integration is the bidirectional flow of data between IoT devices and AI systems. IoT devices, such as wearable sensors, smart medical devices, and health monitoring gadgets, generate vast amounts of real-time data. AI algorithms, equipped with machine learning capabilities, analyze this data to derive meaningful insights, patterns, and predictions. This symbiotic relationship enhances the capabilities of both AI and IoT, creating a dynamic loop of continuous improvement.

This integration shows up in a number of applications in the healthcare field. For example, wearables with internet of things (IoT) sensors can track a patient's blood pressure, heart rate, and other health metrics over time. The real-time analysis of this data by AI algorithms can then provide early abnormality or health risk detection. Predictive analytics is made easier by the smooth integration of AI and IoT, which empowers medical professionals to foresee health problems, customize treatment regimens, and take proactive measures. Furthermore, AI improves IoT-generated data's interpretive potential. For instance, AI systems in medical imaging are capable of analyzing radiological images, spotting anomalies, and offering diagnostic insights. This helps healthcare providers make better decisions by speeding up the diagnostic process and increasing accuracy.

Optimizing healthcare operations is also greatly aided by the integration of AI and IoT. Smart hospitals can improve resource allocation, automate repetitive tasks, and streamline workflows with IoT-connected devices and AI-driven analytics (Batsis and DiMilia, 2020). For example, supply chain optimization can be achieved by inventory management systems that use AI and IoT to make sure that necessary medical supplies are available when and where they are needed. Nonetheless, there are obstacles to the smooth application of AI and IoT in the healthcare industry. Robust solutions and careful consideration are necessary for data security, privacy concerns, and interoperability issues. When these issues are resolved, the potential for a healthcare environment that is more effective, individualized, and sensitive to the changing needs of both patients and healthcare providers is presented by the combined power of AI and IoT.

10.4.1 Seamless Data Exchange

A key component of integrating modern technologies is seamless data exchange, especially in industries like healthcare where effective information flow is critical. Creating a cohesive and interconnected ecosystem in the healthcare industry requires the ability to facilitate seamless data exchange, as various systems and devices generate copious amounts of data. This is especially clear when it comes to the convergence of technologies like AI and IoT, as AI algorithms are used to process and analyze real-time data produced by IoT devices.

The uninterrupted flow of information between different parts of the healthcare infrastructure is made possible by the smooth exchange of data. Healthcare providers have secure access to and sharing of patient data, diagnosis, and treatment plans, which guarantees a thorough and current understanding of a patient's health status. This improves the precision of diagnosis and treatment choices while also supporting a more patient-centered and team-oriented approach to healthcare.

Furthermore, the idea of interoperability is based on seamless data exchange, which enables various healthcare systems, tools, and applications to function together without any issues (Wang and Kung, 2018). For example, regardless of the healthcare facility or system where the data originated, interconnected Electronic Health

Record (EHR) systems allow healthcare providers to access a patient's medical history, test results, and treatment plans. Interoperability promotes continuity of care, cuts down on duplication of effort, and gives medical staff a comprehensive understanding of a patient's medical history.

To maintain the integrity of the smooth data exchange, however, issues like data security, standardization, and privacy concerns must be carefully handled. The benefits of a seamlessly interconnected health information landscape become more evident as healthcare systems adapt to meet these challenges. In addition to optimizing the delivery of healthcare, the seamless sharing, access, and analysis of data opens the door for creative ideas that take full advantage of technology to improve patient outcomes and raise the general effectiveness of healthcare systems.

The smooth transfer of data has major advantages for the patient as well. By giving people access to their own health information, it enables them to actively participate in their healthcare journey (Mittelstadt et al., 2016). More individualized and collaborative care is made possible by patients' ability to share pertinent data with healthcare professionals. Furthermore, seamless data interchange enables the integration of patient-generated data—such as information from wearables or health apps—into the larger healthcare ecosystem, providing a more thorough and ongoing picture of a person's health.

The need for smooth data exchange is becoming more and more important as the healthcare industry changes. Newer technologies that depend on the smooth exchange of data between patients and healthcare providers are telemedicine and remote monitoring. The healthcare sector can fully utilize connected health technologies to create a more effective, patient-centered, and collaborative healthcare ecosystem by tackling the technical, regulatory, and privacy issues related to data exchange,

10.4.2 Real-Time Decision Support

Real-time decision support, which uses cutting-edge technologies to give medical professionals timely and informed insights, is a crucial part of modernizing healthcare (Kvedar et al., 2014). This ability is especially noticeable when it comes to IoT and AI integration in healthcare systems. Healthcare providers now have immediate access to data-driven recommendations that have a big influence on clinical decision-making thanks to real-time data analytics and AI algorithms.

In the field of healthcare, where choices can have far-reaching effects, having access to immediate support is crucial. AI, for example, can analyze a wide range of patient data during patient consultations, such as medical history, ongoing vital signs, and diagnostic results, giving medical professionals quick insights into possible diagnoses, treatment options, and risk assessments. In addition to improving diagnosis speed and accuracy, this dynamic decision support helps clinicians create individualized treatment regimens that are catered to the unique requirements of each patient.

In emergency and critical care scenarios, real-time decision support integration is especially important. Healthcare personnel can make quick, well-informed decisions that can be crucial in emergency situations when they have quick access to pertinent information, such as allergies, prescriptions, and prior medical interventions. This capacity is essential for enhancing patient outcomes as well as for maximizing resource use and guaranteeing the smooth operation of healthcare facilities.

Moreover, real-time decision support helps to advance healthcare practices through continuous learning. Artificial intelligence algorithms are always improving their recommendations as they evaluate results and reactions to interventions in real time. Decision support systems are guaranteed to adapt to new medical knowledge and incorporate the most recent evidence-based practices through an iterative learning process.

While there is much promise in implementing real-time decision support, there are also issues that must be resolved, including data security, ethical issues, and the requirement for open communication between AI systems and healthcare providers. When these obstacles are overcome, real-time decision support has the potential to improve healthcare quality and make the industry more data-driven, flexible, and responsive.

REFERENCES

Batsis, J. A., & DiMilia, P. R. (2020). Effect of COVID-19 on telemedicine and virtual patient monitoring for the management of obesity. *Journal of Telemedicine and Telecare*, 1357633X20960515.

Islam, S. M. R., Kwak, D., Kabir, M. H., Hossain, M., & Kwak, K. S. (2015). The internet of things for health care: a comprehensive survey. *IEEE Access*, 3, 678–708.

Kvedar, J., Coye, M. J., & Everett, W. (2014). Connected health: a review of technologies and strategies to improve patient care with telemedicine and telehealth. *Health Affairs*, 33(2), 194–199.

LeCun, Y., Bengio, Y., & Hinton, G. (2015). Deep learning. *Nature*, 521(7553), 436–444.

Miotto, R., Wang, F., & Wang, S. (2017). Deep learning for healthcare: review, opportunities and challenges. *Briefings in Bioinformatics*, 19(6), 1236–1246.

Mittelstadt, B. D., Allo, P., Taddeo, M., Wachter, S., & Floridi, L. (2016). The ethics of algorithms: mapping the debate. *Big Data & Society*, 3(2), 2053951716679679.

O'Donoghue, J., Herbert, J., & McNeive, E. (2020). Applying the IoT paradigm to healthcare. In *Proceedings of the 2020 International Conference on IoT and Intelligent Systems (IoTIS)* (pp. 32–37). Springer.

Panda, S. K., Reddy, G. S. M., Goyal, S. B., Thirunavukkarasu, K., Bhambri, P., Rao, M. V., Singh, A. S., Fakih, A. H., Shukla, P. K., Shukla, P. K., & others. (2019). Method for management of scholarship of large number of students based on blockchain. IN Patent App. 201,911,034,937 A.

Potluri, S., Tiwari, P. K., Bhambri, P., Obulesu, O., Naidu, P. A., Lakshmi, L., Kallam, S., Gupta, S., & Gupta, B. (2019). Method of load distribution balancing for fog cloud computing in IoT environment. IN Patent App. 201,941,044,511.

Rajkomar, A., Hardt, M., Howell, M. D., Corrado, G., & Chin, M. H. (2019). Ensuring fairness in machine learning to advance health equity. *Annals of Internal Medicine*, 169(12), 866–872.

Rana, R., Chhabta, Y., & Bhambri, P. (2019). A review on development and challenges in wireless sensor network. In *International Multidisciplinary Academic Research Conference* (pp. 184–188). CT University, Ludhiana.

Topol, E. J. (2019). High-performance medicine: the convergence of human and artificial intelligence. *Nature Medicine*, 25(1), 44–56.

Tuli, S., Tuli, S., & Gill, S. S. (2020). Predicting the growth and trend of COVID-19 pandemic using machine learning and cloud computing. *Internet of Things*, 11, 100222.
Wang, H., & Kung, L. (2018). Health data privacy protection through blockchain-based tokenization. *Journal of the American Medical Informatics Association*, 25(2), 157–162.
Wynants, L., Van Calster, B., Collins, G. S., Riley, R. D., Heinze, G., Schuit, E., . . . Steyerberg, E. W. (2020). Prediction models for diagnosis and prognosis of covid-19: systematic review and critical appraisal. *BMJ*, 369.

11 Integrating Sensor, Actuators, and IoT for Smart Healthcare in Post-COVID-19 World

Rachna Rana and Pankaj Bhambri

11.1 INTRODUCTION OF INTEGRATING SENSOR, ACTUATORS, AND IoTs FOR SMART HEALTHCARE

The internet of things (IoTs) discuss the complete system of interrelated processes among computer software and computer hardware which allows interactions among them as well as through the web. The idea of Electronic-Health (E-Health) has evolved from the IoTs as a network of devices gathering information from both close and remote locations. The employment of BANs (Body Area Networks) and ground observation devices has made it possible to gather continuous requirements and provide the necessary trajectory-and-follow supports for epidemic management (Albzeirat et al., 2022, p. xx).

Health data, such as blood pressure, temperature, heart rate, and other measurements, can be gathered using E-Health methods that operate in close proximity. A healthcare provider has access to this information that can be conveniently stored.

In addition, local systems can be utilized to notify the patient about when to seek medical attention and when to obtain medication. For healthcare practitioners to have distant entree to patients and patient information, distant-based E-Health is crucial (Allam and Jones, 2020). For monitoring, frequent transmissions of patient vitals and location can be made to adjacent or distant medical institutions (Rachna et al., 2022).

Monitoring community isolation protocols and effectively supervising patients are crucial during a global pandemic such as the 2019 coronavirus (COVID-19). These two elements play a substantial role in preventing the widespread distribution of the disease. The use of IoT amenities is crucial in preventing the spread of viral pandemics since they have the ability to collect private information and monitor patients. However, they are currently limited in their implementation (Barabas et al., 2020).

In order to effectively control the rapidly spreading respiratory pandemic, health authorities and experts must access to information. Data can be utilized for the purpose of diagnosing COVID-19 infections and monitoring the spread of the disease among the population. The three most crucial pieces of information needed are body temperature, location, and portable history. The system of measurements can alert

 DOI: 10.1201/9781032698519-11

authorities as to whether or not more research and testing are necessary (Chamola et al., 2020).

In the past, health experts employed UV thermometers to directly measure temperature and verbally questioned patients regarding their conditions and whereabouts. Interacting with potentially infected individuals posed a significant risk to health professionals. Contamination rates have been steadily increasing, making it a more complex and challenging issue (Desyansah et al., 2021).

To efficiently monitor and manage the escalating COVID-19 infections, researchers have suggested using a network of things that already exists (Elmousalami et al., 2021). Wearable technology, mobile phones, cameras, and drones are just a few examples of the heterogeneous sensor network that is quickly becoming a part of society. Data gathering and monitoring are now possible across extremely broad distances because to long-range low-power communication protocols (Rachna et al., 2020). This trait becomes a valuable monitoring technique as the virus spreads across different locations and international borders. Software-defined wireless sensor network has significantly improved the guidance of numerous diverse sensors that collect data on position and temperature for government purposes (Greco et al., 2020).

Health personnel may be able to collect information and keep track of the coronavirus spread over several places and sizable populations by utilizing SDWSN in conjunction with low power wide area networking (Greco et al., 2020). The core IoT platforms and communication protocols are expected to undergo changes as they are being utilized to address the COVID-19 pandemic. This is an outcome of continuous modifications made to align with the viral spread pattern and regulatory guidelines for monitoring and adapting, as stated by Rachna et al. (2021).

Modifications to the method examples of adaptations that could lead to the development of IoT include strategies such as smartphones and whines, gathering information, making adjustments to IoT controlling proposals to meet supervisory standards, and advancements by academics to effectively handle a viral pandemic using IoT technology (Hussain et al., 2020).

11.1.1 Placement Services

Healthcare staff can easily identify devices such as wheelchairs, rulers, implanted cardioverter-defibrillators (ICDs), atomizers, expulsion devices, or monitoring devices by connecting them to IoT instruments. The corporal apparatus often becomes misplaced or proves challenging to locate, but through the IoT, personnel will consistently have knowledge of the whereabouts of all such equipment.

11.1.2 Remote Watching

IoT devices allow medical personnel to track the patients who have just experienced an operation or who are getting home healthcare. If a patient presents with a serious illness or requires necessary treatment, they will be notified. In 2018 and beyond, IoT innovation in healthcare is expected to increase. The above-mentioned IoT uses in healthcare are only the beginning.

The implementation of health monitoring systems in healthcare facilities and other health establishments has substantially increased, and many countries worldwide are now highly concerned about portable health monitoring systems with advanced technology. The transition of healthcare from in person consultation to telemedicine is an acknowledgment to the development of IoTs technology (Rani et al., 2023a).

This study proposes an intelligent health system for the IoTs that can continuously display the patient and their critical signs, as well as the condition of the room they are currently in (Rana, 2018; Rana et al., 2019). This system employs five sensors, including the intuition range sensor, organic construction fundamental measure sensor, area fundamental measure sensor, carbon monoxide gas sensor, and carbonic acid gas sensor, to gather data pertaining to the medical facility's surroundings. The proposed system and the error rate are within the given range (5%) for both.

11.2 THE DEVELOPMENT OF IoT-BASED HEALTHCARE PANDEMIC

Utilize scientific principles in urban endeavors, diverse research initiatives, and the implementation of "urban intelligence" in the post-World War II era. Consequently, a number of these endeavors have resulted in the concept of "smart cities." Urban intelligence encompasses three essential competencies: the information resources of local governments, the abilities of scientific computing, and the managerial competence to prepare for and respond to a pandemic (Rana et al., 2021a, 2021b).

For instance, in response to the epidemic, many strategies such as information observation, mine-laying, integration of information, molding, inquiry, and imaging have been utilized (Marais et al., 2020). Urban intelligence refers to the application of computational methodologies and data science frameworks to address specific issues in urban areas.

Recently, as a result of research on the internet of medical things (IoMT) sector, a new paradigm has been proposed for the health system, called intelligent treatment or healthcare IoT. Early research and development of wireless sensor networks (WSN) was the driving force behind IoT research in healthcare. The IoMT primarily uses widely distributed online digitally connected devices with built-in data exchange, detection, and identification capabilities (Mbunge, 2020).

It bridges the gap between patients and their healthcare providers. It goes without saying that smart healthcare is about harnessing innovation in the management of the healthcare system (Rani et al., 2023b).

For example, smart healthcare uses wearable technology, the flexible network and the internet of things to collect information about the people, things, and organizations involved in healthcare, and then use that information to monitor and consider health services (Olatinwo et al., 2019). By efficiently receiving, assimilating, and scrutinising precise, pertinent, and sophisticated messages in real-time, intelligent well-being can effectively halt the spread of illness.

Similarly, smart healthcare can collect data to track new cases of COVID-19 through patient health-based apps. In addition, thanks to wearable technology (sensors worn on the body), patients with COVID-19 can receive healthcare with continuous connected care rather than appointment-based care.

Furthermore, due to the constant influx of data and ongoing development, COVID-19 hotspots have the potential to change often and can be both identified and monitored. Therefore, it is more convenient to prohibit the spread of the infectious agent and take action accordingly. Moreover, the integration of diverse sources of information via intelligent healthcare systems might enhance community security.

We examine current market trends and their applicability in healthcare to better understand the healthcare-based IoT (Raj et al., 2017). By obtaining, desegregating, and analyzing accurate, relevant, and high-quality information in real-time, intelligent well-being can effectively address the spread of diseases.

In addition, the information integrated through smart healthcare can improve community safety. We examine current market trends and their applicability in healthcare to better understand the healthcare-based IoT (Raj et al., 2017).

11.2.1 Healthcare IoT Research and Development Efforts Pre-COVID-19: Healthcare IoT enables the connection and integration of patients, medical professionals, body sensors, well-being devices, and data engineering systems through on-demand internet access.

Implementing healthcare internet of things (HIoT) technology has the potential to enhance patient satisfaction, optimize operational efficiency, and boost employee productivity. The aforementioned advantages finally resulted in cost savings and reduced human error. HIoT devices has physical attributes that play a crucial role in shaping their design and functionality.

Here are some of these characteristics. The topics discussed in Singh et al.'s (2020a) study include surveillance, control, detection, intelligence collection, command, technology, and expansion. Hence, the period preceding COVID-19 and the integration of IoTs in healthcare predominantly revolved around the patient and was characterized by the following attributes.

11.2.1.1 Safety: The utilization of HIoT during the COVID-19 pandemic has resulted in significant benefits for patients and security. IoT enhances patient well-being and safety by combining remote wellness works with individuals in need through real-time health data. Real-time health data management improves the safety of patients by remotely monitoring and predicting their critical movements and current health status (Rani et al., 2023a). Similar to HIoT, it offers public health services and psychopharmacology, both of which are crucial for ensuring the safety of individuals enduring prolonged suffering. In addition, the use of well-being IoT technology allows for the implementation of public well-being insurance and the enforcement of high-quality rules in an epidemic scenario, thereby ensuring public safety.

11.2.1.2 Satisfaction: Through connected continuous care, IoT in healthcare replaces traditional face-to-face interactions in primary or secondary healthcare with interactive virtual healthcare. The positive satisfaction of patients is influenced by the ease of use of telemedicine and the welcoming comments of medical professionals.

11.2.1.3 Engagement: HIoT tracks prescriptions (drug therapy), creates patient-based education (personalized wellness and wellness planning), and organizes wellness choices (care coordination). The utilization of interactive practical world has facilitated the administration of wellbeing information.

11.2.1.4 A Case of COVID-19: Healthcare IoT Research and Development During a Pandemic: There have been three virulent epidemic in the ancient period of time, in 1918, 1957, and 1968, in addition to the latest novel coronavirus, which originated in Wuhan in late 2019. An epidemic is often characterized as an illness that is distributed vastly across many continents and has an unparalleled cultural and system consequence to society (Singh et al., 2020a).

Furthermore, the ongoing economic development resulting from the increasing social progress, human development, and global mobility has transformed several cities into hubs for rapid transmission of the epidemic.

However, the implementation of advanced technology such as IT-supported healthcare, abundant data, and artificial intelligence has enhanced the city's ability to prevent the spread of the pandemic (Singh et al., 2020b). For instance, following the COVID-19 pandemic, several countries worldwide have adopted either a people-centered or technology-centered approach to combat the spread of the virus (Ritu and Bhambri, 2023).

A technology-led strategy uses a sophisticated top-down approach to impose technologies on cities and their residents and force them to adopt smart technologies. However, a people-oriented approach forces cities to adopt the necessary smart technology, empowering, and educating their residents (Siriwardhana et al., 2020).

The joint operation report by the WHO and China commended China's technology-driven policy as a proactive, agile, and forceful reaction to the previous health crisis, and declared that they had effectively controlled the pandemic (Singh et al., 2020b). However, the humanistic approach employed by the United States and Europe had a limited impact on the dispersion and contamination of the prevailing situation. In addition, the person-centred approach has a flexible position towards complex philosophical theories, enabling users to select the specific engineering methods they prefer.

The technology-based approach, on the other hand, adopts an attitude of strict technical philosophical theory, where engineering is seen as a means to solve the problems facing governments (Stojanovic et al., 2020). It offers an integrated IoT platform that processes interactive dashboard information using big data collected from various IoT devices.

The AI subsystem uses a micro-controller together with the IoT scheme to collect user information to study and predict the velocity of micro-organism distribution. The AI system utilizes a panel map to provide users with information regarding the state of ill health in a specific area ("portable ECG monitoring system for smart health care based on IoT," 2023). Otoom et al. has introduced a new IoT system designed to detect and track COVID-19 instances at an early stage.

The projected system consists of five main components: Wearable sensors, a quarantine centre, a machine learning-based computing component, healthcare workers, and a cloud platform. The platform uses eight ML algorithms to efficiently and quickly identify potential cases of COVID-19. Five of these algorithms were found to have more than 90% accuracy ("South Asian Urbanization and Regional Sustainability", 2020).

However, the flow of data is expected to be monitored as virus cases and IoT deployments for COVID-19 rapidly increase. This requires rapid transmission of data to the subsystems responsible for managing and analyzing the COVID-19 data. As a result, performance accuracy and efficiency are improved. 5G has prepared this high-speed, low-latency communication protocol for IoT to provide IoT-based management of COVID-19.

The push towards 5G infrastructure as part of the IoT architecture of smart cities has made this even easier. By allowing high-resolution thermal images to move quickly through the IoT framework, such an infrastructure can keep up with the rapid spread of the virus.

Drones with IoT technology can be used to monitor the outbreak of COVID-19, including tracking individuals who have come into contact with patients with COVID-19. Drones can also be used to enforce quarantine laws, monitor patients who violate them, and enforce the use of face shields.

In Hubei, for example, as well as in Europe and the United States, drones have been used to ensure that residents strictly follow lockdown and social distancing laws. Artificial intelligence based on the internet of things.

Artificial intelligence has the capability to evaluate and analyze both prospective homeowners and the likelihood of infection. In addition, big data algorithms using artificial intelligence can be programmed to recognize, explain, and predict patterns and generate reasonable awareness.

Artificial intelligence technologies have been utilized to track and analyze the mobility patterns of individuals residing in highly polluted regions, subsequently providing reports to the appropriate authorities. In addition to preventing or slowing down the spread of the virus, it is very useful for predicting the onset of the disease. Just as social media spreads a lot of false information about a virus, AI-based systems can be trained to remove false information.

11.2.1 Research and Development Initiatives in Healthcare IoT Following the COVID-19 Pandemic

IoT technology has seen amazing development in the post-COVID period as a consequence of innovators, researchers, and developers being more aware of its potential as a result of the necessity to use it in these crucial times. IoT was mostly recognized for a concept with a much larger scope, such as smart cities, smart automobiles, etc.

This article outlined the several businesses that might profit from IoT after COVID-19 but weren't previously thought of. Both benefits and drawbacks come with IoT adoption. However, considerable progress can be observed shortly if there is noticeable increase in IoT research, development, and application in 2020. Some IoT use cases, including contact tracing and home education, will be primarily motivated by the need to control and adapt to the COVID-19 epidemic (Hegde et al., 2021).

Given that there are estimated to be 20 billion internet-connected devices and objects by 2020 and that the global technology industry will generate close to 1.6 trillion dollars in sales, the term "IoT" has become one of the most often used in business and technology. Integration of IoT with many technologies, including cloud computing and integrating actuators and intelligent sensors, makes it easier to engage with smart objects, enabling access from various places, improving data exchange efficiency, and boosting storage and processing capacity.

11.3 ISSUES WITH IoT

Based on a study that examined several forms of counterattacks and how they are classified, it was found that there is a limited understanding and awareness regarding the safety of internet devices (Yüksel, 2022). As a result of the recent widespread use of computer and internet technology, many organizations and individuals are vulnerable to these criminal activities. Researchers assert that both organizations and institutions must possess comprehensive awareness of digital threats (Turner et al., 2022).

According to a study conducted by several academics, a deeper knowledge of the dangers and assaults against IoT infrastructure is required, and cyber defenses must be treated seriously because they are influencing both our personal and societal life. Hoque points out that in order to protect and stop assaults on networks, it is crucial that we have a thorough awareness of the present systems and tools that are available in the public domain (Agarwal and Prabha, 2021).

The combination of devices with multiple capabilities, vendors, complexities, versions, and functions creates some common security challenges due to the heterogeneous nature, power consumption, scalability, and fragmentation of IoT devices.

11.4 CONCLUSION

IoTs have the potential to improve and perhaps save people's lives in terms of health. We can manage medical emergencies, provide patients with better care, encourage healthy behaviors, and monitor disease rates. The greatly improved healthcare systems brought about by IoT may help save countless lives. These advancements may result in an improvement in the patient's quality of life due to easier access to information and increased two-way communication. In the case of a pandemic like the one brought on by COVID-19, this branch of knowledge will be used to enhance surgical treatment and ensure that people can keep their health. As a result, fewer people will pass away from infectious diseases and other medical issues. The potential for IoT to advance healthcare is enormous. Thanks to IoT, thousands of lives might be saved. Two illustrations of potential applications are the use of IoT inclination to represent and assist patients during pandemics of infectious diseases like COVID-19.

REFERENCES

Agarwal, S., & Prabha, C. (2021). Diseases prediction and diagnosis system for healthcare using IoT and machine learning. In *Smart Healthcare Monitoring Using IoT with 5G* (pp. 197–228). https://doi.org/10.1201/9781003171829-11

Albzeirat, M., Zulkepli, N., & Qaralleh, H. (2022). A vision to face COVID-19 pandemic and future risks through artificial intelligence. *Journal of Basic and Applied Research in Biomedicine*, *6*(1), 15–20. https://doi.org/10.51152/jbarbiomed.v6i1.3

Allam, Z., & Jones, D.S. (2020). On the coronavirus (COVID-19) outbreak and the smart city network: Universal data sharing standards coupled with artificial intelligence (AI) to benefit urban health monitoring and management. *Healthcare*, *8*(1), 46. https://doi.org/10.3390/healthcare8010046

Barabas, J., Zalman, R., & Kochlan, M. (2020). Automated evaluation of COVID-19 risk factors coupled with real-time, indoor, personal localization data for potential disease identification, prevention and smart quarantining. In *2020 43rd International Conference on Telecommunications and Signal Processing (TSP)*. https://doi.org/10.1109/tsp49548.2020.9163461

Chamola, V., Hassija, V., Gupta, V., & Guizani, M. (2020). A comprehensive review of the COVID-19 pandemic and the role of IoT, drones, AI, blockchain, and 5G in managing its impact. *IEEE Access*, *8*, 90225–90265. https://doi.org/10.1109/access.2020.2992341

Desyansah, S.F., Mohammed, M.N., Al-Zubaidi, S., Syamsudin, H., Abdullah, I., & Yusuf, E. (2021). Bradykinesia detection system using IoT based health care system for Parkinson's disease patient. In *2021 IEEE International Conference on Automatic Control & Intelligent Systems (I2CACIS)*. https://doi.org/10.1109/i2cacis52118.2021.9495885

Elmousalami, H.H., Darwish, A., & Hassanien, A.E. (2021). The truth about 5G and COVID-19: Basics, analysis, and opportunities. In *Digital Transformation and Emerging Technologies for Fighting COVID-19 Pandemic: Innovative Approaches* (pp. 249–259). https://doi.org/10.1007/978-3-030-63307-3_16

Greco, L., Percannella, G., Ritrovato, P., Tortorella, F., & Vento, M. (2020). Trends in IoT based solutions for health care: Moving AI to the edge. *Pattern Recognition Letters*, *135*, 346–353. https://doi.org/10.1016/j.patrec.2020.05.016

Hegde, R., Ranjana, S., & Divya, C.D. (2021). Survey on development of smart healthcare monitoring system in IoT environment. In *2021 5th International Conference on Computing Methodologies and Communication (ICCMC)*. https://doi.org/10.1109/iccmc51019.2021.9418405

Hussain, A.A., Bouachir, O., Al-Turjman, F., & Aloqaily, M. (2020). Notice of retraction: AI techniques for COVID-19. *IEEE Access*, *8*, 128776–128795. https://doi.org/10.1109/access.2020.3007939

IoT based portable ECG monitoring system for smart healthcare. (2023). *International Research Journal of Modernization in Engineering Technology and Science*. https://doi.org/10.56726/irjmets39561

Marais, J.M., Abu-Mahfouz, A.M., & Hancke, G.P. (2020). A survey on the viability of confirmed traffic in a LoRaWAN. *IEEE Access*, *8*, 9296–9311. https://doi.org/10.1109/access.2020.2964909

Mbunge, E. (2020). Integrating emerging technologies into COVID-19 contact tracing: Opportunities, challenges and pitfalls. *Diabetes & Metabolic Syndrome: Clinical Research & Reviews*, *14*(6), 1631–1636. https://doi.org/10.1016/j.dsx.2020.08.029

Olatinwo, Abu-Mahfouz, & Hancke. (2019). A survey on LPWAN technologies in WBAN for remote health-care monitoring. *Sensors*, *19*(23), 5268. https://doi.org/10.3390/s19235268

Rachna, Bhambri, P., & Chhabra, Y. (2022). Deployment of distributed clustering approach in WSNs and IoTs. In *Cloud and Fog Computing Platforms for Internet of Things* (pp. 85–98). https://doi.org/10.1201/9781003213888-7

Rachna, Chhabra, Y., & Bhambri, P. (2020). Comparison of clustering approaches for enhancing sustainability performance in WSNSL a study. In *TEQIP-III Sponsored International Conference on Sustainable Development Through Engineering Innovations* (pp. 62–71). Ludhiana Center. ISBN: 978-93-89947-14-4.

Rachna, Chhabra, Y., & Bhambri, P. (2021). Various approaches and algorithms for monitoring the energy efficiency of wireless sensor networks. In *Lecture Notes in Civil Engineering* (pp. 761–770). https://doi.org/10.1007/978-981-15-9554-7_68

Raj, C., Jain, C., & Arif, W. (2017). HEMAN: Health monitoring and nous: An IoT based e-health care system for remote telemedicine. In *2017 International Conference on Wireless Communications, Signal Processing and Networking (WiSPNET)*. https://doi.org/10.1109/wispnet.2017.8300134

Rana, R. (2018, March). A review of the evolution of wireless sensor networks. *International Journal of Advanced Research Trends in Engineering and Technology (IJARTET), 5*(Special issue), ISSN2394-3777 (Print), ISSN2394-3785 (Online). Available online atwww.ijartet.com

Rana, R., Chhabra, Y., & Bhambri, P. (2019). A review on development and challenges in wireless sensor networks. In *International Multidisciplinary Academic Research Conference (IMARC, 2019)* (pp. 184–188). CT University. ISBN: 978-81-942282-0-2.

Rana, R., Chhabra, Y., & Bhambri, P. (2021a). Comparison and evaluation of various QoS parameters in WSNs with the implementation of enhanced low energy adaptive efficient distributed clustering approach. *Webology, 18*(1), 2021. ISSN: 1735-188X.

Rana, R., Chhabra, Y., & Bhambri, P. (2021b). Design and development of distributed clustering approach in wireless sensor network. *Webology, 18*(1), 2021. ISSN: 1735-188X.

Rani, S., Bhambri, P., & Kataria, A. (2023a). Integration of IoT, big data, and cloud computing technologies. In *Big Data, Cloud Computing, and IoT: Tools and Applications* (pp. 1–22). CRC Press, Taylor & Francis Group. https://www.taylorfrancis.com/chapters/edit/10.1201/9781003298335-1/integration-iot-big-data-cloud-computing-technologies-sita-rani-pankaj-bhambri-aman-kataria?context=ubx&refId=dc607001-1c5d-48ed-8754-9ad4a978a12d

Rani, S., Bhambri, P., Kataria, A., & Khang, A. (2023b). Smart city ecosystem: Concept, sustainability, design principles, and technologies. In *AI-Centric Smart City Ecosystems* (pp. 1–20). CRC Press.

Rani, S., Pareek, P. K., Kaur, J., Chauhan, M., & Bhambri, P. (2023c). Quantum machine learning in healthcare: Developments and challenges. Paper presented at the International Conference on Integrated Circuits and Communication Systems, 1–7.

Ritu, P., & Bhambri, P. (2023, February 17). Software effort estimation with machine learning—a systematic literature review. In *Agile Software Development: Trends, Challenges and Applications* (pp. 291–308). John Wiley & Sons, Inc.

Singh, R. P., Javaid, M., Haleem, A., & Suman, R. (2020a). Internet of things (IoT) applications to fight against COVID-19 pandemic. *Diabetes & Metabolic Syndrome: Clinical Research & Reviews, 14*(4), 521–524. https://doi.org/10.1016/j.dsx.2020.04.041

Singh, V., Chandna, H., Kumar, A., Kumar, S., Upadhyay, N., & Utkarsh, K. (2020b). IoT-Q-Band: A low cost Internet of things based wearable band to detect and track absconding COVID-19 quarantine subjects. *EAI Endorsed Transactions on Internet of Things, 6*(21), 163997. https://doi.org/10.4108/eai.13-7-2018.163997

Siriwardhana, Y., De Alwis, C., Gur, G., Ylianttila, M., & Liyanage, M. (2020). The fight against the COVID-19 pandemic with 5G technologies. *IEEE Engineering Management Review, 48*(3), 72–84. https://doi.org/10.1109/emr.2020.3017451

Stojanovic, R., Skraba, A., & Lutovac, B. (2020). A headset like wearable device to track COVID-19 symptoms. In *2020 9th Mediterranean Conference on Embedded Computing (MECO)*. https://doi.org/10.1109/meco49872.2020.9134211

Turner, T., Elliott, J., Tendal, B., Vogel, J.P., Norris, S., Tate, R., & Green, S. (2022). The Australian living guidelines for the clinical care of people with COVID-19: What worked, what didn't and why, a mixed methods process evaluation. *PLOS ONE*, *17*(1), e0261479. https://doi.org/10.1371/journal.pone.0261479

Urbanization and regional sustainability in South Asia. (2020). *Contemporary South Asian Studies*. https://doi.org/10.1007/978-3-030-23796-7

Yüksel, H. (2022). IoT-based smart healthcare monitoring system. In *Healthcare Monitoring and Data Analysis Using IoT: Technologies and Applications* (pp. 71–98). https://doi.org/10.1049/pbhe038e_ch5

12 Design and Implementation of 3D Printed Non-Invasive Mechanical Ventilator Device against COVID-19 Pandemic

Mehmet Cem Catalbas

12.1 INTRODUCTION

Following the 2002 SARS (severe acute respiratory syndrome) and 2012 MERS (Middle East respiratory syndrome) epidemics, the world was once again faced with a worldwide pandemic of zoonotic origin. In December 2019, an outbreak of pneumonia caused by an unknown etiology occurred in Wuhan, China. The pathogen was soon determined by the World Health Organization (WHO) to be a novel coronavirus called 2019-nCoV. While pandemics are uncommon, proper planning for one is vital in order to achieve a successful outcome. Preparing for a pandemic is difficult because it can affect everyone in a society. For this reason, scientists, health personnel and experts in the field of epidemics from around the world have come together to plan and prepare for possible pandemics around the world. Coronavirus disease 2019 (COVID-19) is a new and extremely contagious respiratory disease caused by Coronavirus 2 (SARS-CoV-2), which results in a severe acute respiratory syndrome when contracted. Human-to-human transmission is also a concern with COVID-19 (Chen et al., 2020). People who are severely affected by COVID-19 require respiratory support for their lungs because of breathing difficulties due to the coronavirus. As a life-saving procedure, ventilators are used to provide the proper amount of oxygen (O2) to their lungs while also reducing carbon dioxide (CO2). During this pandemic, one of the vital medical devices required to keep these patients alive has been ventilator devices. The number of people impacted by the COVID-19 pandemic in hospitals and intensive care units (ICUs) around the world has recently increased dramatically. Even at this advanced stage in the pandemic, the demand for ventilator devices is critical, particularly in developing countries.

 DOI: 10.1201/9781032698519-12

12.1.1 COVID-19 Pandemic and Ventilator Device

Individuals infected with COVID-19 were admitted to the ICU in Wuhan, China, as part of the research. At the time of admission, 56 percent of their patients needed non-invasive ventilator, and 76 percent needed invasive mechanical ventilator (Iyengar et al., 2020). Experts estimated that approximately 880,000 ventilator devices would be required globally in April 2020, during the early phases of the pandemic. The number of current and predicted additional respiratory devices according to some countries is shown in Figure 12.1 for the COVID-19 pandemic (STATISTA, 2020).

According to the World Health Organization in April 2020, it is stated that the total number of ventilator devices in 41 countries in Africa is approximately 2000 and these numbers are far from what is required in an effective fight against the COVID-19 pandemic. Even one year after this situation, the ratio of ventilator devices to total COVID-19 cases has not changed significantly in these regions, and this situation has been creating a significant strain on healthcare systems. Even though the need for ventilator devices has decreased at this stage of the pandemic due to increased production capability and strengthening of supply chains of ventilator devices, only half of the ventilator devices required in India can be obtained for COVID-19 patients nowadays. Clinical ventilator devices are quite expensive for developing-country economies, with prices surpassing $50,000.

Researchers have been investigating creative methods to meet the requirement for vital low-cost quick manufactured ventilator devices from the first day of the COVID-19 pandemic. In a comprehensive study on 1042 COVID-19 patients, ventilator devices are one of the most important factors in the fight against the COVID-19 disease and the positive effect of the use of ventilator devices on the death rate is clearly seen (Nicholson et al., 2021). Because of the stated importance of ventilator devices for the COVID-19 pandemic, researchers have been looking for innovative solutions that will reduce ventilator device production costs and speed up production

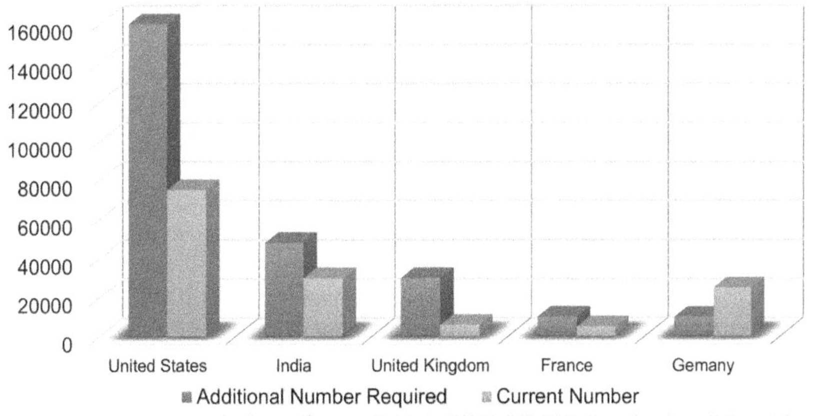

FIGURE 12.1 Number of ventilator devices according to countries.

processes since the beginning of the pandemic. Three dimensional (3D) printer technologies are at the forefront of solutions that provide the desired outcome. In this process, the idea of using additive manufacturing (AM) for local sourcing of equipment that is difficult to access has emerged, and the potential of production has reduced supply chain commitment.

The hospitalization rate is about 15 percent in the United States and this rate is decreasing significantly due to the effects of vaccines (Nakamichi et al., 2021). Even though the rate of COVID-19 related hospitalization has decreased because of vaccines, a shortage of ventilators remains a major issue, particularly in developing countries due to access difficulties to vaccines. These difficulties and COVID-19 variants have raised the demand for COVID-19 patients suffering from severe acute respiratory distress to have access to emergency ventilators that can be deployed quickly and have adequate functioning. Mechanical ventilator devices have become vital equipment in the fight against the COVID-19 pandemic due to these and similar factors that have been ongoing since the pandemic began. A ventilator machine is a device that helps people breathe. It basically transfers air in and out of the lungs. Every breath is in fact a four-phase variable. When inspiration begins (trigger), how flow is given during inspiration (goal), proximal airway pressure (baseline), and when inspiration concludes (cycle) are determined by these phase factors. The phase variable components trigger, target and loop define each ventilator mode. Volume-controlled ventilator (VCV), pressure-controlled ventilator (PCV) and pressure support ventilator (PSV) are the three fundamental ventilator modes. The most important advantage of VCV is that it can give constant tidal volume. While this situation provides stable alveolar ventilator, changes arising from respiratory mechanics can be easily defined by PIP and P_{Plat} values. The constant current may cause asynchronization. Unlike PCV, tidal volume cannot exceed safe limits in the presence of active respiratory effort. In volume-controlled ventilator, the variable breaths that are constant in all breaths is the gas volume (tidal volume) entering and leaving the lungs during breathing. In pressure-controlled modes, non-invasive ventilators have also been employed as invasive ventilators (Pons-Òdena et al., 2020). Ventilator devices are available on the market with varying features, technology and prices, and they can be classified in general way. The ventilators' cost-performance distribution and our target low-cost ventilator devices have been shown in Figure 12.2 (Mohsen Al Husseini et al., 2010).

The SARS-CoV-2 pandemic is putting pressure on healthcare systems around the world, and the global scarcity of ventilators is exacerbating the problem. Due to that, several studies were conducted on the development of low-cost and high-performance ventilator device projects. One of these low-cost ventilator projects, the MADVent Mark V, adds robust safety and functionality to existing solutions for the lack of a single-mode, pressure-controlled, time-terminated emergency ventilator.

It forms a pressure curve up to the set level at a predetermined rise time. A commonly available stepper motor, controller and on-chip system direct the airflow through a simple mechanical system controlled by the computer. Standard PEEP control is provided with a disposable ready valve (Vasan et al., 2020). In a recent study, the MIT E-Vent Team successfully developed a scalable ventilator prototype deemed ready for mass production (MIT E-Vent, 2021). The ventilator comes equipped with pressure-based alerts, including the Spiro Wave device, which, while based on the

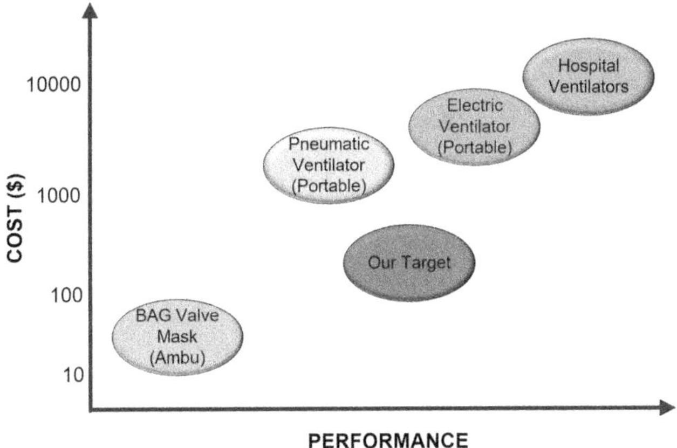

FIGURE 12.2 Cost versus performance of ventilator devices.

MIT E-Vent, has received approval from the US FDA solely for emergency usage. The MIT E-Vent prototype incorporates several key features, such as a manual resuscitator, an external compression mechanism, and a sophisticated control system. This control system allows for the adjustment of crucial parameters, including tidal volumes, inspiratory-expiratory pace, and respiratory rate. Noteworthy additions to the MIT E-Vent include a pressure relief valve and a PEEP valve. These features contribute to the ventilator's overall functionality and effectiveness in addressing respiratory challenges. Volume-controlled ventilator is available in both unassisted and aided modes. With the studies conducted, it is necessary to develop simple, lightweight and inexpensive ventilators that can be produced rapidly with minimum sensitivity to supply chain disruptions (Raymond et al., 2020; Pearce, 2020). The overall objective of this research study is to design, test and produce an inexpensive, lightweight, rapidly deployable mechanical ventilator that is specifically designed to battle COVID-19 and other pandemics with similar symptoms. To precisely control the airflow rate, the proposed ventilator design includes pressure sensors and Pulse Width Modulation (PWM) control mechanisms.

12.2 MECHANICAL VENTILATOR DESIGN

In modern generation ventilators, closed-loop ventilator control is commonly used. Under changing circumstances, resistance or compliance, closed-loop control systems are used in ventilator devices to provide steady pressure and desired flow waveforms (Hess and Kacmarek, 2018). The mode of ventilator is the link between breath types and phase factors. As seen in Figure 12.3, mechanical ventilator devices consist of many components (Sayın, 2017).

The designed system was revealed in the light of these components. The main aims of our 3D printing mechanical ventilator device project are low-cost and

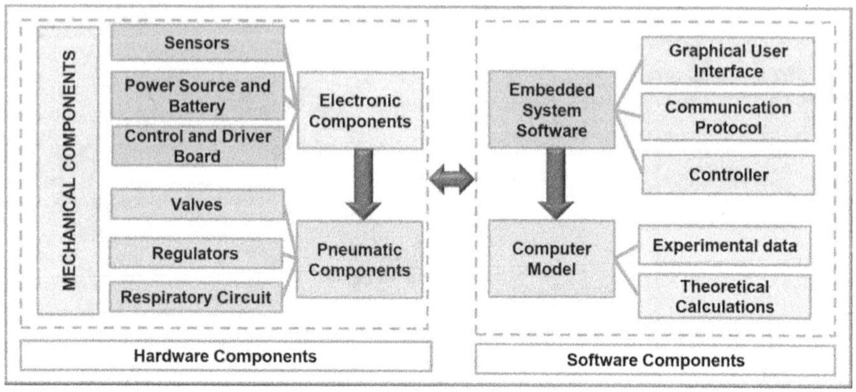

FIGURE 12.3 Internal structure of the mechanical ventilator.

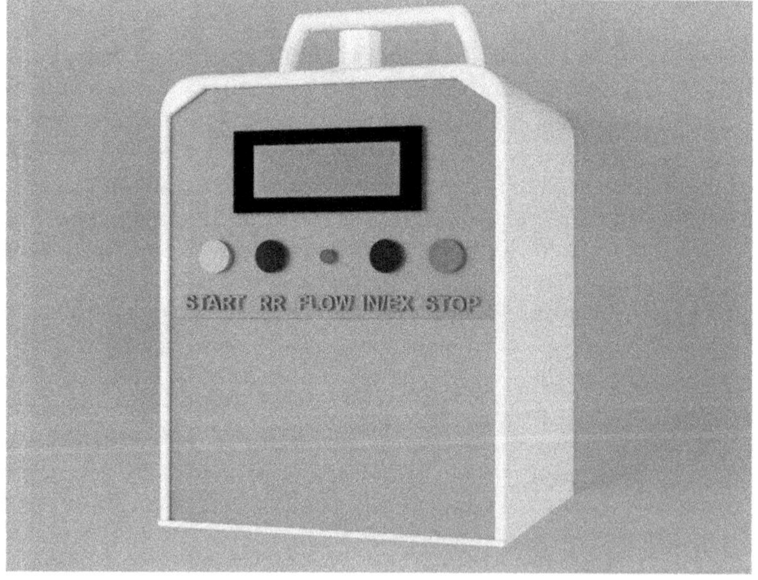

FIGURE 12.4 3D model of the ventilator device.

suitability to rapid manufacturing. The 3D model of the designed ventilator device is given in Figure 12.4.

Compatibility with portable use of Li-ion batteries is one of the design criteria of the ventilator equipment. There is a 4 x 20 LCD user information screen in order to control important values such as respiratory rate (RR), flow rate, inspiration/expiration (I/E) ratio and to show possible malfunction in the working process (Shuttleworth and Dodds, 2019). The energy required for the operation of the ventilator device is provided in two different ways. The ventilator device is powered by a battery consisting of nine 3.7V 3000mAh 18650 model Li-ion cells or by connecting directly to the grid via plugs (Franco, 2015). The parameters regarding the designed ventilator have been identified according to the MIT E-vent project. Thus, rates have been determined to meet the urgent need of an adult person during the COVID-19 pandemic. Arduino Uno microcontroller device was used to control the device and it has six analog to digital converter (ADC) with ten bit (Cameron, 2021). These ADC inputs are used to adjust flow ratio and detect pressure anomaly in the ventilator device for this work. A pressure sensor is built into the airway to determine possible faults in the ventilator device and the model of the used pressure sensor is MPXV5050GP in this work (El Majid et al., 2020). It has been determining pressure level with a maximum 2.5 percent error between zero and 50kpA measurement range. With this pressure sensor, the device gives a warning via a buzzer as a result of a possible airway obstruction or blocking of oxygen entry and this error is shown on Liquid Crystal Display (LCD) with the information (Shrivastava et al., 2021). PWM motor driving technique has been used to control the blower on the ventilator device. In this way, a relationship has been established between the duty cycle of the generated PWM signal and the amount of flow generated. In addition, buttons are used to start the ventilator device and stop it in case of emergency. DTH11 temperature and humidity sensor has been added to the ventilator system in order to instantly observe the temperature and humidity information of the environment on the LCD panel. An optional Covidien electrostatic filter has been added between the NIV mechanical ventilator mask and the air connection to reduce the risk of disease transmission through the air released into the environment by the COVID-19 patient (Ari et al., 2016). Thanks to these filters, the heat and humidity needed in the respiratory tract are created.

12.2.1 3D Printer Technologies and NIV Mechanical Ventilator Design

The body frame and hose connections of the ventilator device in this study were created with a 3D printer and it is suitable for improvement. Fused Deposition Modeling (FDM) 3D printing technique has been used for the NIV mechanical ventilator devices against COVID-19 for this work (Mwema and Akinlabi, 2020). The process of producing all components of a ventilator device with a 3D printer takes approximately 16 hours (Singh and Bhambri, 2023). The operation of the proposed low-cost ventilator device has been tested for approximately 600 hours and it has been observed that it works successfully in this process. These values were obtained with a conventional 3D printer produced for a home user. The ventilator device produced consists of several components and its case structure and connection points of blowers were produced via 3D printing technology (Bhambri et al., 2023). The diameter of the hose connections in the device are designed as 22 mm and they are suitable for the standard ventilator circuits. 3D-printed stabilizers were used to keep the components stable inside and prevent their movement during transport. As a result, a light construction with a stiff body and composed of 3D recyclable material has been created. The designed ventilator device consists of many components, and these are given in Figure 12.5.

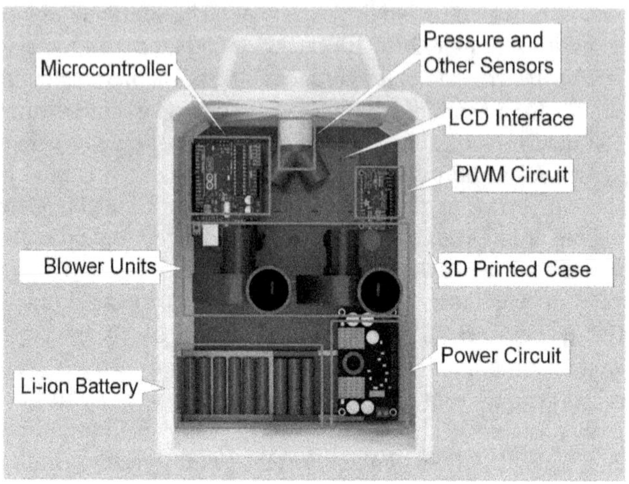

FIGURE 12.5 Components of the manufactured ventilator device.

TABLE 12.1
Technical Specifications of Ventilator Device

IN/EX Ratio	**1:2 1:3 1:4**
Respiratory Rate (min)	10-12-15
Flow Rate	0-120 L/Min
Power Consumption	30 Watts per hour
Dimensions: Width x Height x Depth	180 mm x 220 mm x 180 mm
Battery type (Li-Ion)	12.6 V 9000 mAH
Charged Usage Time	240 Minutes
3D Printing Material	PLA (polylactic acid)

The technical specifications of the designed 3D printed ventilator system are given in Table 12.1. While determining the technical parameters of the proposed ventilator device, MIT E-Vent and other ventilator device design studies in the literature were examined and the parameters were selected according to these works.

12.2.2 PWM and Airflow Control Model

During the first stage of device implementation, the operating characteristics of the device were analyzed with the simulation results of the difference RR. At this step, flow rate analyses were performed first (Rana et al., 2024). While doing this, a time parameter was determined in software in the microcontroller device, and the desired RR were obtained precisely by increasing or decreasing this time parameter with the relevant interface. Furthermore, an additional time parameter is defined in software

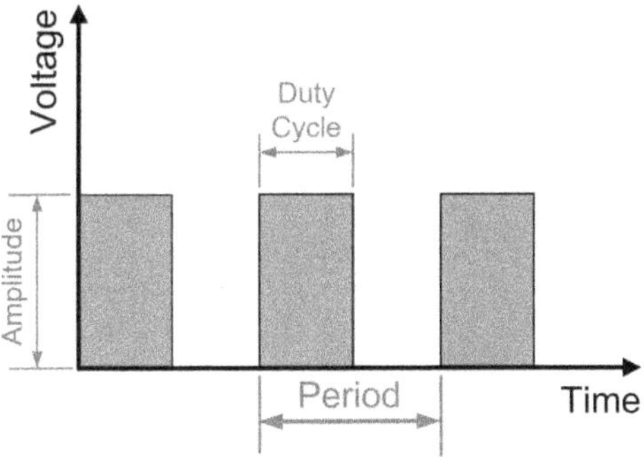

FIGURE 12.6 The basic parameters of PWM signal.

for I:E ratios, which is another parameter that users can adjust. Users can obtain the appropriate RR and I:E ratio by adjusting these two separate time parameters (Shanmuga and Bhambri, 2024). These created time parameters are used in collaboration with the microcontroller-based fixed one-minute timer. The parameters of the PWM signal control these time parameters, which affect the airflow rate, RR, and I:E ratios. The basic parameters of the PWM signal are given in Figure 12.6.

For the control of the ventilator device, a meaningful relationship was established between the period and duty cycle parameters of the PWM signal applied to the blower units and the RR, I:E ratios and airflow in this work. The linear fitting model approach is preferred when developing this meaningful relationship between PWM parameters and airflow rates (Faraway, 2016). The actual airflow rates corresponding to the different duty cycles of the PWM signals were measured in real-time for 30 different test points and these test points can be defined as ventilator device calibration points for this work. The measurement results and the linear fitting model are given in Figure 12.7. Thanks to this model, a significant relationship between PWM duty cycle and airflow rate has been established and RR, I:E ratios and airflow rate parameters can be controlled effectively and precisely via the user interface of the ventilator device.

The coefficients for the proposed linear fitting model are given in Equation 12.1.

$$\begin{aligned} y_i &= b_0 + b_1 x_i \\ y_i &= 1.393 + 1.185 x_i \end{aligned} \tag{12.1}$$

where, x_i is the PWM duty cycle and y_i is the flow (L/min). The success of the created model was also observed with the $R^2 = 0.997$ parameter. To prevent rapid changes in the system parameters set by the users and to ensure that the device works more reliably, software-defined exponential filters were applied to the system input parameters such as airflow rate. The exponential filter is the basic linear recursive filter, and it is providing a suitable smoothing effect on variable signals. The output waveforms of the exponential filter for the different α parameters are given in Figure 12.8 and the α parameter which is the smoothing factor is selected as $\alpha = 0.3$ for this work.

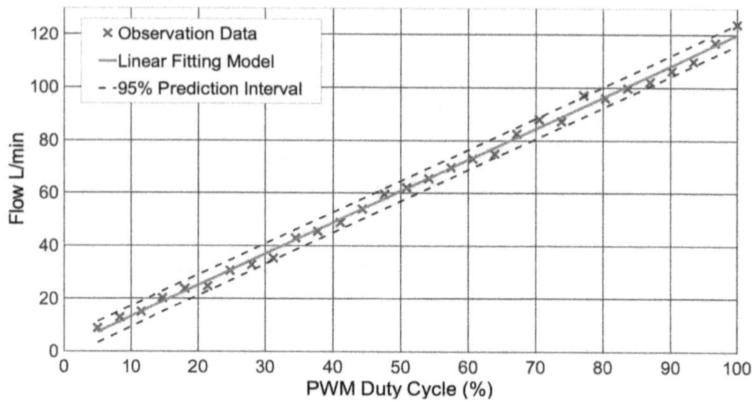

FIGURE 12.7 Linear fitting model and measurements results.

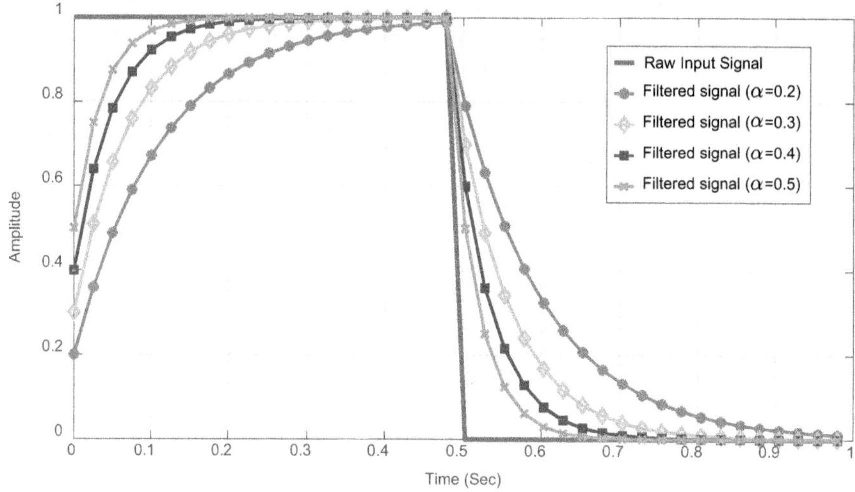

FIGURE 12.8 The output waveforms of exponential filter according to different α parameters.

12.3 PERFORMANCE ANALYSIS OF 3D PRINTED MECHANICAL VENTILATOR DEVICE

Following the design processes, the device's airflow, volume and pressure waveforms were obtained for different RR and I:E ratios. The flow waveforms according to different RR is given in Figure 12.9 for the proposed system.

In Figure 12.10, the change of volume according to time for different RR has been given.

The pressure waveform of proposed ventilator device is given in Figure 12.11.

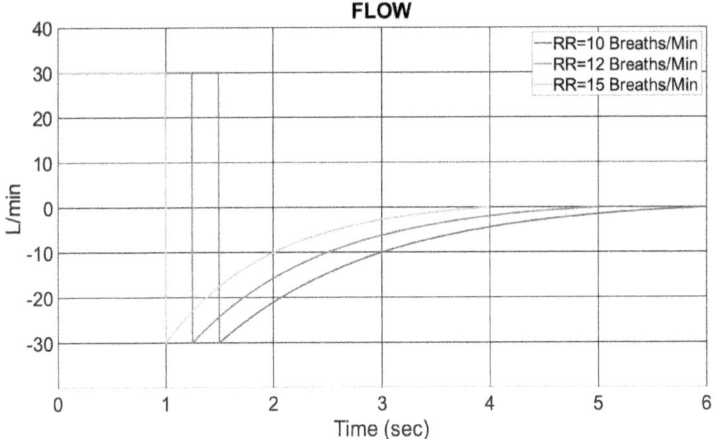

FIGURE 12.9 The waveform of flow rate according to different RR.

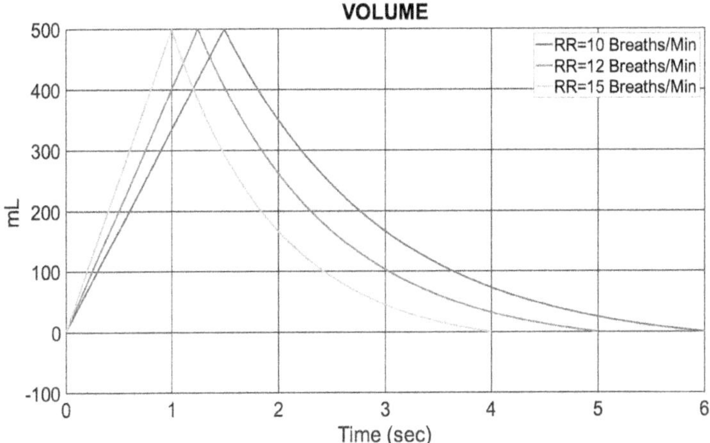

FIGURE 12.10 The waveform of volume change according to different RR.

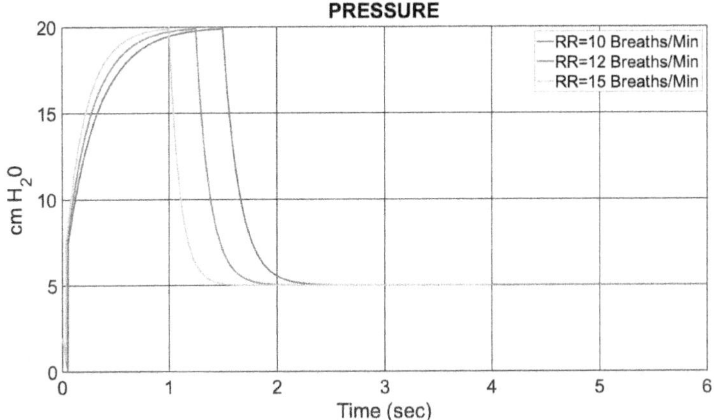

FIGURE 12.11 The waveform of pressure about ventilator device.

The change in waveform of volume according to pressure has been given in Figure 12.12. Positive end expiratory pressure (PEEP) of the proposed system has been provided via an external valve system as a fixed value at 5 cm H_20 (Chang et al., 2021).

The flow signal for different I:E ratios for the ventilator device has been given in Figure 12.13.

At the end of design process, the differences between the airflow rates set by the user and the actual flow rates were measured in real-time. During the performance test of the proposed ventilator device, the user increased the value of the airflow at

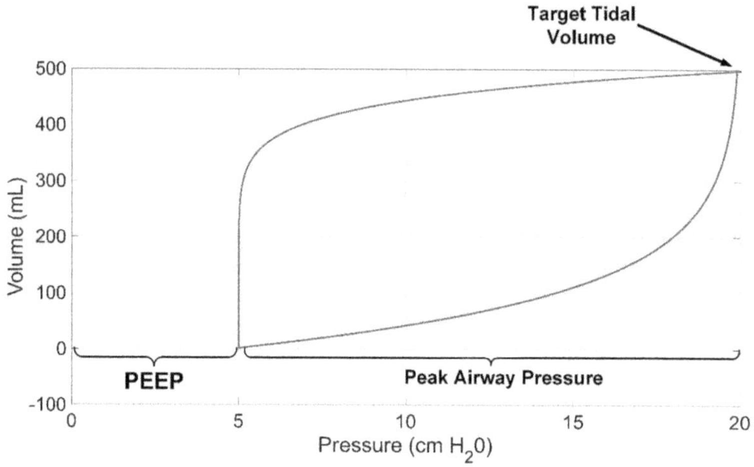

FIGURE 12.12 The waveform of volume versus pressure.

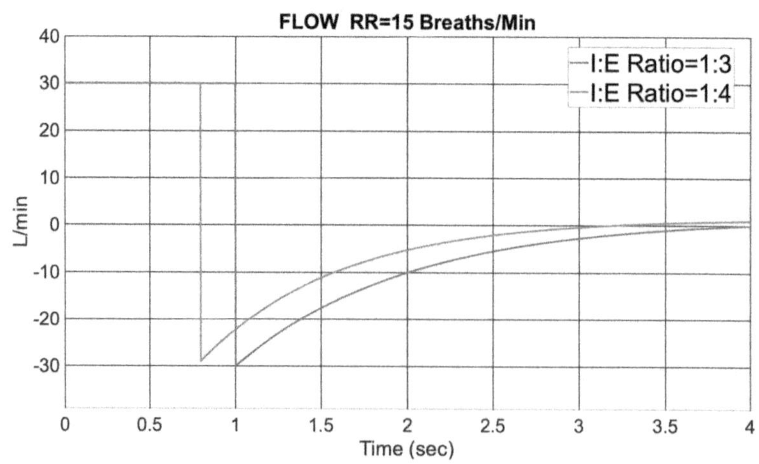

FIGURE 12.13 Flow waveform for different I:E ratios.

equal intervals from the minimum to the maximum value, and the airflow produced by the ventilator device was measured 30 times during this procedure. The measurement results obtained because of this test process are given in Table 12.2.

As shown in the table, the mean error between created flow rate and real flow rate is 1.434 L/min. As a result, the realized ventilator device provides the needed flow with a high success rate. By linearizing the relationship between the PWM signal controlling the blower and the flow rate and increasing the correlation between them, the precision of the I:E and RR increased significantly (Kazmierkowski et al., 2003). The prototype output of the low-cost portable ventilator device produced within the scope of this study is given in Figure 12.14.

TABLE 12.2
Error on Flow Rates (L/min)

Max Error	4.336
Min Error	0.011
Mean Error	1.434
Standard Deviation of Error	1.134

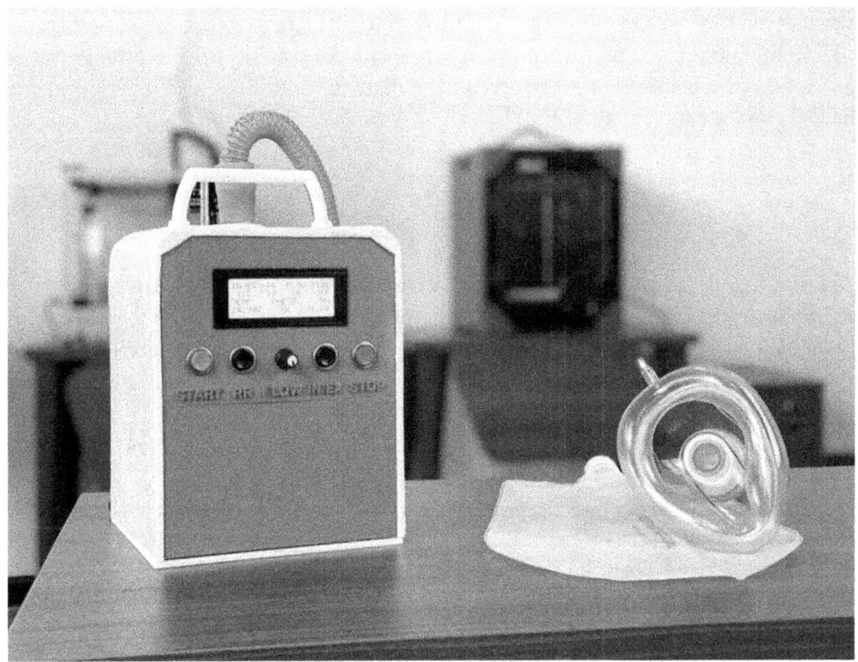

FIGURE 12.14 NIV 3D printed mechanical ventilator device against COVID-19.

12.4 CONCLUSION

In this work, NIV 3D printed mechanical ventilator devices have been produced. The main purpose of this study is to design a low-cost and rapid manufacturing ventilator device against the COVID-19 pandemic. It was ensured that the cost of the manufactured device was approximately 250 US dollars. A basic linear model was used to reduce the error between the air produced by the device's blower and the actual airflow, thereby reducing the difference to an average of 1.434 L/min for 30 test points. The device is supported by Li-ion batteries in order for it to be portable. All waveforms of the device have been simulated and the actual performance of these simulations has been analyzed over 30 real test points. The production time of all components of this device, which is produced with the FDM technique, is approximately 16 hours with a conventional 3D printing device. In this device, a pressure sensor is used to observe possible error conditions. There is an LCD screen and audible warning structures to communicate these errors to the user. The RR, I:E ratio or flow rates can be adjusted easily with created user interface in this device, and it can be shown in LCD. A device has been designed to reduce the effects of the lack of ventilator devices, which is considered one of the most important problems during the COVID-19 pandemic. There are some ways that can be performed to improve the device's performance. The airflow rate error obtained in one minute can be easily reduced to less than 0.5 L by updating the used estimation model with a nonlinear high-order predicting model instead of a linear structure. In addition, increasing the test points used in the calibration process will significantly reduce this flow rate error. The quality of airflow rate and total life span can be easily enhanced by replacing the low-cost blower units utilized in this study with more expensive and reliable components. The airflow waveform and other basic information about the devices may be easily monitored from long distances with the modification of low-cost IoT devices such as the ESP32.

12.5 ACKNOWLEDGEMENT

This study was supported by OSTIM Technical University, Institute of Scientific Research (BAP)/TURKEY in frame of the project code of BAP0014 as researchers, we thank the OSTIM Technical University Institute of Scientific Research/TURKEY.

REFERENCES

Ari, A., Fink, J. B., & Pilbeam, S. P. (2016). Secondhand aerosol exposure during mechanical ventilator with and without expiratory filters: An in-vitro study. *Indian Journal of Respiratory Care*, *5*(1).

Bhambri, P., Singh, S., Jain, S., & Dhanoa, S. I. (2023). Plants recognition using leaf image pattern analysis with focus on advanced smart computing technologies. In *AIP Conference Proceedings* 2916, 020003 (2023). https://doi.org/10.1063/5.0179534

Cameron, N. (2021). Electronics projects with the ESP8266 and ESP32. In *Electronics Projects with the ESP8266 and ESP32*. https://doi.org/10.1007/978-1-4842-6336-5

Chang, J., Acosta, A., Benavides-Aspiazu, J., Reategui, J., Rojas, C., Cook, J., Nole, R., Giampietri, L., Pérez-Buitrago, S., Casado, F. L., & Castaneda, B. (2021). Masi: A mechanical ventilator based on a manual resuscitator with telemedicine capabilities for patients with ARDS during the COVID-19 crisis. *HardwareX*, *9*. https://doi.org/10.1016/j.ohx.2021.e00187

Chen, N., Zhou, M., Dong, X., Qu, J., Gong, F., Han, Y., Qiu, Y., Wang, J., Liu, Y., Wei, Y., Xia, J., Yu, T., Zhang, X., & Zhang, L. (2020). Epidemiological and clinical characteristics of 99 cases of 2019 novel coronavirus pneumonia in Wuhan, China: A descriptive study. *The Lancet*, *395*(10223). https://doi.org/10.1016/S0140-6736(20)30211-7

El Majid, B., El Hammoumi, A., Motahhir, S., Lebbadi, A., & El Ghzizal, A. (2020). Preliminary design of an innovative, simple, and easy-to-build portable ventilator for COVID-19 patients. *Euro-Mediterranean Journal for Environmental Integration*, *5*(2). https://doi.org/10.1007/s41207-020-00163-1

Faraway, J. J. (2016). Extending the linear model with R. In *Extending the Linear Model with R*. https://doi.org/10.1201/b21296

Franco, A. A. (2015). Rechargeable lithium batteries: From fundamentals to applications. In *Rechargeable Lithium Batteries: From Fundamentals to Applications*. https://doi.org/10.1016/C2013-0-16455-0

Hess, D. R., & Kacmarek, R. M. (2018). *Essentials of Mechanical Ventilator* (4th edition). McGraw-Hill Education.

Iyengar, K., Bahl, S., Vaishya, R., & Vaish, A. (2020). Challenges and solutions in meeting up the urgent requirement of ventilators for COVID-19 patients. *Diabetes & Metabolic Syndrome: Clinical Research & Reviews*, *14*(4), 499–501. https://doi.org/10.1016/j.dsx.2020.04.048

Kazmierkowski, M. P., Krishnan, R., & Blaabjerg, F. (2003). Control in power electronics: Selected problems. In *Control in Power Electronics: Selected Problems*. https://doi.org/10.1016/B978-0-12-402772-5.X5000-5

MIT E-Vent. (2021). *E-VENT*. https://emergency-vent.mit.edu/

Mohsen Al Husseini, A., Ju Lee, H., Negrete, J., Powelson, S., Tepper Servi, A., & Slocum, A. H. (2010). Design and prototyping of a low-cost portable mechanical ventilator. *Journal of Medical Devices, Transactions of the ASME*, *4*(2). https://doi.org/10.1115/1.3442790

Mwema, F. M., & Akinlabi, E. T. (2020). Basics of fused deposition modelling (FDM). In *SpringerBriefs in Applied Sciences and Technology*. https://doi.org/10.1007/978-3-030-48259-6_1

Nakamichi, K., Shen, J. Z., Lee, C. S., Lee, A., Roberts, E. A., Simonson, P. D., Roychoudhury, P., Andriesen, J., Randhawa, A. K., Mathias, P. C., Greninger, A. L., Jerome, K. R., & Van Gelder, R. N. (2021). Hospitalization and mortality associated with SARS-CoV-2 viral clades in COVID-19. *Scientific Reports*, *11*(1). https://doi.org/10.1038/s41598-021-82850-9

Nicholson, C. J., Wooster, L., Sigurslid, H. H., Li, R. H., Jiang, W., Tian, W., Lino Cardenas, C. L., & Malhotra, R. (2021). Estimating risk of mechanical ventilator and in-hospital mortality among adult COVID-19 patients admitted to Mass General Brigham: The VICE and DICE scores. *EClinicalMedicine*, *33*. https://doi.org/10.1016/j.eclinm.2021.100765

Pearce, J. M. (2020). A review of open source ventilators for COVID-19 and future pandemics. *F1000Research*, *9*. https://doi.org/10.12688/f1000research.22942.2

Pons-Òdena, M., Valls, A., Grifols, J., Farré, R., Cambra Lasosa, F. J., & Rubin, B. K. (2020). COVID-19 and respiratory support devices. In *Paediatric Respiratory Reviews* (Vol. 35). https://doi.org/10.1016/j.prrv.2020.06.015

Rana, R., Bhambri, P., & Chhabra, Y. (2024). Evolution and the future of industrial engineering with the IoT and AI. In *Integration of AI-Based Manufacturing and Industrial Engineering Systems with the Internet of Things* (pp. 19–37). CRC Press.

Raymond, S. J., Wesolowski, T., Baker, S., Liu, Y., Edmunds, J. L., Bustamante, M. J., Ley, B., Free, D., Maharbiz, M., van Wert, R., Cornfield, D. N., & Camarillo, D. B. (2020). A low-cost, rapidly scalable, emergency use ventilator for the COVID-19 crisis. *MedRxiv*, August.

Sayın, F. S. (2017). *Neonatal Intensive Care And Transport Ventilator (Artificial Respiration Device) Design*. Marmara.

Shanmuga, S. M., & Bhambri, P. (2024). Bone marrow cancer detection from leukocytes using neural networks. In P. Bhambri, S. Rani, & M. Fahim (Eds.), *Computational Intelligence and Blockchain in Biomedical and Health Informatics* (1st ed., pp. 307–319). CRC Press. https://doi.org/10.1201/9781003459347

Shrivastava, A., Rizwan, A., Kumar, N. S., Saravanakumar, R., Dhanoa, I. S., Bhambri, P., & Singh, B. K. (2021, November 30). VLSI Implementation of Green Computing Control Unit on Zynq FPGA for Green Communication. *Wireless Communications and Mobile Computing*, 2021, 4655400. https://doi.org/10.1155/2021/4655400

Singh, G., & Bhambri, P. (2023). Simulation Analysis of AODV and DSDV Routing Protocols for Secure and Reliable Service in Mobile Adhoc Networks (MANETs). In *Integration of AI-Based Manufacturing and Industrial Engineering Systems with the Internet of Things* (pp. 205–216). CRC Press.

Shuttleworth, D., & Dodds, N. (2019). Ventilators and breathing systems. In *Maths, Physics and Clinical Measurement for Anaesthesia and Intensive Care*. https://doi.org/10.1017/9781108758505.010

STATISTA. (2020). *Current Number of Ventilators and Additional Number Required in Select Countries as of April 2020.* www.statista.com/statistics/1122713/current-ventilators-and-additional-number-required-select-countries/

Vasan, A., Weekes, R., Connacher, W., Sieker, J., Stambaugh, M., Suresh, P., Lee, D. E., Mazzei, W., Schlaepfer, E., Vallejos, T., Petersen, J., Merritt, S., Petersen, L., & Friend, J. (2020). MADVent: A low-cost ventilator for patients with COVID-19. *Medical Devices & Sensors*, *3*(4), 1–14. https://doi.org/10.1002/mds3.10106

13 Emotional Sentiment Analysis by Machine Learning from EEG of Brainwave Data

Pankaj Bhambri and Manpreet Singh

13.1 INTRODUCTION

Electroencephalogram (EEG) data, which records electrical activity in the brain, serves as a unique source of information for understanding emotional states. This research involves the development of machine learning algorithms capable of analyzing EEG data patterns associated with different emotions (Chanel et al., 2006). By identifying distinct neural signatures linked to specific emotional states, the system can classify and interpret the emotional sentiments of an individual in real-time (Singh et al., 2021a).

An important benefit of this approach is its capacity to offer a more impartial and straightforward assessments of emotions in contrast to conventional methods like self-reporting. EEG records the nuanced electrical impulses produced by the brain, providing a neurophysiological viewpoint that is less prone to biases or mistakes seen in subjective accounts (Vijayalakshmi et al., 2021). Moreover, the utilization of machine learning enables the development of prediction models that can consistently acquire knowledge and adjust, hence enhancing the precision of emotion recognition as time progresses. The application of this technology could extend beyond individual emotional analysis to fields like mental health, human-computer interaction, and neuromarketing (Babu et al., 2021).

However, challenges and ethical considerations must be addressed in the development and deployment of this technology. Ensuring the privacy and consent of individuals contributing EEG data is paramount, and researchers must navigate the ethical implications of accessing and analyzing such sensitive information. Moreover, the interpretability of machine learning models in this context is crucial to building trust and understanding the basis for emotional predictions (Bakshi et al., 2021). In order to fully exploit the possibilities of Emotional Sentiment Analysis through machine learning via EEG of brainwave data, it is crucial for neuroscientists, data analysts, and ethicists to collaborate. This collaboration is necessary to ensure the protection of the well-being and rights of the individuals involved in this field, which is constantly changing.

DOI: 10.1201/9781032698519-13

13.2 OVERVIEW OF EMOTIONAL SENTIMENT ANALYSIS

Emotional Sentiment Analysis, often referred to as sentiment analysis or opinion mining, is a branch of natural language processing that focuses on extracting and understanding emotions and sentiments expressed in text data (Lin et al., 2010). This computational technique aims to discern the subjective information embedded in written or spoken language to determine the emotional tone or attitude conveyed by the speaker. The main objective is to classify the emotion of the text as good, negative, or neutral, so offering useful insights to public opinion, consumer feedback, and social media attitudes.

Emotional Sentiment Analysis is performed using a range of machine learning, as well as deep learning methods. These methodologies utilize labeled datasets to train models to recognize patterns and nuances in language associated with different emotional states. Some common features used for analysis include word frequency, context, and syntactic structures (Chanel et al., 2008). As the field progresses, researchers are exploring more advanced approaches, such as sentiment analysis based on multimodal data, incorporating visual and auditory cues alongside text to achieve a more comprehensive understanding of emotional expressions. The applications of Emotional Sentiment Analysis are widespread, ranging from business and marketing strategies to social media monitoring, enabling organizations to make data-driven decisions and respond effectively to the sentiments expressed by their audience.

13.2.1 Importance in Healthcare

Emotional Sentiment Analysis employs machine learning and natural language processing approaches to identify and comprehend human emotions conveyed through text or speech. This technology plays a crucial role in healthcare by providing a means to gauge and respond to the emotional well-being of patients (Kaur and Kumar, 2020). Analyzing sentiments in patient feedback, social media posts, or even clinical notes allows healthcare providers to gain valuable insights into the emotional states of individuals. Recognizing patterns of emotional distress or positive sentiments enables timely interventions, personalized care, and improved patient outcomes (Liu et al., 2012). Additionally, Emotional Sentiment Analysis can aid in monitoring mental health trends on a broader scale, contributing to the development of preventive strategies and more effective public health initiatives. The integration of this technology in healthcare not only enhances patient care but also underscores the significance of addressing emotional well-being as an integral component of overall health management (Sharma et al., 2019).

13.2.2 Applications and Use Cases

Emotional Sentiment Analysis has a wide range of applications across various industries and domains, leveraging its ability to extract valuable insights from human emotions. Some notable applications and use cases include:

- Customer Feedback and Sentiment Analysis: Businesses can analyze customer reviews, feedback, and comments to gauge the sentiment surrounding their products or services (AlZoubi et al., 2018). This enables companies to identify areas for improvement, understand customer satisfaction levels, and tailor their offerings based on consumer sentiments.
- Social Media Monitoring: Social media platforms are rich sources of user-generated content expressing opinions and emotions. Emotional Sentiment Analysis can be employed to monitor social media channels, helping businesses and organizations understand public perception, track brand sentiment, and respond to emerging trends or crises in real-time.
- Market Research: In market research, Emotional Sentiment Analysis can be used to analyze responses to surveys, interviews, or focus group sessions (Devadutta et al., 2020). This allows researchers to gain deeper insights into consumer attitudes, preferences, and emotional responses to different products or marketing strategies.
- Human Resources and Employee Engagement: Organizations can apply sentiment analysis to evaluate the contentment, involvement, and welfare of their employees. Through the examination of employee input, HR departments can discern possible difficulties, boost workplace conditions, and elevate the general business culture.
- Healthcare and Mental Health Monitoring: In healthcare, Emotional Sentiment Analysis can assist in monitoring mental health conditions (Yannakakis and Hallam, 2009). Analyzing verbal or written expressions can help healthcare professionals assess patients' emotional states, providing valuable information for diagnosis and treatment planning.
- Educational Technology: Educational platforms can employ Emotional Sentiment Analysis to understand students' engagement levels and emotional responses to learning materials. This information can be used to tailor educational content, identify areas of improvement, and enhance the overall learning experience.
- Virtual Assistants and Human-Computer Interaction: Integrating Emotional Sentiment Analysis into virtual assistants allows for more personalized and empathetic interactions. These systems can adapt their responses based on the user's emotional state, creating a more intuitive and supportive user experience.
- Law Enforcement and Security: Sentiment analysis can be applied in security and law enforcement to monitor social media and other online platforms for potential threats or public sentiment shifts (Mendes et al., 2016). This can aid in proactive risk assessment and crisis management.
- Entertainment and Gaming: In the entertainment industry, Emotional Sentiment Analysis can enhance user experiences in gaming and interactive content by adapting storylines or game dynamics based on players' emotional reactions.
- Fraud Detection and Cybersecurity: By analyzing user behavior and communication patterns, Emotional Sentiment Analysis can contribute to fraud detection and cybersecurity efforts (Katsigiannis and Ramzan, 2018).

Unusual emotional responses in communication may indicate potential security threats or fraudulent activities.

13.2.3 Challenges and Opportunities

Emotional Sentiment Analysis holds great promise, but overcoming its challenges requires a concerted effort from researchers, technologists, and ethicists to ensure its responsible and effective integration into various aspects of society (Lin et al., 2011). Challenges and opportunities abound in the field of Emotional Sentiment Analysis, reflecting the complexity of understanding and interpreting human emotions through technological means. The major challenges are:

- Subjectivity and Ambiguity: Human emotions are multifaceted and often context-dependent, leading to challenges in defining clear boundaries between different emotional states (Koelstra et al., 2012). The subjective nature of emotions poses difficulties in creating standardized datasets for training machine learning models.
- Cultural Variations: Emotions are expressed and interpreted differently across cultures. Training models on datasets that are biased towards specific cultural norms may result in limited generalizability. Cross-cultural variations in emotional expressions and perceptions need to be considered for accurate sentiment analysis.
- Dynamic Nature of Emotions: Emotions are dynamic and can change rapidly. Real-time emotional analysis faces the challenge of capturing and interpreting evolving emotional states accurately (Singh et al., 2021b). Continuous adaptation of models to reflect the changing emotional landscape is crucial.
- Lack of Ground Truth Labels: Obtaining labeled emotional data for training models is challenging, as emotions are often subjective and can vary between individuals (Joshi and Ahmed, 2019). The absence of a universally agreed-upon "ground truth" for emotional states makes it difficult to validate and fine-tune sentiment analysis models.
- Multimodal Challenges: Integrating multiple modalities such as text, speech, and facial expressions for comprehensive sentiment analysis adds complexity (Singh et al., 2020). Aligning information from diverse sources and ensuring their consistency present challenges in creating holistic emotional models.

The major Opportunities in the discipline of Emotional Sentiment Analysis are:

- Interdisciplinary Collaboration: Emotional Sentiment Analysis benefits from collaboration between experts in psychology, neuroscience, linguistics, and computer science (Soleymani et al., 2012). Combining insights from these diverse fields can enhance the accuracy and depth of emotion recognition models.
- Advancements in Neural Networks: With the evolution of deep learning and neural network architectures, there's an opportunity to build more

sophisticated models capable of learning intricate patterns in emotional data. These advancements contribute to improved feature extraction and model performance.

- Real-world Applications: Emotional Sentiment Analysis has practical applications across various industries, including customer service, marketing, mental health, and human-computer interaction. Developing tailored solutions for specific domains can unlock opportunities for widespread implementation.
- Ethical Considerations: Addressing ethical concerns, such as user privacy and consent, ensures responsible development and deployment of sentiment analysis technologies. Establishing ethical guidelines and standards helps build trust with users and stakeholders.
- Continuous Learning Models: Implementing machine learning models that can adapt and learn from new data over time allows for continuous improvement. This adaptability is crucial for capturing changes in language, cultural norms, and individual expression of emotions.

13.3 EEG DATA IN EMOTIONAL SENTIMENT ANALYSIS

EEG data plays a pivotal role in advancing Emotional Sentiment Analysis (ESA) by providing a direct and real-time measure of neural activity associated with emotional states (Koelstra et al., 2012). EEG recordings capture electrical potentials generated by the brain, offering insights into the temporal dynamics of emotional responses. In the context of ESA, EEG data enables the identification and classification of distinct neural patterns correlated with various emotional states, such as happiness, sadness, or anxiety. Analyzing EEG signals in emotional sentiment analysis not only enhances the accuracy of emotion recognition models but also provides a deeper understanding of the neural mechanisms underlying emotional experiences. This integration of neurophysiological data into sentiment analysis holds promise for applications in fields ranging from human-computer interaction to mental health monitoring, facilitating a more nuanced and comprehensive understanding of the interplay between emotions and cognition.

13.3.1 Brainwave Patterns and Emotions

Understanding the intricate relationship between brainwave patterns and emotions is pivotal in the realm of ESA, especially when utilizing EEG data. EEG records the electrical activity of the brain, and distinct brainwave patterns are associated with various emotional states. For instance, beta waves are commonly linked to alertness and concentration, while alpha waves are associated with relaxation. Delta waves are prominent during deep sleep, and theta waves are often observed in meditative or reflective states. These patterns form the neurophysiological basis for emotional experiences, as different emotions are correlated with specific combinations of these brainwave frequencies. As individuals experience emotions, their brainwave patterns exhibit unique signatures that can be detected and analyzed through EEG, providing valuable insights for emotional sentiment analysis.

In the context of EEG data in emotional sentiment analysis, researchers and data scientists leverage machine learning algorithms to interpret these intricate brainwave patterns. By employing pattern recognition techniques, EEG data can be analyzed to discern the emotional states of individuals, offering a non-invasive and objective means of understanding emotions. The integration of machine learning models with EEG data allows for the development of emotion classifiers that can accurately identify and categorize emotional states based on the detected brainwave patterns. This interdisciplinary approach holds immense potential for applications in fields such as human-computer interaction, mental health assessment, and personalized user experiences (Sharma et al., 2018). As our understanding of brainwave patterns and emotions deepens, the synergy between neuroscience and machine learning in emotional sentiment analysis continues to unlock new avenues for enhancing our comprehension of human emotional experiences.

13.3.2 Acquisition and Preprocessing of EEG Data

The acquisition and preprocessing of EEG data play pivotal roles in the realm of ESA. EEG, a non-invasive neuroimaging technique, captures electrical activity generated by the brain, providing valuable insights into emotional states (Mower Provost et al., 2001). To obtain relevant data for ESA, electrodes are strategically placed on the scalp to record voltage fluctuations associated with emotional responses. The acquisition process involves careful consideration of factors such as electrode placement, signal sampling rates, and noise reduction techniques to ensure data quality. Once acquired, EEG data undergo preprocessing steps to enhance its utility for emotional sentiment analysis (Soleymani et al., 2012). Preprocessing involves tasks such as filtering, artifact removal, and segmentation to isolate meaningful brainwave patterns associated with emotional states. This meticulous process not only ensures the reliability of the data but also facilitates the extraction of features relevant to emotional sentiment analysis, ultimately contributing to the effectiveness and accuracy of emotion recognition systems.

13.3.3 Challenges in EEG Data Analysis for Emotion Detection

Analyzing EEG data for emotion detection poses several challenges due to the complex and dynamic nature of both brain signals and emotions (Bhambri, 2020). EEG is a valuable tool in understanding the neural correlates of emotions, but extracting meaningful information for emotional sentiment analysis requires overcoming specific obstacles (Koelstra et al., 2010). Here are some challenges associated with EEG data analysis for emotion detection in the context of emotional sentiment analysis:

- Temporal Dynamics of Emotions: Emotions are dynamic and evolve over time. EEG signals capture fast and dynamic neural processes, making it challenging to precisely identify the temporal characteristics associated with different emotional states. Analyzing the temporal dynamics of emotions in EEG data requires advanced signal processing techniques to capture rapid changes.

- Inter-Subject Variability: Individuals exhibit variations in their brain responses to emotional stimuli (Cecotti and Graser, 2011). Inter-subject variability in EEG signals makes it difficult to establish a universal set of features or patterns that reliably represent specific emotions. Personalized models or adaptive approaches may be necessary to account for these individual differences.
- Ambiguity of Emotional States: Emotions are multifaceted, and a single emotion can manifest differently across individuals. The ambiguity in defining emotional states poses a challenge in creating precise and generalizable EEG-based models for emotion detection. Integrating other modalities, such as facial expressions or physiological signals, may enhance the accuracy of emotion classification.
- Noise and Artifacts: EEG signals are susceptible to various types of noise and artifacts, including muscle artifacts, eye movements, and environmental interference. Proper preprocessing techniques are essential to minimize these artifacts and enhance the signal-to-noise ratio, ensuring that the extracted features are genuinely reflective of brain activity related to emotions.
- Limited Spatial Resolution: EEG has lower spatial resolution compared to other neuroimaging techniques like fMRI. This limitation makes it challenging to precisely localize the brain regions responsible for specific emotional processes. Combining EEG with other imaging modalities or leveraging source localization techniques can help address this challenge to some extent.
- Subject Compliance and Comfort: EEG data collection often requires subjects to wear electrodes and stay relatively still, which may impact the natural expression of emotions. Ensuring subject compliance and comfort is crucial for obtaining reliable and ecologically valid EEG data for emotion detection.
- Large-Scale Data Collection: Building robust models for emotional sentiment analysis requires large and diverse datasets. However, collecting labeled EEG datasets with a sufficient number of samples for various emotions is a resource-intensive task. Collaboration across research groups and standardization in data collection protocols can help address the issue of limited data.
- Ethical and Privacy Concerns: EEG data, being a direct measure of brain activity, raises ethical concerns regarding privacy and informed consent. Ensuring ethical practices in data collection, storage, and sharing is crucial. Researchers must consider the implications of using neural data for emotional sentiment analysis and implement appropriate safeguards.

13.4 MACHINE LEARNING IN EMOTIONAL SENTIMENT ANALYSIS

Machine Learning (ML) plays a pivotal role in Emotional Sentiment Analysis, leveraging computational models to discern and interpret the emotional content embedded in textual, visual, or physiological data (Ritu and Bhambri, 2022). Through the application of various ML techniques such as Natural Language Processing (NLP), deep learning, and ensemble methods, algorithms can learn patterns and features indicative of different emotional states. These models are trained on labeled datasets, enabling them to generalize and predict emotional sentiment in unseen data (Sumathi et al., 2021). ML facilitates the automation of sentiment classification tasks, offering scalability and efficiency in processing large volumes of information. Continuous advancements in ML, coupled with the integration of multimodal data sources, contribute to the refinement and sophistication of Emotional Sentiment Analysis models, empowering applications across diverse domains such as customer feedback analysis, social media monitoring, and mental health assessment.

13.4.1 Role of Machine Learning in Healthcare

Machine learning plays a transformative role in healthcare, bringing about significant changes in multiple areas of research, medical practice, and administration. Machine learning algorithms process extensive patient data, ranging from digital health records to imaging studies, in order to detect trends, forecast disease outcomes, and tailor treatment approaches (Picard, 1997). These algorithms enhance diagnostic accuracy, allowing for earlier detection of diseases, and aid in the identification of optimal treatment strategies. Additionally, machine learning contributes to the improvement of operational efficiency in healthcare systems, streamlining administrative tasks, resource allocation, and patient management (Bhambri, 2021). By harnessing the power of data-driven insights, machine learning not only facilitates evidence-based decision-making but also holds the potential to revolutionize preventive care, drug discovery, and the overall delivery of healthcare services, ultimately leading to more efficient, personalized, and accessible healthcare solutions.

13.4.2 Machine Learning Algorithms for EEG Data Analysis

Unsupervised as well as supervised approaches are both important in the field of machine learning algorithms to analyze EEG data. These approaches are essential for obtaining valuable information from the intricate brain signals. Supervised learning is a process where a model is trained with labeled data, allowing the algorithm to learn how to associate input properties with predetermined labels for output (Liu et al., 2011). In the context of EEG data analysis, supervised learning is often applied for tasks such as emotion detection, where the algorithm is trained on EEG recordings associated with specific emotional states. Features extracted from EEG signals, such as power spectral density or event-related potentials, serve as input for the model (Huang et al., 2006). The trained algorithm can then classify new, unlabeled EEG data into predefined emotional categories, contributing to our understanding of the neural correlates of emotions and facilitating applications such as affective computing or brain-computer interfaces.

On the other hand, unsupervised learning approaches are valuable when dealing with unlabeled or exploratory EEG datasets, where the objective is to uncover hidden patterns or structures within the data. Clustering algorithms, such as k-means or hierarchical clustering, are frequently employed in EEG data analysis to group similar patterns of neural activity without prior knowledge of the emotional states involved (Lin et al., 2010). Unsupervised learning is particularly useful for identifying natural subgroups within a population or discovering novel patterns that may not be predefined. In the context of EEG, unsupervised learning contributes to the exploration of brain dynamics, revealing inherent structures and relationships that may not be apparent through manual inspection. By combining both supervised and unsupervised learning approaches, researchers can gain a comprehensive understanding of the underlying neural processes and advance the field of EEG-based machine learning applications in areas like emotion recognition and cognitive state monitoring.

13.4.3 Challenges and Considerations in Machine Learning for Emotional Sentiment Analysis

Machine learning for emotional sentiment analysis faces various challenges and considerations that impact the development and deployment of robust models. One significant challenge is the inherent subjectivity and variability in human emotions, making it difficult to create universally applicable models. The interpretation of emotions may differ across individuals and cultures, introducing biases and reducing the generalizability of models. Another critical consideration is the need for diverse and well-annotated datasets that adequately represent the complexity of human emotions in different contexts. Data privacy concerns and ethical considerations surrounding the use of personal emotional data also pose challenges (Sharma et al., 2019). Additionally, achieving real-time processing capabilities and addressing interpretability issues in complex machine learning models are crucial for practical deployment in applications such as sentiment analysis in social media or customer feedback. Balancing model accuracy with transparency and fairness, while considering the dynamic nature of emotions, requires a thoughtful approach to ensure that machine learning applications in emotional sentiment analysis are both reliable and ethically sound.

13.5 FRAMEWORKS AND TOOLS FOR EEG DATA ANALYSIS

Several frameworks and tools are employed for EEG data analysis, facilitating the processing, visualization, and interpretation of complex neural signals (Liu et al., 2011). Open-source platforms like EEGLAB and MNE-Python offer comprehensive toolboxes for preprocessing, source localization, and statistical analysis, providing a wide array of functions for researchers and practitioners. MATLAB-based EEGLAB is renowned for its user-friendly interface, extensive plugin support, and robust signal processing capabilities. MNE-Python, on the other hand, is a Python-based library that leverages the scientific computing capabilities of Python for EEG data analysis, offering flexibility and compatibility with other machine learning and data analysis libraries. Commercial software options, such as BrainVision Analyzer and NeuroScan, provide user-friendly interfaces and advanced features for both novice and expert users. These frameworks and tools empower researchers to handle diverse EEG analysis tasks, from basic preprocessing steps to sophisticated machine learning applications, contributing significantly to the advancement of neuroscience and the development of EEG-based applications in various domains.

13.5.1 Overview of Existing EEG Data Analysis Frameworks

Existing EEG data analysis frameworks provide a structured and systematic approach to processing, interpreting, and extracting valuable information from electroencephalogram recordings. These frameworks typically encompass a range of methods and tools for preprocessing raw EEG data, including artifact removal, filtering, and feature extraction. They often integrate machine learning algorithms for tasks such as emotion recognition, cognitive state classification, or brain-computer interface applications. Popular EEG analysis frameworks, such as EEGLAB, MNE-Python, and FieldTrip, offer a wide array of functionalities, enabling researchers to explore temporal and spatial patterns in neural activity (Kuzhaloli et al., 2020). These frameworks contribute to standardizing analysis pipelines, fostering collaboration across research groups, and accelerating advancements in neuroscience and related fields. As EEG technology continues to evolve, so do these frameworks, playing a pivotal role in advancing our understanding of the brain and facilitating the development of innovative applications for healthcare, human-computer interaction, and cognitive neuroscience.

13.5.2 Tools for Feature Extraction and Selection

Frameworks and tools for EEG data analysis encompass a variety of methods for feature extraction and selection, crucial steps in translating raw neural signals into meaningful information. Feature extraction tools aim to identify relevant characteristics within EEG data that capture important aspects of brain activity. Popular techniques include time-domain features like amplitude and latency of event-related potentials, as well as frequency-domain features such as power spectral density (AlZoubi et al., 2018). Moreover, spatial features, extracted through methods like independent component analysis (ICA) or dipole source localization, offer insights into the specific brain regions contributing to the observed signals. Feature selection tools then play a pivotal role in reducing dimensionality by identifying the most informative features, preventing model overfitting and enhancing algorithm efficiency. Widely used tools such as scikit-learn in Python or MATLAB's Signal Processing Toolbox provide a rich set of functions for feature extraction and selection, facilitating the integration of advanced machine learning algorithms in EEG data analysis frameworks. The effective combination of these tools empowers researchers to extract relevant information from EEG signals, improving the accuracy and interpretability of machine learning models in applications ranging from emotion recognition to cognitive state assessment.

13.5.3 Integration with AI and IoT Platforms

By incorporating AI (Artificial Intelligence) algorithms into EEG data analysis frameworks, researchers can enhance the accuracy and efficiency of tasks such as feature extraction, classification, and interpretation of complex neural patterns. Additionally, connecting EEG frameworks to IoT (Internet of Things) platforms enables real-time monitoring and seamless data exchange, facilitating remote patient monitoring and personalized healthcare applications (Kroupi and Charisis, 2016). This integration not only streamlines the analysis pipeline but also opens avenues for the development of intelligent, adaptive systems that can respond dynamically to changes in brain activity, thereby paving the way for innovative solutions in neurotechnology and brain-computer interfaces. The synergy between EEG data analysis frameworks, AI, and IoT platforms offers a holistic approach, fostering advancements in both research and practical applications for neurological and psychiatric disorders.

13.6 CASE STUDIES AND APPLICATIONS

In human-computer interaction, the integration of EEG-based emotional sentiment analysis has been explored to enhance user experience (Salido-Ruiz et al., 2021). Case studies involving interactive systems, gaming interfaces, and virtual reality platforms have demonstrated the ability to adapt in real-time based on users' emotional states, creating more immersive and responsive environments. For instance, EEG-driven interfaces can dynamically adjust the difficulty level of a game or tailor content delivery in educational applications based on the learner's emotional engagement.

Moreover, in affective computing, companies have employed machine learning algorithms on EEG data to gauge customer reactions and sentiment towards products or advertisements (Singh et al., 2021a). These case studies involve monitoring participants' neural responses while exposed to stimuli, such as advertisements or product prototypes, to predict consumer preferences and optimize marketing strategies.

Furthermore, the field of neurofeedback and cognitive enhancement has seen applications of emotional sentiment analysis from EEG data (Bose et al., 2021). By providing real-time feedback on individuals' emotional states, neurofeedback systems aim to enhance emotional regulation and well-being. Case studies involving stress reduction programs and mindfulness applications have demonstrated the potential of EEG-based sentiment analysis in promoting emotional self-awareness and resilience.

13.6.1 Real-World Examples of Emotional Sentiment Analysis using EEG

Here are a few real-world instances that showcase the potential of EEG-based emotional sentiment analysis:

- Mental Health Monitoring: Researchers and healthcare professionals have been exploring EEG-based emotional sentiment analysis to monitor mental health conditions such as depression and anxiety. By analyzing patterns in brainwave data, studies aim to identify neural markers associated with emotional states, providing insights into individuals' mental well-being.

- Human-Computer Interaction: Applications in human-computer interaction involve adapting interfaces based on users' emotional states to improve user experience (Jabeen et al., 2021). For instance, EEG data can be used to detect frustration or engagement levels, leading to real-time adjustments in gaming interfaces or educational software for a more personalized and engaging interaction.
- Neurofeedback and Stress Reduction: Some real-world applications focus on using EEG-based emotional sentiment analysis for neurofeedback interventions. By providing individuals with real-time feedback on their emotional states, these applications aim to help users regulate stress levels and achieve emotional well-being. This could be applied in stress reduction programs, mindfulness applications, and other wellness initiatives.
- Marketing and Consumer Research: Companies have explored EEG-based emotional sentiment analysis to understand consumer reactions to products, advertisements, or brand experiences. This approach provides insights into consumer preferences and emotional responses, enabling businesses to tailor marketing strategies for improved engagement and satisfaction.
- Emotion Recognition in Human-Robot Interaction: EEG data has been employed in real-world scenarios involving human-robot interaction. By detecting and understanding human emotions through brainwave patterns, robots can adapt their behavior or responses to create more empathetic and socially intelligent interactions, making them more suitable for various applications, including healthcare and customer service.
- Affective Computing in Education: In educational settings, EEG-based emotional sentiment analysis has been applied to gauge students' engagement and frustration levels during learning activities. Adaptive learning systems can use this information to customize content delivery, providing a more tailored and effective educational experience.

13.6.2 Impact on Patient Care and Well-Being

The integration of emotional sentiment analysis through machine learning from EEG brainwave data has the potential to significantly impact patient care and well-being across various healthcare domains. Here are several ways in which this technology can contribute to improving patient outcomes and well-being:

- Early Detection and Monitoring of Mental Health Conditions: Emotional sentiment analysis from EEG data can play a crucial role in the early detection and continuous monitoring of mental health conditions such as depression, anxiety, and stress. By identifying specific neural markers associated with emotional states, healthcare professionals can intervene early, providing timely and targeted interventions to support patients in managing their mental health.
- Personalized Treatment Plans: Machine learning algorithms analyzing EEG data can contribute to the development of personalized treatment plans for individuals with mental health disorders. By understanding the unique

neural signatures of patients, healthcare providers can tailor therapeutic approaches, medication regimens, or behavioral interventions to better align with the specific emotional and cognitive needs of each patient.

- Neurofeedback for Emotional Regulation: EEG-based emotional sentiment analysis enables the implementation of neurofeedback interventions, where patients receive real-time feedback on their emotional states. This can empower individuals to actively participate in the regulation of their emotions, contributing to stress reduction, improved mood, and overall well-being. Neurofeedback has shown promise in various applications, including anxiety management and emotional resilience training.
- Enhanced Therapeutic Relationships: Integrating emotional sentiment analysis into patient care can enhance the therapeutic relationship between healthcare providers and patients. Understanding the emotional states of patients through objective EEG data can improve communication, empathy, and treatment planning, leading to a more patient-centered approach to care.
- Optimizing Cognitive Rehabilitation: In cases of neurological disorders or brain injuries, emotional sentiment analysis from EEG data can inform cognitive rehabilitation strategies. By assessing emotional responses and cognitive states, rehabilitation programs can be tailored to address specific cognitive and emotional deficits, improving overall rehabilitation outcomes and quality of life for patients.
- Monitoring Stress and Burnout in Healthcare Professionals: Healthcare professionals themselves can benefit from emotional sentiment analysis to monitor their stress levels and emotional well-being. This technology can be employed to implement proactive measures for stress management and burnout prevention, ultimately contributing to the overall mental health of healthcare providers and the quality of patient care.

13.7 CONCLUSION

The exploration of emotional sentiment analysis through machine learning from EEG brainwave data presents a promising frontier in the understanding of human emotions and their applications in healthcare. This book chapter has delved into the intricate interplay between neuroscience, machine learning, and healthcare, showcasing how advancements in EEG-based emotional sentiment analysis can transform patient care and well-being. From early detection and personalized treatment plans for mental health conditions to the implementation of neurofeedback interventions, the integration of EEG data analysis into clinical practice holds immense potential. By unraveling the neural correlates of emotions, healthcare professionals can adopt a more targeted, individualized approach to patient care, ushering in a new era of precision medicine with a focus on the emotional well-being of individuals.

These advancements also bear profound implications for the evolution of smart healthcare systems. The integration of emotional sentiment analysis from EEG data can contribute to the development of intelligent, responsive healthcare environments. Smart healthcare systems equipped with machine learning algorithms can adapt in real-time to patients' emotional states, optimizing treatment modalities, and fostering a more empathetic and patient-centered care paradigm. Furthermore, these systems can extend beyond clinical settings, providing continuous monitoring and support for mental health in daily life. As technology continues to advance, the convergence of emotional sentiment analysis, machine learning, and smart healthcare systems holds the promise of revolutionizing the landscape of healthcare delivery, ultimately enhancing the holistic well-being of individuals and communities.

REFERENCES

AlZoubi, O., Chaware, L., & Patra, J. C. (2018). EEG-based emotion recognition using a novel feature selection method. *Cognitive Neurodynamics*, 12(2), 133–142.

Babu, G. C. N., Gupta, S., Bhambri, P., Leo, L. M., Rao, B. H., & Kumar, S. (2021). A semantic health observation system development based on the IoT sensors. *Turkish Journal of Physiotherapy and Rehabilitation*, 32(3), 1721–1729.

Bakshi, P., Bhambri, P., & Thapar, V. (2021). A review paper on wireless sensor network techniques in internet of things (IoT). *Wesleyan Journal of Research*, 14(7), 147–160.

Bhambri, P. (2020). Green compliance. In S. Agarwal (Ed.), *Introduction to Green Computing* (pp. 95–125). Chennai, Tamil Nadu: AGAR Saliha Publication. ISBN: 978-81-948141-5-3.

Bhambri, P. (2021). Electronic evidence. In *Textbook of Cyber Heal* (pp. 86–120). Chennai, Tamil Nadu: AGAR Saliha Publication. ISBN: 978-81-948141-7-7.

Bose, M. M., Yadav, D., Bhambri, P., & Shankar, R. (2021). Electronic customer relationship management: Benefits and pre-implementation considerations. *Journal of Maharaja Sayajirao University of Baroda*, 55(01(VI)), 1343–1350. The Maharaja Sayajirao University of Baroda.

Cecotti, H., & Graser, A. (2011). Convolutional neural networks for P300 detection with application to brain-computer interfaces. *IEEE Transactions on Pattern Analysis and Machine Intelligence*, 33(3), 433–445.

Chanel, G., Kronegg, J., Grandjean, D., & Pun, T. (2006). Emotion assessment: Arousal evaluation using EEG's and peripheral physiological signals. In *Affective Computing and Intelligent Interaction* (pp. 125–136). London: Springer.

Chanel, G., Rebetez, C., Bétrancourt, M., & Pun, T. (2008). Emotion assessment from physiological signals for adaptation of game difficulty. *IEEE Transactions on Systems, Man, and Cybernetics, Part A: Systems and Humans*, 39(4), 830–841.

Devadutta, K., Bhambri, P., Gountia, D., Mehta, V., Mangla, M., Patan, R., Kumar, A., Agarwal, P. K., Sharma, A., Singh, M., & Gadicha, A. B. (2020). *Method for Cyber Security in Email Communication among Networked Computing Devices* [Patent application number 202031002649]. India.

Huang, G. B., Zhu, Q. Y., & Siew, C. K. (2006). Extreme learning machine: Theory and applications. *Neurocomputing*, 70(1–3), 489–501.

Jabeen, A., Pallathadka, H., Pallathadka, L. K., & Bhambri, P. (2021). E-CRM successful factors for business enterprises case studies. *Journal of Maharaja Sayajirao University of Baroda*, 55(01(VI)), 1332–1342. The Maharaja Sayajirao University of Baroda.

Joshi, J., & Ahmed, B. (2019). Real-time EEG-based human emotion recognition using extreme learning machines. *Procedia Computer Science*, 165, 123–130.

Katsigiannis, S., & Ramzan, N. (2018). DREAMER: A database for emotion recognition through EEG and ECG signals from wireless low-cost off-the-shelf devices. *IEEE Journal of Biomedical and Health Informatics*, 23(6), 2344–2351.

Kaur, N., & Kumar, A. (2020). A comprehensive review of emotion recognition from EEG signals. *Cognitive Computation*, 12(5), 1137–1161.

Koelstra, S., Muhl, C., Soleymani, M., Lee, J. S., Yazdani, A., Ebrahimi, T., . . . Patras, I. (2012). Deap: A database for emotion analysis; using physiological signals. *IEEE Transactions on Affective Computing*, 3(1), 18–31.

Koelstra, S., Yazdani, A., Soleymani, M., Mühl, C., Lee, J. S., Nijholt, A., & Pun, T. (2010). *Single Trial Classification of EEG and Peripheral Physiological Signals for Recognition of Emotions Induced by Music Videos.* Proceedings of the 2nd International Workshop on EMOTION, 7–14.

Kroupi, E., & Charisis, V. (2016). Affective learning: Empathetic agents with emotional facial and tone of voice expressions. *Procedia Computer Science*, 83, 276–283.

Kuzhaloli, S., Devaneyan, P., Sitaraman, N., Periyathanbi, P., Gurusamy, M., & Bhambri, P. (2020). *IoT based Smart Kitchen Application for Gas Leakage Monitoring* [Patent application number 202041049866A]. India.

Lin, Y. P., Wang, C. H., Jung, T. P., Wu, T. L., Jeng, S. K., Duann, J. R., & Chen, J. H. (2011). EEG-based emotion recognition in music listening. *IEEE Transactions on Biomedical Engineering*, 58(12), 3167–3176.

Lin, Y. P., Wang, C. H., Wu, T. L., Jeng, S. K., & Chen, J. H. (2010). An EEG-based affective computing system with self-adapting neuro-fuzzy classifiers. *IEEE Transactions on Affective Computing*, 1(4), 190–202.

Liu, Y., Sourina, O., Nguyen, M. K., & Wang, L. (2011). *Real-time EEG-Based Human Emotion Recognition and Visualization.* Proceedings of the International Conference on Cyberworlds, 19–26.

Liu, Y., Sourina, O., Nguyen, M. K., & Wang, L. (2012). Real-time EEG-based human emotion recognition and visualization. In *Advances in Visual Computing* (pp. 91–100). London: Springer.

Mendes, J. V., Anastácio, A. P., & Silva Cunha, J. P. (2016). Emotion recognition using brain-computer interface: A comprehensive survey. *Journal of Artificial Intelligence and Systems*, 2(1), 1–11.

Mower Provost, E., Kort, B., & Reilly, R. (2001). *Socially Intelligent Computing: Perspectives on Intelligent Agents for Social Agents.* New York: MIT Press.

Picard, R. W. (1997). *Affective Computing.* New York: MIT Press.

Ritu, & Bhambri, P. (2022). *A CAD System for Software Effort Estimation.* Paper presented at the International Conference on Technological Advancements in Computational Sciences, 140–146. IEEE. DOI: 10.1109/ICTACS56270.2022.9988123.

Salido-Ruiz, R. A., García-Vázquez, J. P., García-Hernández, M. D., & Palacio-Caballero, D. (2021). Emotion recognition system using EEG signals: A systematic review. *Biomedical Signal Processing and Control*, 66, 102416.

Sharma, K., Sharma, S., & Sharma, N. (2018). Emotion recognition using EEG: A review. In *2018 9th International Conference on Computing, Communication and Networking Technologies (ICCCNT)* (pp. 1–7). New York: IEEE.

Sharma, K., Sharma, S., & Sharma, N. (2019). EEG-based emotion recognition: A review. In *Advances in Signal Processing and Intelligent Recognition Systems* (pp. 3–13). London: Springer.

Singh, G., Singh, M., & Bhambri, P. (2020). Artificial intelligence based flying car. In *Proceedings of the International Congress on Sustainable Development through Engineering Innovations* (pp. 216–227). Ludhiana Center. ISBN 978-93-89947-14-4.

Singh, M., Bhambri, P., Dhanoa, I. S., Jain, A., & Kaur, K. (2021a). Data mining model for predicting diabetes. *Annals of the Romanian Society for Cell Biology*, 25(4), 6702–6712.

Singh, M., Bhambri, P., Lal, S., Singh, Y., Kaur, M., & Singh, J. (2021b). Design of the effective technique to improve memory and time constraints for sequence alignment. *International Journal of Applied Engineering Research (Netherlands)*, 6(2), 127–142. Roman Science Publications and Distributions.

Soleymani, M., Lichtenauer, J., Pun, T., & Pantic, M. (2012). A multimodal database for affect recognition and implicit tagging. *IEEE Transactions on Affective Computing*, 3(1), 42–55.

Sumathi, N., Thirumagal, J., Jagannathan, S., Bhambri, P., & Ahamed, I. N. (2021). A comprehensive review on bionanotechnology for the 21st century. *Journal of the Maharaja Sayajirao University of Baroda*, 55(1), 114–131.

Vijayalakshmi, P., Shankar, R., Karthik, S., & Bhambri, P. (2021). Impact of work from home policies on workplace productivity and employee sentiments during the Covid-19 pandemic. *Journal of Maharaja Sayajirao University of Baroda*, 55(01(VI)), 1314–1331. The Maharaja Sayajirao University of Baroda.

Yannakakis, G. N., & Hallam, J. (2009). Entertainment modeling through physiology in physical play. *International Journal of Human-Computer Studies*, 67(5), 450–466.

14 Marvel of Biosensors in Smart Healthcare and Application of Internet of Medical Things for Diagnosis

Unveiling Benefits, Challenges and Futuristic Approach

Bhupinder Singh and Christian Kaunert

14.1 INTRODUCTION

The intersection of cutting-edge technologies in healthcare has ushered in a new era of diagnostic capabilities, enhancing patient care, and treatment outcomes. Among these technologies, biosensors and the internet of medical things (IoMT) have emerged as transformative forces, revolutionizing the landscape of smart healthcare. Biosensors, intricate devices that detect and quantify biological signals, have found unprecedented applications in healthcare, particularly in the realm of diagnostics (Phan et al., 2022). Simultaneously, the IoMT, a network of interconnected medical devices and applications, has paved the way for a seamless and data-driven healthcare ecosystem. This research delves into the marvel of biosensors and the application of IoMT in the context of smart healthcare, unraveling their multifaceted benefits, intricate challenges, and futuristic approaches (Blazek et al., 2022).

In recent years, biosensors have evolved beyond traditional laboratory settings, finding their way into wearable devices, implantable gadgets, and point-of-care diagnostic tools (Pateraki et al., 2020). These biosensors, often equipped with micro- or nanoscale components, enable real-time monitoring of physiological parameters, facilitating early disease detection and personalized medicine (Bose et al., 2021). The integration of biosensors into smart healthcare systems has transcended the boundaries of conventional healthcare, empowering individuals to actively participate in their well-being through continuous health monitoring. This paradigm shift from reactive

DOI: 10.1201/9781032698519-14

to proactive healthcare has the potential to mitigate the burden of chronic diseases and improve overall healthcare outcomes (Dwivedi et al., 2022).

The IoMT's role in diagnostics is particularly noteworthy, as it facilitates the rapid transmission of health data to healthcare providers, enabling quicker and more informed decision-making. As a result, the IoMT has become an indispensable tool in the diagnostic toolkit, enhancing the efficiency and effectiveness of healthcare delivery (Manickam et al., 2022).

Real-time data collection and analysis empower healthcare professionals to make informed decisions, tailor treatments to individual patient needs, and intervene promptly in critical situations (Jangra and Gupta, 2018). Emerging technologies, such as advanced biosensor designs and the integration of artificial intelligence, hold the promise of pushing the boundaries of diagnostics even further (Stone et al., 2022).

14.1.1 Concept of Biosensors and IoMT in Context of Smart Healthcare

The concept of biosensors and IoMT forms the bedrock of a transformative paradigm in the realm of smart healthcare. Biosensors, intricate devices designed to detect and quantify biological signals, represent a technological breakthrough in healthcare diagnostics. These devices, often employing biologically sensitive elements coupled with transducers, enable the real-time monitoring of physiological parameters. Whether embedded in wearable devices, implanted in the human body, or integrated into point-of-care diagnostic tools, biosensors empower individuals and healthcare professionals alike with continuous and personalized health insights (Irkham et al., 2023).

The synergy of biosensors and the IoMT thus lays the foundation for a dynamic and responsive smart healthcare system, wherein the proactive monitoring of health parameters and the swift transmission of data redefine the standards of patient care. This conceptual integration stands poised to revolutionize healthcare, offering a holistic approach to diagnostics and treatment that is data-driven, patient-centric, and technologically advanced (Johnson, 2020).

14.1.2 Objectives of Paper

This paper aims to delve into the synergistic realm of biosensors in smart healthcare and the application of IoMT for diagnosis. The primary objectives include:

- Explore biosensor technologies via investigate and analyze various biosensor technologies used in smart healthcare, understanding their principles, and applications in monitoring physiological parameters.
- Examine IoT applications in medical diagnosis and evaluate the role of IoMT in medical diagnosis, exploring how connected devices and sensors contribute to real-time health monitoring and diagnostic capabilities.
- Identify and elucidate the advantages of integrating biosensors and IoMT in smart healthcare, emphasizing improvements in early diagnosis, personalized treatment, and overall healthcare efficiency.

- Investigate challenges associated with the adoption of biosensors and IoMT, including data security, privacy concerns, and ethical implications, and propose strategies for mitigating these challenges.
- Provide insights into the futuristic possibilities of biosensors and IoMT in healthcare, exploring potential advancements, novel applications, and emerging technologies that could shape the future landscape of medical diagnosis and healthcare delivery.

14.1.3 Significance of Research and its Potential Impact on Healthcare

The significance of research in healthcare cannot be overstated, as it serves as the catalyst for advancements that shape the future of medical practices, patient care, and overall public health. Research acts as the guiding force in understanding the complexities of diseases, unraveling the intricacies of biological processes, and developing innovative interventions. In the context of biosensors and IoMT, ongoing research has the potential to revolutionize healthcare delivery. By delving into the development and integration of biosensors, researchers can unlock novel diagnostic tools, enabling early detection of diseases and fostering personalized treatment strategies (Bhambri et al., 2021). Simultaneously, the exploration of IoMT applications offers opportunities to create interconnected healthcare ecosystems, facilitating seamless data exchange and enhancing remote patient monitoring. The impact of such research is profound, promising improved patient outcomes, optimized resource utilization, and a more efficient and responsive healthcare system.

The potential impact of research in biosensors and IoMT on healthcare is far-reaching. It spans from the empowerment of individuals through continuous health monitoring to the enhancement of diagnostic accuracy and the evolution of personalized treatment plans. So, the significance of paper in biosensors and IoMT lies in its ability to shape the trajectory of healthcare, paving the way for a future where advanced technologies contribute to healthier societies and improved quality of life.

The diverse use of biosensors into healthcare practices aligns with the broader trend of digital health, fostering a more patient-centric and data-driven model. Despite the immense potential, challenges such as data security, standardization, and ethical considerations must be carefully navigated to ensure the responsible and equitable integration of biosensors into the healthcare ecosystem (Singh et al., 2021). Overall, the potential impact of biosensors in healthcare is poised to redefine diagnostics, treatment, and patient engagement, contributing to a more efficient, personalized, and proactive healthcare system.

14.2 BIOSENSORS IN HEALTHCARE

Biosensors represent a revolutionary frontier in healthcare, offering compact and sensitive devices that detect specific biological markers. These devices, often utilizing biological elements like enzymes or antibodies, convert biological signals into measurable electrical signals. Biosensors find diverse applications in healthcare, from rapid diagnostic tests to continuous monitoring of physiological parameters.

Wearable devices and point-of-care tools allows for real-time health data acquisition, enabling early disease detection and personalized treatment strategies (Verma et al., 2022). Biosensors play a pivotal role in ushering in a new era of precision medicine and proactive healthcare, where timely and accurate information empowers both individuals and healthcare professionals in the quest for improved health outcomes.

The widespread adoption of biosensors in healthcare is not without challenges. Concerns related to data security, privacy, and the ethical implications of continuous monitoring need careful consideration. As technology continues to advance, the integration of biosensors into routine medical practice holds the promise of not only improving the efficiency of healthcare services but also empowering individuals to take an active role in managing their health. The ongoing research and development in biosensor technologies underscore their significance in shaping the future landscape of healthcare, contributing to a more proactive, personalized, and patient-centric approach to medicine (Mbunge et al., 2021).

14.2.1 Biosensors and their Role in Healthcare

Biosensors represent a groundbreaking innovation in healthcare, with their role extending across a diverse spectrum of applications. In diagnostics, biosensors offer rapid and precise identification of pathogens, biomolecules, and changes in physiological parameters. For instance, they play a crucial role in glucose monitoring for diabetes management, ensuring timely adjustments in treatment plans. Biosensors also shine in infectious disease detection, providing quick and accurate results for timely intervention. The key contribution of biosensors lies in their ability to usher in a new era of personalized medicine (Sharma and Singh, 2022).

The real-time data provided by biosensors enables early disease detection, allowing for timely interventions and personalized treatment plans. From glucose monitoring in diabetes to identifying infectious diseases, biosensors contribute to more efficient and targeted healthcare (Sangwan Singh et al., 2021). Their portability, cost-effectiveness, and ability to provide continuous monitoring make them invaluable tools in modern healthcare, empowering both healthcare professionals and individuals to make informed decisions about health management. As technology continues to advance, biosensors are poised to become even more integral to diagnostics and personalized medicine, shaping the future of healthcare. Biosensors contribute significantly to the emerging field of precision medicine, where treatments are customized based on an individual's unique genetic makeup and other factors. This paradigm shift towards personalized healthcare is made possible by the accurate and real-time data generated by biosensors (Saba et al., 2020).

14.2.2 Types of Biosensors used in Medical Applications

Biosensors play a pivotal role in modern medical diagnostics, offering a diverse array of types tailored to specific applications. Enzyme-based biosensors utilize enzymes as recognition elements, often employed in glucose monitoring for diabetes. DNA-based biosensors leverage DNA strands for applications such as genetic testing. Immunoassay biosensors utilize antibodies or antigens, commonly employed in clinical diagnostics for protein and pathogen detection. Microbial biosensors use whole microbial cells, valuable in environmental monitoring and medical diagnostics (Srivastava et al., 2022).

Optical biosensors, relying on light-based detection, find applications in label-free medical diagnostics and biomolecular interaction studies. Piezoelectric biosensors measure changes in mass or density, crucial in detecting molecular interactions. Electrochemical biosensors measure changes in electrical properties, commonly used in point-of-care diagnostics. Nanomaterial-based biosensors leverage nanomaterials for enhanced sensitivity and selectivity in various applications. These diverse biosensor types highlight the adaptability of this technology, offering a range of solutions for precise and targeted medical diagnostics, catering to the intricacies of different healthcare needs (Cutitoi, 2022).

14.2.3 Examples of Biosensors in Real-World Healthcare Scenarios

Biosensors have demonstrated their versatility in real-world healthcare scenarios, providing innovative solutions for diagnostics, monitoring, and personalized care. In glucose monitoring for diabetes management, enzyme-based biosensors are widely employed, with devices like continuous glucose monitors (CGMs) offering real-time readings, empowering individuals to manage their blood sugar levels more effectively.

In infectious disease diagnostics, immunoassay biosensors play a crucial role. Rapid diagnostic tests (RDTs) for diseases like HIV and malaria utilize antibodies as recognition elements to provide quick and reliable results, enabling timely interventions and reducing the spread of infections (Parihar et al., 2023). DNA-based biosensors find application in genetic testing and personalized medicine. For instance, in cancer diagnostics, DNA biosensors can identify specific genetic mutations or biomarkers associated with certain cancers, guiding oncologists in tailoring treatment strategies based on the individual's genetic profile. Optical biosensors, such as surface plasmon resonance (SPR) sensors, are used in studying biomolecular interactions. Researchers and healthcare professionals leverage these biosensors to understand the binding kinetics of molecules, aiding in drug discovery and the development of targeted therapies (Rachna et al., 2022).

Electrochemical biosensors, particularly in point-of-care devices, are employed for cholesterol monitoring. Portable devices utilizing electrochemical sensors allow for quick and on-the-spot assessment of cholesterol levels, facilitating preventive care measures to mitigate the risk of cardiovascular diseases.

In microbial biosensors, the application extends to environmental monitoring. Biosensors with microbial components are utilized to detect pollutants or contaminants in water sources, ensuring the safety of drinking water and environmental health. Nanomaterial-based biosensors are making strides in various applications, including detecting specific biomarkers for neurodegenerative diseases. Nanoparticle-based biosensors offer enhanced sensitivity, allowing for early detection and monitoring of conditions like Alzheimer's or Parkinson's disease.

These examples underscore the tangible impact of biosensors in addressing critical healthcare challenges, from chronic disease management to infectious disease control and personalized treatment approaches. As technology advances, biosensors continue to evolve, offering increasingly sophisticated tools to improve patient outcomes and contribute to the advancement of healthcare practices.

14.3 INTERNET OF MEDICAL THINGS (IoMT) MEDICAL DEVICES AND TECHNOLOGY IN HEALTHCARE

The internet of medical things (IoMT) represents a transformative integration of medical devices and technology into healthcare systems. IoMT connects a network of medical devices, sensors, and applications, facilitating the seamless exchange of health-related data. This interconnected ecosystem enables real-time monitoring, remote patient management, and data-driven insights for healthcare professionals. From wearable devices that monitor vital signs to smart medical implants and telemedicine platforms, IoMT enhances the efficiency of healthcare delivery, improves patient outcomes, and contributes to the shift towards proactive and personalized medicine (Singh, 2022).

The widespread adoption of IoMT also poses challenges related to data security, interoperability, and ethical considerations, underscoring the need for robust regulations and innovative solutions in this rapidly evolving landscape. IoMT represents a transformative paradigm in healthcare, revolutionizing the way medical devices and technology interact and contribute to patient care. IoMT involves the interconnectivity of medical devices and applications through networks, allowing for the seamless exchange of health data and information. Embracing this interconnected future of medical devices and technology holds the promise of a more responsive, integrated, and patient-centered healthcare landscape.

14.3.1 IoMT and its Relevance in Healthcare Industry

IoMT holds profound relevance in the healthcare industry, reshaping traditional paradigms and ushering in an era of enhanced patient care and operational efficiency. IoMT leverages interconnected medical devices, wearables, and health applications to create a network that facilitates the seamless exchange of critical health data (Tiwari and Sharma, 2022). This connectivity enables real-time monitoring and tracking of patient health metrics, offering healthcare professionals unprecedented insights into individual well-being. Remote patient monitoring, a cornerstone of IoMT, allows for timely interventions and proactive management of chronic conditions, thereby reducing hospitalizations and healthcare costs.

IoMT plays a pivotal role in preventive medicine and personalized healthcare. Wearable devices and health apps empower individuals to actively engage in their health management by providing continuous monitoring and personalized insights. This shift towards preventive and personalized care aligns with the industry's broader goals of improving health outcomes and reducing the overall burden on healthcare systems (Turner and Pera, 2021). IoMT is a transformative force in the healthcare industry, offering a pathway to more effective and patient-centric care. Its ability to harness the power of data, improve connectivity, and foster innovation positions IoMT as a cornerstone of the future healthcare landscape, promising better health outcomes, improved operational efficiency, and a more resilient and responsive healthcare system (Al-Turjman et al., 2020).

14.3.2 Integration of Biosensors into the IoMT

The integration of biosensors into IoMT marks a significant advancement in healthcare technology. Biosensors, with their ability to detect and quantify biological signals, seamlessly become a crucial component within the IoMT ecosystem. These sensors, embedded in wearables, medical devices, and point-of-care tools, enable real-time monitoring of physiological parameters and facilitate the continuous collection of health data. The IoMT harnesses this data from biosensors to create a connected healthcare environment, where information flows seamlessly between devices, networks, and data analytics platforms. This integration empowers healthcare professionals with timely, accurate insights into patients' health status, enabling personalized interventions and contributing to a more proactive and efficient healthcare system. However, it also necessitates careful attention to data security, privacy, and interoperability to ensure the responsible and effective use of biosensor-generated health information within the IoMT framework.

14.4 BENEFITS OF BIOSENSORS AND IoMT IN HEALTHCARE

The application of biosensors and IoMT in healthcare brings forth a myriad of benefits, transforming the landscape of patient care and diagnostics. Biosensors, with their ability to provide real-time, continuous monitoring of physiological parameters, offer a revolutionary approach to disease management. For instance, in the context of chronic conditions like diabetes, biosensors enable individuals to track their blood glucose levels seamlessly, facilitating proactive adjustments in treatment plans and reducing the risk of complications. This proactive approach not only improves patient outcomes but also reduces the burden on healthcare facilities, preventing unnecessary hospitalizations and lowering overall healthcare costs. The amalgamation of biosensors and IoMT contributes to the paradigm shift towards personalized medicine. The continuous stream of data generated by biosensors, when analyzed through IoMT platforms, enables healthcare professionals to tailor treatment plans based on individual patient profiles. This personalized approach enhances treatment efficacy and minimizes adverse effects, marking a departure from one-size-fits-all healthcare strategies.

The benefits extend beyond individual patient care to the optimization of healthcare workflows. The interconnected nature of IoMT devices streamlines data collection, promotes collaboration among healthcare professionals, and improves the overall efficiency of healthcare delivery. Moreover, biosensors and IoMT contribute valuable data for medical research, fostering advancements in understanding diseases, developing new therapies, and enhancing public health strategies.

14.4.1 Biosensors: Improved Patient Monitoring, Early Disease Detection and Personalized Medicine

Biosensors play a pivotal role in revolutionizing patient care by significantly enhancing monitoring capabilities, enabling early disease detection, and fostering personalized medicine. The real-time data provided by biosensors facilitates improved patient monitoring, allowing healthcare professionals to track vital signs and biomarkers continuously. This continuous monitoring not only enhances the quality of care but also enables early detection of deviations from normal health parameters, enabling timely interventions and preventing the progression of diseases.

Biosensors contribute to the paradigm of personalized medicine by providing precise and individualized health information. These devices allow for the monitoring of specific biomarkers and physiological parameters tailored to each patient, supporting healthcare providers in designing treatment plans that align with the unique characteristics of an individual's health profile. This shift towards personalized medicine ensures that interventions are targeted, maximizing efficacy while minimizing adverse effects. It represents a cornerstone in the evolution of healthcare, offering a pathway to proactive and personalized patient care. Improved monitoring, early detection, and personalized medicine collectively contribute to more effective healthcare strategies, ultimately leading to better patient outcomes and an enhanced quality of life.

14.5 CHALLENGES IN IMPLEMENTING BIOSENSORS AND IoMT: INTEGRATING BIOSENSORS AND IoMT INTO HEALTHCARE SYSTEMS

The implementation of biosensors and the internet of medical things (IoMT) in healthcare is not without challenges. Technical hurdles pose significant obstacles, ranging from device interoperability issues to the need for standardized data formats. Ensuring seamless communication among diverse biosensors and IoMT devices is critical for a cohesive healthcare ecosystem.

The ethical and privacy concerns also loom large because the continuous and interconnected nature of IoMT raises questions about patient data security and privacy. Safeguarding sensitive health information becomes paramount to build and maintain public trust. So, developing robust regulatory frameworks addresses these concerns while fostering innovation is a delicate yet crucial task. These regulatory and compliance issues add complexity to the implementation process. Navigating diverse regulatory landscapes across regions and ensuring that biosensors and IoMT devices adhere to established standards demand concerted efforts from industry stakeholders and policymakers. The rapid evolution of biosensors and IoMT technologies necessitates ongoing training for healthcare providers to keep pace with the latest developments. Additionally, patients must be informed about the benefits and risks of these technologies, ensuring their active participation in their own healthcare journey. So, addressing these challenges requires a collaborative effort involving healthcare professionals, technology developers, regulatory bodies, and policymakers. Only through a comprehensive and multidimensional approach can the full potential of biosensors and IoMT be harnessed for the betterment of healthcare delivery.

14.5.1 Issues Related to Data Security, Privacy, and Regulatory Compliance

The integration of biosensors and IoMT into healthcare raises critical issues related to data security, privacy, and regulatory compliance. Ensuring the security of health data generated by biosensors and transmitted through IoMT devices is paramount. The interconnected nature of these technologies exposes potential vulnerabilities that could be exploited by malicious actors. Robust encryption, authentication mechanisms, and secure data storage are imperative to safeguard patient information from unauthorized access or cyber threats. Health systems must invest in state-of-the-art cybersecurity measures to protect sensitive medical data and maintain the trust of both healthcare professionals and patients.

The continuous monitoring facilitated by biosensors and IoMT devices brings forth significant privacy concerns. Patients may be apprehensive about the collection, storage, and sharing of their health information. Addressing these concerns requires transparent communication about data practices, clear consent mechanisms, and the implementation of privacy-by-design principles. Anonymization and aggregation of data, where possible, can mitigate privacy risks while still allowing for valuable insights from large datasets. The healthcare industry is subject to a complex web of regulations and compliance standards. Implementing biosensors and IoMT devices necessitates adherence to these regulations. Achieving regulatory compliance involves meticulous attention to data handling practices, consent management, and cybersecurity measures. Non-compliance not only risks legal consequences but also erodes public trust, which is foundational to successful healthcare technology adoption.

14.6 FUTURISTIC APPROACHES AND INNOVATIONS

Futuristic approaches in the integration of biosensors and IoMT hold the promise of transforming healthcare in unprecedented ways. One key avenue is the exploration of advanced biosensor designs, including the incorporation of nanotechnology and novel materials. Nanoscale biosensors offer enhanced sensitivity and specificity, enabling the detection of biomarkers at even lower concentrations. This could revolutionize early disease detection and monitoring, particularly in conditions like cancer, where early intervention is critical.

The advancements in implantable biosensors are also poised to play a transformative role. These devices, capable of continuous monitoring within the body, could provide invaluable insights into organ function, medication effectiveness, and disease progression. This could revolutionize the management of chronic conditions and significantly improve the quality of life for patients.

As it looks to the future, the integration of biosensors and IoMT will likely extend beyond traditional healthcare settings. Smart homes equipped with biosensor-driven technologies could create an environment that actively supports health and wellness, detecting early signs of health issues and adjusting the living space accordingly. These futuristic approaches also bring forth ethical considerations, including privacy concerns, the responsible use of AI, and ensuring equitable access to these technologies. Striking a balance between innovation and ethical implementation will be crucial in realizing the full potential of these futuristic approaches, ensuring that they contribute to a healthcare landscape characterized by enhanced diagnostics, personalized care, and improved patient outcomes.

14.6.1 Emerging Trends and Technologies in Biosensors and IoMT for Healthcare

Emerging trends and technologies in biosensors and IoMT are reshaping the landscape of healthcare. Nanotechnology is playing a pivotal role in refining biosensor designs, allowing for enhanced sensitivity and precision in detecting biomarkers. The integration of biosensors with artificial intelligence (AI) is a transformative trend, enabling advanced data analytics for more accurate diagnostics and predictive insights. Implantable biosensors are emerging as a cutting-edge technology, offering continuous monitoring within the body and providing valuable data for chronic disease management.

14.6.2 Potential Future Developments and Their Impact on Healthcare Delivery

The potential future developments in healthcare are driven by emerging technologies, hold the promise of transformative impacts on healthcare delivery. Precision medicine, empowered by advanced genomic and biomarker research, may revolutionize treatment strategies, tailoring interventions to individual genetic profiles. The integration of artificial intelligence (AI) and machine learning in diagnostics and treatment planning is poised to enhance accuracy and efficiency, enabling more personalized and effective healthcare. Telemedicine, further refined and expanded, has the potential to bring healthcare to remote areas, improving accessibility and reducing healthcare disparities. Wearable technologies and the internet of medical things (IoMT) may evolve to become even more integral, enabling continuous monitoring and proactive health management. Additionally, breakthroughs in regenerative medicine and gene therapies hold promise for innovative treatments and even potential cures for certain conditions. While these developments offer unprecedented opportunities, ethical considerations, data security, and the equitable distribution of these advancements will be crucial to ensuring that the future of healthcare benefits all segments of society.

14.7 CONCLUDING OBSERVATIONS AND FUTURE SCOPE

Biosensors and IoMT represent a pivotal shift in healthcare, offering unprecedented opportunities and challenges. The continuous monitoring facilitated by biosensors, coupled with the interconnectedness of IoMT, holds immense potential for proactive and personalized healthcare. Real-time data acquisition, early disease detection, and improved patient outcomes are just a glimpse of the transformative impacts witnessed thus far. Though, as with any technological advancement, careful considerations must be given to ethical, privacy, and regulatory concerns. The responsible use of patient data, transparent communication, and the establishment of robust security measures are essential to foster trust among patients and healthcare stakeholders.

The future scope of biosensors and IoMT is boundless. Advancements in nanotechnology, artificial intelligence, and telemedicine are poised to amplify the capabilities of these technologies. The emergence of smart homes, implantable biosensors, and further integration with wearable devices open new frontiers for continuous health monitoring and disease management. So, future developments in healthcare will likely be characterized by precision medicine, driven by the convergence of biosensors, genomic research, and personalized treatment strategies. The potential for regenerative medicine and gene therapies to redefine treatment modalities is on the horizon.

REFERENCES

Al-Turjman, F., Nawaz, M. H., & Ulusar, U. D. (2020). Intelligence in the internet of medical things era: A systematic review of current and future trends. *Computer Communications*, *150*, 644–660.

Bhambri, P., Singh, M., Jain, A., Dhanoa, I. S., Sinha, V. K., & Lal, S. (2021). Classification of the GENE expression data with the aid of optimized feature selection. *Turkish Journal of Physiotherapy and Rehabilitation*, *32*(3), 1158–1167.

Blazek, R., Hrosova, L., & Collier, J. (2022). Internet of medical things-based clinical decision support systems, smart healthcare wearable devices, and machine learning algorithms in COVID-19 prevention, screening, detection, diagnosis, and treatment. *American Journal of Medical Research*, *9*(1), 65–80.

Bose, M. M., Yadav, D., Bhambri, P., & Shankar, R. (2021). Electronic customer relationship management: Benefits and pre-implementation considerations. *Journal of Maharaja Sayajirao University of Baroda*, *55*(01(VI)), 1343–1350.

Cuţitoi, A. C. (2022). Remote patient monitoring systems, wearable internet of medical things sensor devices, and deep learning-based computer vision algorithms in COVID-19 screening, detection, diagnosis, and treatment. *American Journal of Medical Research*, *9*(1), 129–144.

Dwivedi, R., Mehrotra, D., & Chandra, S. (2022). Potential of internet of medical things (IoMT) applications in building a smart healthcare system: A systematic review. *Journal of Oral Biology and Craniofacial Research*, *12*(2), 302–318.

Irkham, I., Ibrahim, A. U., Pwavodi, P. C., Al-Turjman, F., & Hartati, Y. W. (2023). Smart graphene-based electrochemical nanobiosensor for clinical diagnosis. *Sensors*, *23*(4), 2240.

Jangra, P., & Gupta, M. (2018, August). A design of real-time multilayered smart healthcare monitoring framework using IoT. In *2018 International Conference on Intelligent and Advanced System (ICIAS)* (pp. 1–5). IEEE.

Johnson, A. (2020). Medical wearables and biosensor technologies as tools of internet of things-based health monitoring systems. *American Journal of Medical Research*, *7*(1), 7–13.

Manickam, P., Mariappan, S. A., Murugesan, S. M., Hansda, S., Kaushik, A., Shinde, R., & Thipperudraswamy, S. P. (2022). Artificial intelligence (AI) and internet of medical things (IoMT) assisted biomedical systems for intelligent healthcare. *Biosensors*, *12*(8), 562.

Mbunge, E., Muchemwa, B., & Batani, J. (2021). Sensors and healthcare 5.0: Transformative shift in virtual care through emerging digital health technologies. *Global Health Journal*, *5*(4), 169–177.

Parihar, A., Yadav, S., Sadique, M. A., Ranjan, P., Kumar, N., Singhal, A., & Srivastava, A. K. (2023). Internet-of-medical-things integrated point-of-care biosensing devices for infectious diseases: Toward better preparedness for futuristic pandemics. *Bioengineering & Translational Medicine*, e10481.

Pateraki, M., Fysarakis, K., Sakkalis, V., Spanoudakis, G., Varlamis, I., Maniadakis, M., & Koutsouris, D. (2020). Biosensors and internet of things in smart healthcare applications: Challenges and opportunities. *Wearable and Implantable Medical Devices*, 25–53.

Phan, D. T., Nguyen, C. H., Nguyen, T. D. P., Tran, L. H., Park, S., Choi, J., & Oh, J. (2022). A flexible, wearable, and wireless biosensor patch with internet of medical things applications. *Biosensors*, *12*(3), 139.

Rachna, Bhambri, P., & Chhabra, Y. (2022). Deployment of distributed clustering approach in WSNs and IoTs. In *Cloud and Fog Computing Platforms for Internet of Things* (pp. 85–98). Chapman and Hall/CRC.

Saba, T., Haseeb, K., Ahmed, I., & Rehman, A. (2020). Secure and energy-efficient framework using internet of medical things for e-healthcare. *Journal of Infection and Public Health*, *13*(10), 1567–1575.

Sangwan Singh, Y., Lal, S., Bhambri, P., Kumar, A., & Dhanoa, I. S. (2021). Advancements in social data security and encryption: A review. *Natural Volatiles & Essential Oils*, *8*(4), 15353–15362.

Sharma, A., & Singh, B. (2022). Measuring impact of E-commerce on small scale business: A systematic review. *Journal of Corporate Governance and International Business Law*, *5*(1).

Singh, B. (2022). Relevance of agriculture-nutrition linkage for human healthcare: A conceptual legal framework of implication and pathways. *Justice and Law Bulletin*, *1*(1), 44–49.

Singh, M., Bhambri, P., Dhanoa, I. S., Jain, A., & Kaur, K. (2021). Data mining model for predicting diabetes. *Annals of the Romanian Society for Cell Biology*, *25*(4), 6702–6712.

Srivastava, J., Routray, S., Ahmad, S., & Waris, M. M. (2022). Internet of medical things (IoMT)-based smart healthcare system: Trends and progress. *Computational Intelligence and Neuroscience, 2022*.

Stone, D., Michalkova, L., & Machova, V. (2022). Machine and deep learning techniques, body sensor networks, and internet of things-based smart healthcare systems in COVID-19 remote patient monitoring. *American Journal of Medical Research*, *9*(1), 97–112.

Tiwari, S., & Sharma, N. (2022). Idea, architecture, and applications of 5G enabled IoMT systems for smart health care system. *ECS Transactions*, *107*(1), 5499.

Turner, D., & Pera, A. (2021). Wearable internet of medical things sensor devices, big healthcare data, and artificial intelligence-based diagnostic algorithms in real-time COVID-19 detection and monitoring systems. *American Journal of Medical Research*, *8*(2), 132–145.

Verma, D., Singh, K. R., Yadav, A. K., Nayak, V., Singh, J., Solanki, P. R., & Singh, R. P. (2022). Internet of things (IoT) in nano-integrated wearable biosensor devices for healthcare applications. *Biosensors and Bioelectronics: X*, *11*, 100153.

15 An Application of Hybrid Machine Learning Framework to Predict the Heart Diseases in Smart Healthcare Systems

Biswajit Tripathy, Sujit Bebortta, Subhranshu Sekhar Tripathy and Tien Anh Tran

15.1 INTRODUCTION

As the incidence of illnesses rises (caused by complex interactions between genetic and lifestyle factors) [1], the use of highly specialized technologies to analyze clinical data is becoming more important than ever. Heart disease is one of the most significant threats to one's health, despite the fact that there are many other health issues. It is the main cause of death on a global scale. The World Health Organization (WHO) considers coronary artery heart disease (CAHD) to be a public health problem because it is responsible for the deaths of about millions of people each year. In its most basic form, heart disease is characterized by an obstruction in the regular functioning of the heart [2, 3]. One of the potential causes of heart disease is the constriction or complete obstruction of the coronary arteries, which are responsible for delivering blood to the heart muscle [4–6]. One even more alarming facet of coronary artery heart disease is that up to twenty-five percent of victims can suddenly die without any outward sign whatsoever [7]. This demonstrates how challenging it is to treat the illness, which is why it is important to place an emphasis on prevention. If left untreated, CAHD greatly compromises heart health and increases the risk of deadly heart attacks. Early detection of illness signs and prompt diagnosis can significantly lessen the effects of CAHD [4].

Numerous variables that raise the chance of developing heart disease have been found by researchers. The following are primary risk factors include hypertension, diabetes mellitus, raised blood cholesterol, smoking, and tobacco use [8]. Furthermore, acknowledged as risk factors, alcohol and stress are known to contribute, however it is unclear how much of a role they play or how often they are. It is crucial to emphasize that some of these risk variables may be changed, providing a way to control and intervene [9].

DOI: 10.1201/9781032698519-15

In light of the difficulties associated with predicting cardiovascular illness, machine learning (ML) becomes a crucial tool for utilizing the vast quantities of data produced by the healthcare industry in order to enhance forecasting precision and guide decision-making [10]. Much research in the domain of AI highlights the effectiveness of methods for improving the precision of categorization issues, particularly in the realm of medicine [11]. A statistical computational intelligence method called logistic regression (LR) is ideally suited for predictive analysis, particularly when dealing with binary dependent variables. Its uses cover a wide range of medical issues and difficulties.

A standard method to computational intelligence in contemporary research is the use of support vector machines (SVMs). In supervised learning, SVMs perform exceptionally well in regression and classification problems, as well as in the identification of outliers. This is the best application for SVMs. The results are outstanding in a number of different categories, such as the classification of pictures or the study of bioinformatics; the classification of handwriting and textual content; and the classification of handwriting. When one is dealing with huge training datasets and a high number of input variables, a model known as random forest (RF) begins to emerge. This model is comprised of a collection of decision trees that have not been trimmed. The way it operates is very much like that of a classifier. It takes the output of several decision trees and then produces one overall class number, which is simply the average of each tree's output. But it is more likely that this would happen when the dataset is large and the variables being input are also numerous [12].

In the current stage of research, it is well known that with the powerful computation intelligence and wide applications, the Gradient Boosting classifier (GBC) is an extremely effective technique. Most of the applications for GBC are in the area of supervised learning. It is especially superior to the other approaches in solving classification difficulty, regression problems, and outlier detection. As well as using it for sorting pictures, it could also be used in bioinformatics, text classification, and the classification of content generated by people. Even more importantly, its widespread use has also been put into important applications in the field of medicine such as diagnosing or predicting heart disease. It has also been widely applied. This is an intriguing result since the GBC shows a tendency to perform better than other classification methods. It is a very flexible and accurate predictor in an unfamiliar world of cardiovascular health prediction modeling [13]. The effectiveness of artificial intelligence techniques is investigated from four different points of view in this study including: LR, SVM, GBC, DT. Given how difficult it is to predict heart disease, the researchers went one step further and designed a hybrid classifier. This new approach also incorporates a stacking strategy to increase the accuracy of prediction. By combining the best parts of several different models into an ensemble method. In addition, there is a specialized method that combines Level 0 models (stacking LR, SVM, and GBC) with Random Forest classifier at Level 1 to increase the accuracy of prediction. For the purpose of improving CAHD prediction, this stacking method along with the use of different model advantages within a layered framework are employed.

The results of the research also clearly demonstrate that the suggested hybrid model is effective. Its accuracy rate can achieve as high as 82.608 percent. Moreover, precision and sensitivity measurements for the model are 80.7 percent and 92.3 percent respectively, making its correctness even more securely grounded. This compelling data nevertheless shows that hybrid classifiers can help predict coronary artery heart disease to a high level of accuracy. So, this is a critical juncture between machine learning and medical analytics.

15.1.1 Contributions

This study is to determine whether our proposed model is efficient in predicting heart illness, with comparison to four widely used machine learning models: LR, SVM, DT, and GBC. The aim of this study is to perform a thoroughly comparison between proposed hybrid techniques and traditional benchmark methodologies.

15.1.2 Benchmark Techniques

This comparative analysis contrasts the proposed hybrid machine learning approach with four benchmark approaches, each utilizing a different model for making predictions [14]. Among the widely used benchmark machine learning classifiers, we have used SVM, DT, GBC, and LR, which are relatively less complex and more comprehensible. Thus, they serve as a method of testing the effectiveness of this new hybrid technique.

15.1.3 Innovation

This work surpasses a basic benchmark and introduces an unparalleled machine learning stacking approach. The primary objective of this innovative approach is to enhance the precision and efficacy in forecasting cardiovascular ailments. The comparative study explicitly evaluates the novel stacking model in relation to each benchmark approach, allowing us to ascertain the specific areas in which it can enhance prediction results for cardiovascular health.

15.1.4 Organization

The article is organized in the following manner:

Section 15.2: We take a look at the research that is being conducted on heart disease by a number of different academics in this section.

Section 15.3: This section clarifies the machine learning techniques used in this study and offers a thorough discussion of the technical and basic components.

Section 15.4: In this part, the whole methodology—including data preparation and collection—is described. It looks at the analysis of experimental results in great detail.

Section 15.5: This part carefully looks at the results that arise from the assessments of the experiments. It provides a comparison of the accuracy of several models, including the suggested model.

Section 15.6–15.8: A thorough summary of the main findings and conclusions wraps up the study. It also highlights the beneficial effects of this research on healthcare support systems and offers suggestions for future research endeavors, outlining possible directions for more study.

15.2 RELATED WORK

The health of people depends greatly on medical research. Even tiny errors could lead to gravely serious consequences or even death [15, 16]. The most crucial component and major barrier is the accurate diagnosis and classification of disorders (such as heart disease or other conditions). Many have studied how to best use machine learning (ML) models as diagnostic aides in the identification of coronary heart disease. Preprocessing techniques combined with the Random Forest (RF) classification algorithm were used by Gupta et al. [17], and they managed an excellent score of 96.9 percent on the Cleveland dataset. Its contribution helps emphasize the importance of robust prediction models in healthcare. Guan et al. [18] constructed a system entirely based on SVM that could accurately identify cardiac disease. By this alternative approach, the 76.5 percent accuracy rate was attained. This study examines different Support Vector Machine (SVM) algorithms, stressing that disease classification involves a subtle understanding of model selection. Dwivedi [19], used LR in their classification model on the Cleveland dataset to achieve an accuracy of 85 percent. This reflects the many techniques of machine learning employed in diagnosing cardiac disease. Classification system Kumar and Inbarani [20] used Particle Swarm Optimization (PSO) as a novel approach to detect coronary heart disease. Rabbi et al. [21] obtained several ranges of accuracy by applying different machine learning techniques and optimizing features. The highest accuracy of 91.94 percent was reached by the backpropagation method. SVM, KNN, and ANN were compared in their study to evaluate their performance. As it turns out, SVM performed better than the other two methods with its accuracy rate of 85 percent. This points to the need for care in evaluating different machine learning models when applied in healthcare. Amin et al. [22] achieved an even more impressive accuracy of 87.4 percent by employing a new hybrid technique that couples Naïve Bayes and LR. By bringing attention to outstanding features, the process of improving diagnostic accuracy continues.

By using a variety of feature selection methods and classification strategies, Shilaskar and Ghatol [23] showed that SVM, when combined with optimization approaches, greatly increased accuracy to over 85 percent. With an astounding 92 percent accuracy, Ali et al. [24] presented a stacked SVM-based authority system for heart failure analysis. Their two-step model, which combines prediction with feature reduction, demonstrates the power of advanced ML architectures. Using the Cleveland and Statlog datasets, Fitriyani et al. [25] investigated the use of XGBOOST and DBSCAN in a classification model, obtaining excellent accuracy of 98 percent and 95 percent, respectively. Their research emphasizes how dataset selection affects model performance.

Using majority voting methodologies, Bashir et al. [26] created a system that uses SVM, Naïve Bayes, and DT with Gini Index (DT-GI) with the intention of predicting cardiac illness and reached a remarkable accuracy mark of 82 percent. Disease prediction models gain subtlety from the focus on ensemble approaches and preprocessing processes. Superior data analysis methods were shown by Islam et al. [27] in different research, with logistic regression offering the best accuracy at 86.25 percent. This study clarifies the continuous investigation of several machine learning techniques in the analysis of healthcare data. Together, these works add to the growing body of research on machine learning applications in medicine by emphasizing the significance of feature optimization, model selection, and the never-ending pursuit of increased diagnostic accuracy [28].

15.3 MACHINE LEARNING PROCEDURES

15.3.1 Logistic Regression (LR)

With its insightful and predictive powers, LR is a crucial tool in the diagnosis and prognosis of illness [29]. LR functions on actual-valued input vectors as a discriminative categorical method, making it easier to retrieve important statistical data from the model. LR is used in the context of cardiac disease to forecast a person's chance of developing the illness. Logistic regression involves a binary dependent variable, which represents data that is coded as one to indicate the occurrence of an event, such as success, and as zero to indicate its absence, such as failure. The main goal of logistic regression analysis is to estimate the logarithmic probability of the occurrence of an event.

From a mathematical perspective, the multiple linear regression functions (specified as follows) are estimated in the context of the LR model.

$$\text{Log odds} = \beta_0 + \beta_1 X_1 + \beta_2 X_2 + \cdots + \beta_n X_n$$

In this case, n is the number of features, and $\beta_0, \beta_1, \beta_2, \ldots, \beta_n$ are the coefficients corresponding to the features $X_0, X_1, X_2, \ldots, X_n$.

15.3.2 Support Vector Machine (SVM)

The main goal of the supervised learning approach SVM is to minimize generalization errors in regression and classification tasks [30]. Its categorization ability consists of dividing data into two different classes by drawing a hyperplane. Interestingly, SVM performs quite well in high-dimensional domains, demonstrating its resilience to dimensions larger than the total number of samples. All of these SVM qualities contribute to the extraordinary performance in the medical field, especially in the area of illness prediction. SVM is very effective when it comes to predicting heart disease, but it needs at least one categorical variable in the training sample in order to make it easier to assign new category values to the predicted result. SVM uses linear characteristics as a non-likelihood binary classifier to identify patterns in the data. SVM's versatility goes beyond classification and regression; it can also be used for outlier detection, which makes it a good fit for situations involving high-dimensional data.

A training vector variable in SVM is defined mathematically as:

$$X_i \in R^p, \; for \; i = 1, 2, 3, \ldots, n$$

In this case, X_i stands for a training observation, and R^p denotes the predictor vector space and real-valued p-dimensional feature space.

15.3.3 Decision Tree (DT)

Decision Trees are a well-known and comprehensible machine learning technology that provides a clear and hierarchical modeling approach for cardiovascular health parameters in the field of heart disease prediction [31, 32]. Decision trees are mathematical constructs that relate observations (X) about an object to inferences (Y) about the item's goal value. These models successfully capture complex interactions between many parameters impacting cardiovascular health in the context of heart disease prediction.

Algorithm for DT Using Heart Disease Data:

Heart Disease Data, a dataset with binary outcomes (Y) and characteristics (X), is the input.
Create Decision Tree (decision_tree = DecisionTreeClassifier())
Fit the model using (decision_tree. fit(Data on Heart Disease))
Forecast Using Decision Tree (forecast = predict(NewObservation))

Because decision trees can provide healthcare professionals with a clear structure by means of input data, making it easier for them to understand the predictions made by the model [33]. Decision Trees can help physicians identify important predictors of heart disease by drawing out decision routes relying on such variables as age, blood pressure, cholesterol levels, and lifestyle choices.

This is because cardiac illnesses are very complicated, and factors such as lifestyle choices, family history, and clinical markers play key roles. The adaptability of decision trees therefore become extremely important. For a variety of patient data, decision trees are very flexible: They can handle both numerical and categorical information mathematically. To build a tree-like structure, the decision tree method breaks down the analyzed data according to input attributes [34]. The dataset is divided into smaller groups; decisions are made at each internal node based on different features. The process continues until a stopping requirement is satisfied, producing leaf nodes that indicate the final categorization. They also could help medical practitioners to decide which is the most effective form of therapy by highlighting essential characteristics and ranking their significance in predicting cardiac disease. The problem is overfitting causes them to record noise instead of true patterns. These effects can be reduced by regularization and pruning procedures, but with respect to the particular task of predicting cardiac disease, we need a more rigorous evaluation as to how effective they are compared with other computational intelligence techniques.

15.3.4 Gradient Boosting Classifier (GBC)

For the prediction of heart disease, GBC, introduced by Friedman [35], is a new kind of ensemble learning method in which error correction between weak learners combines to produce accuracy. The GBC process is a mathematical series of iterative processes designed to gradually enhance the model's performance:

1. Initialization: For each observation X, let $F_0\ (X)$ be the initial prediction, which is often a straightforward weak learner. The residuals are calculated as $r_0 = Y - F_0\ (X)$, where Y is the binary outcome variable that denotes the presence or absence of cardiac disease.
2. Sequential Model Building: Create a new weak learner, $h_n\ (X)$, for every iteration n in order to forecast the residuals, r_{n-1}. To update the model, add the forecasts together: The learning rate, denoted as v, is a hyperparameter that governs the influence of every weak learner—$F_n(X) = F_{n-1}\ (X) + v \times h_n\ (X)$ is obtained.
3. Gradient Descent:

   —The pseudo-residuals are defined as $R_n = \dfrac{\delta K\left(Y, F_{n-1}(X)\right)}{\delta F_{n-1}(X)}$, In this case,

   K symbolizes the loss function that quantifies the variation between the anticipated and exact values.
   —Adjust a struggling student to the pseudo-residuals:

   $$h_n(X) = arg\ \min_h \sum_j K\left(Y_j, F_{n-1}(X_j)\right) + h_n(X_j).$$

   —Revise the model: $F_n\ (X) = F_{n-1}\ (X) + v \times h_n\ (X)$.
4. Iteration: The Gradient Descent and Sequential Model Building methods must be repeated for a given number of times or until the convergence condition is satisfied.

Using the GBC has many advantages in heart disease prediction. It's really good at finding intricate relationships between patient data and is able to provide a pretty complete picture of the causes, with how different factors are related to the chances of heart disease. Because the algorithm has an iterative structure, it not only makes its predicted accuracy excellent but also allows it to handle complex relationships and prevent overfitting. Using GBC's intrinsic feature significance measurement, healthcare practitioners can discern the important factors influencing prognosis for heart disease. In short, the GBC is a powerful tool in the arsenal of predictive modeling for heart disease. The model can make more effective predictions, and the whole is better than its parts. It uses ensemble learning [32].

15.3.5 Random Forest Classifier

The Random Forest classifier is a particularly effective and flexible machine learning technique that is especially suitable for predicting cardiovascular disease. The Random Forest approach creates a number of decision trees, and takes the average of their results to make predictions more accurate, like an ensemble of decision trees. As for prognosis of cardiac disease, this method has several advantages. It manages the crowded relations between age, blood pressure, cholesterol, and other risk variables of cardiovascular. Random Forest avoids overfitting by averaging the predictions of many decision trees, making a model more robust and widely usable. Furthermore, the algorithm provides a natural means for measuring feature contribution. Medical experts can then decide how much each parameter contributes to predicting heart disease. The feature importance displayed by the Random Forest classifier also makes it possible to provide more accurate and understandable predictions for effective clinical decision-making, as well as handling nonlinear relationships and missing data. This thus makes it a good analytical tool in the field of cardiovascular health [35].

15.3.6 User Classification Based on Stacking Classifier

When using machine learning to forecast cardiac disease, there are many processes required in putting a stacking model into practice [36]. Another ensemble learning method known as stacking combines many models to improve its overall predictive power. Here we will explain how to build a stacking model with RF at Level 1 and DT, Logistic Regression, and Support Vector Machine as Level 0 models.

Step 1: Data Preparation

1.1 Data Collection: Collect a complete data set containing all relevant characteristics in connection with heart health, including risk factors and medical history.

1.2 Data Cleaning: Deal with outliers, missing numbers, and any other aberrations in the dataset. Also, be concerned with data consistency.

1.3 Feature Scaling: Normalize or standardize the numerical characteristics to get a single scale.

Step 2: Data Splitting

2.1 Train-Test Split: The dataset must be split into separate training and testing sets to test the effectiveness of any model on data which has not previously been observed.

Step 3: Training for Level 0 Models:

3.1 Logistic Regression (LR) Training for Level 0 Models: To predict heart disease, train the initial base model LR using training data.

3.2 Support Vector Machine (SVM): Train SVM to recognize complex structures in the data and classify examples according to their features.

3.3 Decision Tree (DT): A decision tree can be used to determine whether there are any non-linearities and interactions in a data set.
3.4 Gradient Boosting classifier (GBC): Teach GBC to assemble a weak learner ensemble that corrects previous errors one by.

Step 4: Prediction of Level 0 Models

4.1 LR Prediction: With the trained LR model, predict on test set.
4.2 SVM Prediction: With the same test set, make predictions from SVM model.
4.3 DT Prediction: Here we use the DT model to predict test set results.
4.4 GBC Prediction: Using the GBC, generate forecasts based on the test set.

Step 5: Level 1 Model Training

5.1 Feature Engineering: Add the initial features with the Level 0 models' predictions to produce enhanced feature set.
5.2 Random Forest (RF): Get more features. Add the Level 0 model predictions to a larger feature set and train your Random Forest classifier.

Step 6: Predict the Level 1 Model (RF Prediction Set)

Using what we learned from Level 0 model, take RF classifier trained before and make predictions on test set.

Step 7: Stack Model Assessment

Test the effectiveness of the stacking model using appropriate evaluation metrics, such as precision, accuracy, recall, and F1 score.

The main stages for using a stacking model in machine learning to evaluate heart illness are described in this process. It places a strong emphasis on integrating many models at various scales in order to maximize their combined predictive ability and improve overall accuracy.

15.4 METHODOLOGY

In this research we have divide the experiments into following four steps

15.4.1 Data Collection

Originally obtained from the UCI machine learning repository database, the Cleveland Clinic Heart Disease Dataset was utilized in this study. It was acquired via the open-source Kaggle website. There are 14 characteristics in all in this dataset, which includes data from 303 patients. The age range of the patient population is 29 to 77 years old, with 206 men and 97 females. Table 15.1 shows the attribute information for the dataset considered in the study.

TABLE 15.1
Attribute Information for the Dataset Considered in the Study

	Attributes Name	Description
1.	Age in years	Falls between 29 and 77.
2.	Sex	• The value of one is representative of the male gender, whereas the value of zero corresponds to the female gender.
3.	Chest Pain(cp) type	• There are four classifications for chest pain symptoms: 1) classic angina, 2) atypical angina, 3) non-anginal pain, and 4) asymptomatic.
4.	Hospital admission resting blood pressure (trestbps) in millimeter-Hg	Ranges from 94–200.
5.	serum cholesterol (chol) in mg/dl	Ranges from 126–564.
6.	The fasting blood sugar (FBS) level is more than 120 mg/dL	• The value of one represents a state of truth, whereas a value of zero represents a state of falsehood.
7.	Resting electrocardiographic results (restecg)	• The customary value is zero. • A value of one indicates the presence of abnormal ST-T wave patterns, characterized by T wave inversions and/or ST segment elevation or depression above 0.05 mV. • According to Estes' criterion, a value of two indicates the presence of probable or conclusive left ventricular hypertrophy.
8.	Peak heart rate attained (thalach)	Varies between 71 and 202.
9.	Exercise induced angina (exang)	• The value of one represents an affirmative response, whereas the value of zero signifies a negative response.
10.	Exercise-induced ST depression compared to rest (oldpeak)	Ranges from 0.0 to 6.2.
11.	The gradient of the peak workout ST section (slope)	• The value of one indicates an upward slope, whereas the value of two indicates a level surface. • The term "3 means down sloping" refers to a phenomenon characterized by a downward trend or slope.
12.	Quantity of main blood vessels (ca) seen with fluoroscopy	Varies between zero and three.
13.	Results of nuclear stress test (thal)	• Three means usual value, that is, normal. • Six means fixed defect. • Seven means reversable defect.
14.	The variable of interest that indicates the diagnosis of heart illness in any major artery (angiographic disease state) (num)	• Zero which means < 50% diameter narrowing. • One which means > 50% diameter narrowing.

15.4.2 Performance Measure

One helpful matrix for illustrating the efficacy of computational intelligence techniques is a confusion matrix. This matrix has four major categorization performance indices, each with a unique definition: Cases that are correctly rejected are indicated by False Positive (fps), cases that are incorrectly rejected are indicated by False Negative (fns), and instances that are correctly recognized are indicated by True Positive (tps). A comprehensive assessment of these characteristics is a step in the system performance evaluation process [37, 38].

15.4.3 Accuracy

One key indicator of a classification model's overall soundness is its correctness. The computation involves the division of the entire number of occurrences, containing both accurate and faulty predictions, by the sum of the tps and tns values. The mathematical formula for calculating accuracy is (tps + tns)/(tps + tns+ fps+ fns). This expression gives a thorough assessment of the model's predictive power across all classes [37].

15.4.4 Precision

Precision is the most important feature of a model, in terms of its positive estimates. It is calculated by dividing the tps count by the sum of tps and fns. If the cost of a false positive is high, then precision becomes an important aspect because it indicates how precisely the model reduces its estimated number of false positives. Precision: tps/(tps + fps) [37, 38].

15.4.5 Sensitivity/Recall

Sensitivity specifies how well a model captures each and every case that is positive in a dataset. Sometimes, it is called recall or true positives rate. The result comes from dividing the tps count by the sum of tps and fns. In situations in which overlooking good things can have enormous repercussions, sensitivity is critical. This can be expressed mathematically as tps/(tps + fns) [38].

15.4.6 Specificity

The specificity of a model indicates how well it can detect negative examples. The tns is obtained by dividing it into the sum of the two numbers: True negative and false positive. If the goal is to reduce or minimize false positives, specificity becomes important. The concept of specificity can be mathematically expressed as tns/(tns + fps).

15.4.7 F1 Score

A comprehensive indicator which bridges the gap between sensitivity and precision, F1 score provides a complete assessment of a model's overall performance. It is most useful in cases where classes are unevenly distributed. The F1 score is constructed using the formula, 2 * (precision*sensitivity)/(precision+ sensitivity), which emphasizes both precision and sensitivity measurements in a single figure [38].

15.4.8 ROC Curve

A number of visual representations that demonstrate the efficacy for a categorization model over different discriminating thresholds is, for example, the Receiver Operating Characteristic (ROC) curve. For problems involving dichotomous classification it is most helpful. The ROC curve shows the relationship between sensitivity (real positive rate) and one—specificity (false positive rate), at different thresholds of discrimination. With this graphic representation, we can examine the class-specificity of a model in some depth, as well as gaining useful information about the trade-offs involved in sacrificing sensitivity for specificity. The larger the area under the ROC curve (AUC), the better discriminating performance is, and thus indicates greater ability to correctly classify occurrences.

15.4.9 Data Preprocessing

These data contain numerous missing and unwanted variables, raising the specter of incorrect analytical results. To minimize the consequences, a proactive strategy was adopted to deal with the missing data marked by NaN. Missing values were replaced by the average of those obtained from corresponding columns. This systematic approach was designed to make the dataset more complete, which in turn would ensure that the analytical results were reliable.

Additionally, the dataset's class distribution attributes (also known as label attributes) were analyzed. These qualities also have values ranging from zero to three, interestingly enough. It was decided to standardize the labels in order to speed up work on categorization and make for a more concentrated examination. One was always substituted for all values during this standardization of procedure, except zero. The purpose of this change was to create a two-category classification system: Normal (Label 0) versus possible heart disease risk (Label 1). This tactical adjustment not only improved the study of heart disease prediction in terms of its effectiveness and readability, but also increased the efficiency with which predictions could be made.

15.5 THE FINDINGS AND FURTHER ANALYSIS

15.5.1 Experimental Configuration

The programming language used for the experimental processes was Python version 3.10.9. The studies were run on a single computing machine to guarantee a thorough and precise explanation of the outcomes. In particular, a Lenovo 7 computer system with a 12th Generation Intel(R) Core (TM) i7–1260P CPU clocked at 2.10 GHz was used for these investigations. The machine demonstrated improved processing speed along with logical capabilities owing to its significant 16 GB of RAM. The machine learning algorithms were implemented, and the outcomes were then evaluated in a stable and favorable environment thanks to the Windows 11 operating system, which was used for the trials. The purpose of this comprehensive setup is to guarantee repeatability and contextual comprehension of the experimental results by being transparent about the computer environment.

15.5.2 Results Analysis

The correlation matrix pertaining to different attributes of the considered heart disease dataset is shown in Figure 15.1.

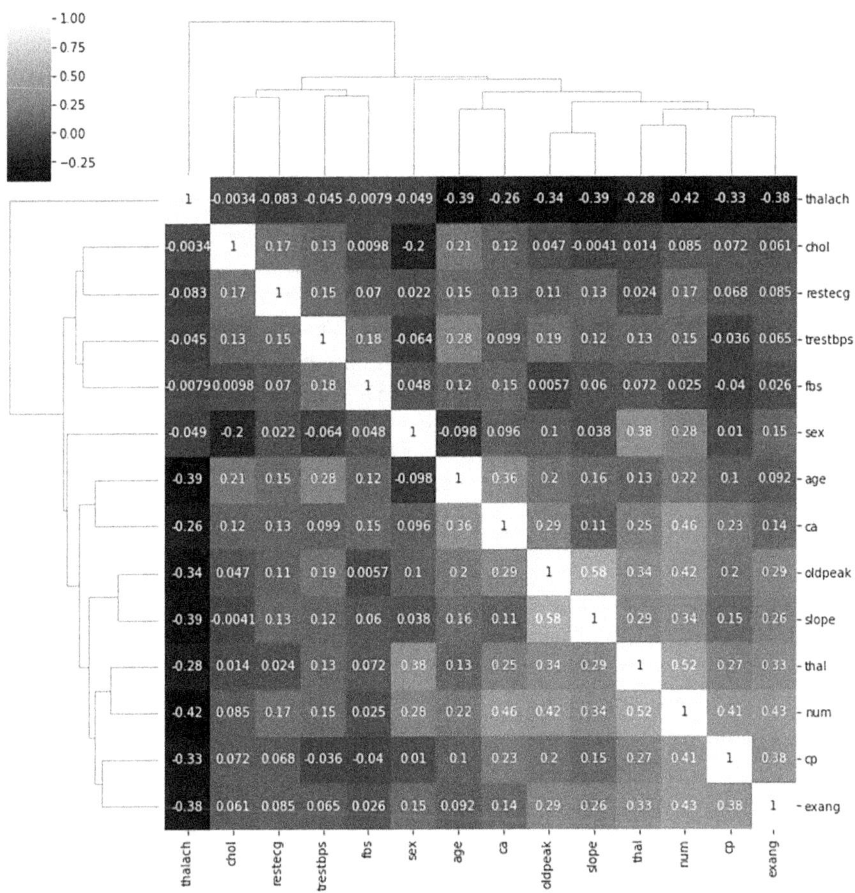

FIGURE 15.1 Correlation matrix for different attributes of the dataset.

15.5.3 Performance Evaluation of Classification Models

The findings shown in Table 15.2 appear to reflect the machine learning models' performance measures when used to forecast cardiac disease. Let's dissect the conversation:

- Logistic regression seems to function rather effectively in every metric. The model has strong precision and recall balance together with great accuracy.
- In comparison to logistic regression, the Decision Tree classifier exhibits somewhat lower accuracy and appears to have a higher recall at the price of precision. It appears that this model may not be the greatest match for the data based on the negative R2 score.
- Concerning about precision and R2 score, the SVC seems to be performing below par. The model is not effectively capturing the variation in the data, as indicated by the negative R2 score.
- The Gradient Boosting classifier has strong performance, exhibiting a solid balance between precision and recall, along with a reasonably high accuracy. However, the R2 score is still negative, showing that there could be space for improvement.

The particular objectives and specifications of the application determine which model is best. For example, even at the expense of precision, the model with the highest recall—that is, the one that accurately identifies people with heart disease—might be chosen. Additional refinement and optimization of hyperparameters may improve these models' performance. Considerations for cross-validation and feature engineering are also crucial. Interpreting these findings in light of the dataset and the unique difficulties associated with heart disease prediction is essential. Engaging in consultations with subject matter experts can yield significant insights for refining the models and comprehending the therapeutic significance of the outcomes. Therefore, even if the models exhibit different degrees of effectiveness, there is still opportunity for development and a need to carefully weigh the particular objectives and trade-offs within the framework of predicting cardiac disease. Precision-Recall curves for the considered dataset for benchmark ML models are shown in Figure 15.2. ROC curves for the considered dataset for benchmark ML models are shown in Figure 15.3.

TABLE 15.2
Performance Comparison of Benchmark Classification Models

	LR	DT Classifier	SVC	GBC
Accuracy	0.78260	0.71739	0.58695	0.73913
Precision	0.78571	0.72413	0.60606	0.73333
Recall	0.84615	0.80769	0.76923	0.84615
R^2 Score	0.11538	–0.15000	–0.68076	–0.06153
F1 Score	0.81481	0.76363	0.67796	0.78571

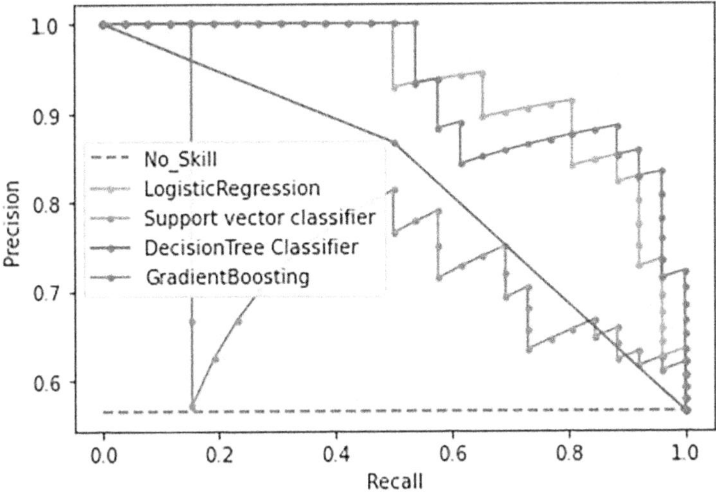

FIGURE 15.2 Precision-Recall curves for the considered dataset for benchmark ML models.

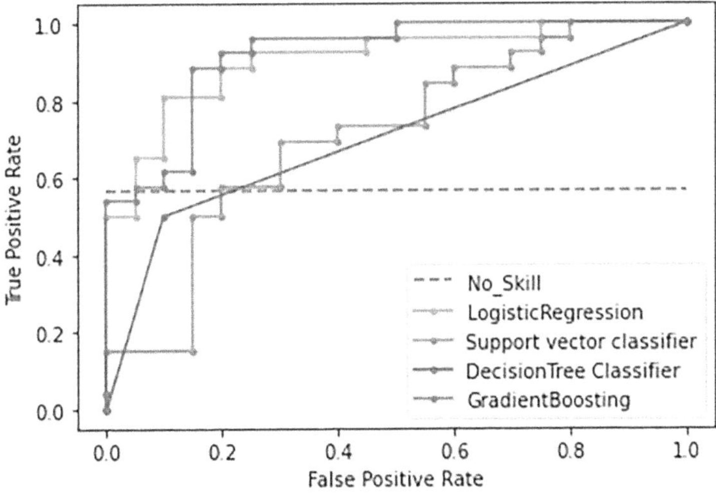

FIGURE 15.3 ROC curves for the considered dataset for benchmark ML models.

15.5.4 Performance Evaluation of Proposed Models

As shown in Table 15.3, stacking seems to be a promising option for predicting heart disease, since it provides a comprehensive enhancement over individual models for accuracy, precision, recall, and R2 score.

In Table 15.3, it is clear that, the Stacking model performs better than any other single model. It exhibits the best F1 score, memory, accuracy, and precision. Additionally, the R^2 score shows that a sizable amount of the data's volatility is

TABLE 15.3

Contrasting the Suggested Algorithm's Performance Metrics with Those of Benchmark Algorithms

	LR	DT Classifier	SVC	GBC	Stacking
Accuracy	0.78260	0.71739	0.58695	0.73913	0.82608
Precision	0.78571	0.72413	0.60606	0.73333	0.8
Recall	0.84615	0.80769	0.76923	0.84615	0.92307
R^2 Score	0.11538	−0.15000	−0.68076	−0.06153	0.29230
F1 Score	0.81481	0.76363	0.67796	0.78571	0.85714

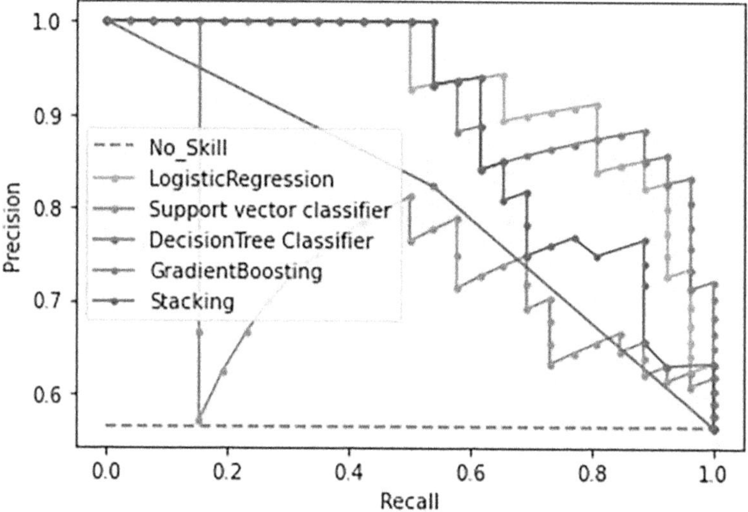

FIGURE 15.4 Precision-Recall curves over the considered dataset for proposed stacking algorithm compared with benchmark ML models.

captured. It is well known that stacking may combine the best features of several models; in this case, it seems to take advantage of the complimentary features of each model to produce better prediction performance. An important factor in a medical setting is the ability to properly identify people with heart disease, and the stacking model shows a considerable increase in memory in this regard. The combined model appears to explain more of the variation in the data, as indicated by the R^2 score for stacking, which shows a significant improvement above the separate models. Even if stacking produces encouraging results, it's crucial to evaluate the model on more datasets and take overfitting into account. The efficacy of the stacking ensemble also greatly relays on the models selected and their hyperparameters. Precision-Recall curves over the considered dataset for proposed stacking algorithm compared with benchmark ML models are shown in Figure 15.4. ROC curves over the considered dataset for proposed stacking algorithm compared with benchmark ML models are shown in Figure 15.5. Bar plot for comparison of different performance metrics obtained using the considered dataset for proposed stacking algorithm compared with benchmark ML models is shown in Figure 15.6.

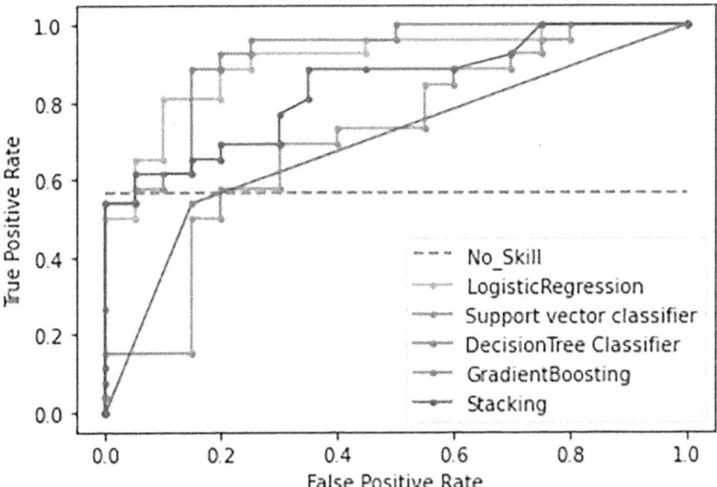

FIGURE 15.5 ROC curves over the considered dataset for proposed stacking algorithm compared with benchmark ML models.

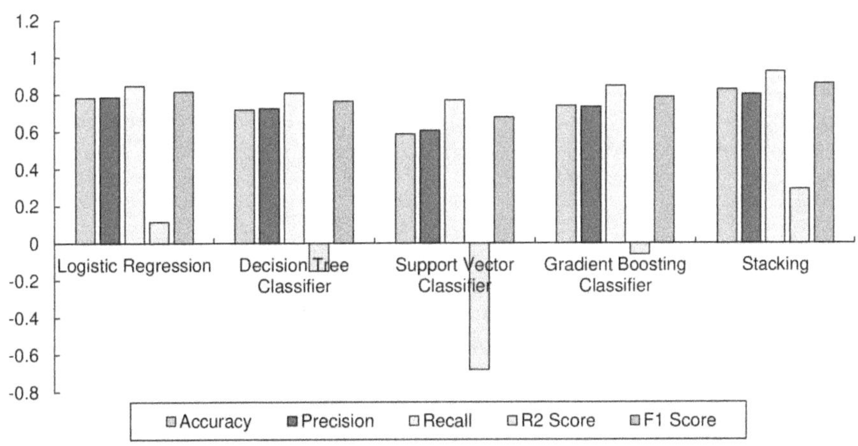

FIGURE 15.6 Bar plot for comparison of different performance metrics obtained using the considered dataset for proposed stacking algorithm compared with benchmark ML models.

15.6 LIMITATIONS

It is important to recognize several limitations that should be taken into account, even if the study provides insightful information on utilizing machine learning models and computational intelligence in the prediction of coronary artery heart disease. First off, the use of a single dataset—the Cleveland Clinic heart disease dataset—may limit the findings generalizability. The suggested hybrid model's suitability for various demographic groups and healthcare environments is still up for debate, since healthcare datasets can differ greatly in terms of clinical procedures, patient demographics, and data quality. This drawback emphasizes the necessity of more study to confirm the model's efficacy in a wider range of circumstances [32, 35].

Second, the suggested hybrid model and four well recognized techniques—LR, SVM, DT, and GBC—are the main subjects of the research. Although these techniques offer a strong basis for comparison, novel algorithms and approaches are introduced by the machine learning field, which is continually changing. The investigation of novel approaches that could supplement or surpass current methods could broaden the study's purview. A more thorough examination of cutting-edge machine learning algorithms may improve our comprehension of the best methods for predicting cardiovascular illness [36].

Furthermore, although acknowledging the difficulty of predicting cardiovascular illness in clinical data analysis, the study does not go into great detail about the models' interpretability [30]. A major disadvantage of predictive models can be their lack of interpretability, particularly in the healthcare industry where trust-building and the ease of integrating them into clinical practice depend heavily on a comprehension of the reasoning behind predictions. Enhancing the hybrid model's explainability might be beneficial for future study, since it would allow medical experts to trust and comprehend the predictions [31].

In conclusion, the research presents a hybrid classifier that employs an ensemble model with stacking, exhibiting encouraging outcomes for accuracy, precision, and sensitivity. Nevertheless, there is a lack of detailed discussion of the computational complexity and resource needs of these models. More research is necessary to determine if these models can be implemented practically and scalably in healthcare systems with different infrastructures and resource limitations. By addressing these issues, the suggested hybrid classifiers for coronary artery heart disease prediction will become more reliable and applicable in the actual world.

15.7 CHALLENGES

1. Dominance of Heart Disease: It highlights the fact that heart disease is the more prevalent and more dangerous than other illnesses, underscoring the need of treating this specific problem.
2. Global Effects of Heart Disease: The article emphasizes how heart disease affects people all over the world and is among the top causes of death, underscoring the need for efficient preventative efforts.
3. Complexity in Cardiovascular Disease Prediction: The paper highlights the challenges associated with clinical data analysis and recognizes the

complexity of predicting cardiovascular illnesses, highlighting the necessity for sophisticated methods such as machine learning.

4. Application of Machine Learning: It highlights the potential of ML in resolving healthcare issues and presents the importance of ML in the realm of healthcare, particularly in facilitating the process of making decisions and forecasting from the huge volumes of data produced by the sector.
5. Proposal for Hybrid Classifier: The article presents a unique strategy that aims to improve prediction accuracy beyond conventional methods. It does this by proposing a hybrid classifier that makes use of an ensemble model and stacking strategy.
6. Performance Assessment and Superiority: The study compares the proposed hybrid model with benchmark methods using the heart disease dataset. The study specifies that the suggested model determines higher performance in relation to the other models, outperforming them with 82.608 percent accuracy, 80.000 percent precision, and 92.307 percent sensitivity. This highlights the usefulness of the suggested hybrid classifiers for enhancing prediction outcomes.

15.8 FUTURE SCOPE

1. Advancements in Hybrid Models: The research indicated a possible opportunity to further investigate and enhance hybrid models in illness prediction using machine learning. In order to improve the accuracy of predictions, it is recommended to focus more on the ensemble model, particularly by using stacking and maybe including more sophisticated techniques or algorithms. This may include using adaptive learning algorithms or investigating the incorporation of advanced machine learning methods to enhance the resilience of the hybrid classifier across various healthcare datasets.
2. The incorporation of real-time data streams and the internet of things (IoT) in healthcare settings is a promising field for future study. The integration of dynamic predictive algorithms, which are regularly refreshed with patient data, enables the capacity to proactively and individually address evolving health issues. The use of real-time analytics has the capacity to enhance the velocity and precision of forecasting, rendering it more relevant and valuable in the swiftly changing healthcare environment.
3. Generalization to Diverse Populations: The literature explores the use of the heart disease dataset to assess the effectiveness of the suggested model. To broaden the reach and practicality of this study, it is recommended to prioritize the expansion of the demographic and healthcare contexts being examined in future studies. This will need the careful examination of the effectiveness of hybrid classifiers on datasets from various demographics, geographical locations, and healthcare systems, thereby guaranteeing the dependability and applicability of the model.
4. The need of explainability and interpretability in the predictions of machine learning models becomes more crucial as their complexity continues to increase. This is especially vital in industries like healthcare where precise

judgments are essential. Given this information, future research should emphasize improving the comprehensibility of hybrid classifiers as suggested in the study report. This entails the creation of techniques to comprehend the model's determinations and provide healthcare practitioners with discernment into the aspects that impact the forecasts. The efficacy and acceptance of these prediction models in actual clinical environments are highly dependent on the clarity and comprehension of their functioning.

15.9 CONCLUSION

In summary, this study examines an important prognostic aspect of the disease, with particular emphasis on the prevalence and high-risk area of cardiovascular disease. The results reveal complex interactions among genetic, lifestyle, and other variables that contribute to disease, which is a major health problem worldwide and cardiovascular disease, in particular stands, out as a major risk factor, as one of the prominent global causes of death. The study recognizes the complexity of cardiovascular disease prediction in clinical data analysis and the critical role of machine learning (ML) in the management of large amounts of medical information.

The effectiveness of four computer intelligence methods—GBC, DT, SVM, and LR—for prediction of cardiomyopathy can be better understood by comparing and contrasting them. The work presents a unique approach with hybrid classification that uses ensemble models and stacking strategies to address the need for increased predictive accuracy. With an impressive 82.608 percent accuracy, 80.000 percent precision, and 92.307 percent sensitivity, this novel model exemplifies the value of hybrid classifiers in the realm of predicting coronary heart disease. Rigorous evaluation approaches are used to enhance the validity of the proposed model.

The effectiveness of the suggested hybrid model motivates more research and development of similar strategies, which may open the door to the development of more precise and trustworthy forecasts in the intricate field of cardiovascular illnesses. This research shows how cutting-edge computational intelligence approaches have the potential to transform healthcare practices and ultimately improve patient outcomes as we continue to harness the power of machine learning.

REFERENCES

1. Verma, P., Tiwari, R. Hong, W. -C., Upadhyay, S., & Yeh, Y.-H. (2022). FETCH: A Deep Learning-Based Fog Computing and IoT Integrated Environment for Healthcare Monitoring and Diagnosis. *IEEE Access*, *10*, 12548–12563. doi: 10.1109/ACCESS.2022.3143793.
2. Talaat, F. M. (2022). Effective Prediction and Resource Allocation Method (EPRAM) in Fog Computing Environment for Smart Healthcare System. *Multimedia Tools and Applications*, *81*(6), 8235–8258.
3. Islam, S. M. R., Kwak, D., Kabir, M. H., Hossain, M., & Kwak, K.-S. (2015). The Internet of Things for Health Care: A Comprehensive Survey. *IEEE Access*, *3*, 678–708.
4. Rahmani, A. M., Gia, T. N., Negash, B., Anzanpour, A., Azimi, I., Jiang, M., & Liljeberg, P. (2018, January). Exploiting Smart e-Health Gateways at the Edge of Healthcare

Internet-of-Things: A Fog Computing Approach. *Future Generation Computer Systems, 78*, 641–658.
5. European Research Cluster on the Internet of Things (2014). IoT semantic interoperability: Research challenges, best practices, solutions and next steps, IERC AC4 Manifesto. *Present and Future*.
6. Xu, B., Xu, L. D., Cai, H., Xie, C., Hu, J., & Bu, F. (2014). Ubiquitous Data Accessing Method in IoT-Based Information System for Emergency Medical Services. *IEEE Transactions on Industrial Informatics, 10*(2), 1578–1586.
7. Jiang, L., Xu, L. D., Cai, H., Jiang, Z., Bu, F., & Xu, B. (2014). An IoT-Oriented Data Storage Framework in Cloud Computing Platform. *IEEE Transactions on Industrial Informatics, 10*(2), 1443–1451.
8. Faust, O., Hagiwara, Y., Hong, T. J., Lih, O. S., & Acharya, U. R. (2018). Deep Learning for Healthcare Applications Based on Physiological Signals: A Review. *Computer Methods and Programs in Biomedicine, 161*, 1–13.
9. Tuli, S., Basumatary, N., & Buyya, R. (2019). Edgelens: Deep Learning Based Object Detection in Integrated IoT, Fog and Cloud Computing Environments. In *Proceedings of the 4th IEEE International Conference on Information Systems and Computer Networks, ISCON 2019*, Mathura, India, November 21–22, IEEE Press, USA.
10. Dietterich, T. G. (2000). Ensemble Methods in Machine Learning. In *International Workshop on Multiple Classifier Systems* (pp. 1–15). Berlin, Heidelberg: Springer.
11. Tuli, S., Mahmud, R., Tuli, S., & Buyya, R. (2019, August). Fog Bus: A Blockchain-Based Lightweight Framework for Edge and Fog Computing. *Journal of Systems and Software, 154*, 22–36.
12. Wang, Y., Nazir, S., & Shafiq, M. (2021). An Overview on Analyzing Deep Learning and Transfer Learning Approaches for Health Monitoring. *Computational and Mathematical Methods in Medicine, 2021*, 1–10.
13. Ali, S., & Ghazal, M. (2017, April). Real-Time Heart Attack Mobile Detection Service (RHAMDS): An IoT Use Case for Software Defined Networks. In *Proceedings of the IEEE 30th Canadian Conference on Electrical and Computer Engineering (CCECE)*, 1–6.
14. Azimi, I., Takalo-Mattila, J., Anzanpour, A., Rahmani, A. M., Soininen, J.-P., & Liljeberg, P. (2018, September). Empowering Healthcare IoT Systems with Hierarchical Edge-Based Deep Learning. In *Proceedings of the IEEE/ACM International Conference on Connected Health: Applications, Systems, and Engineering Technologies*, 63–68.
15. Singh, M., Bhambri, P., Dhanoa, I. S., Jain, A., & Kaur, K. (2021). Data Mining Model for Predicting Diabetes. *Annals of the Romanian Society for Cell Biology, 25*(4), 6702–6712.
16. Bhambri, P., Singh, M., Jain, A., Dhanoa, I. S., Sinha, V. K., & Lal, S. (2021). Classification of the GENE Expression Data with the Aid of Optimized Feature Selection. *Turkish Journal of Physiotherapy and Rehabilitation, 32*(3), 1158–1167.
17. Gupta, A., Kumar, R., Arora, H. S., & Raman, B. (2019, December 27). MIFH: A Machine Intelligence Framework for Heart Disease Diagnosis. *IEEE Access, 8*, 14659–14674.
18. Guan, W., Gray, A., & Leyffer, S. (2009, December 2). Mixed-Integer Support Vector Machine. In *NIPS Workshop on Optimization for Machine Learning*. http://opt.kyb.tuebingen.mpg.de/papers/OPT2009-Guan.pdf
19. Dwivedi, A. K. (2018, May). Performance Evaluation of Different Machine Learning Techniques for Prediction of Heart Disease. *Neural Computing and Applications*, 29, 685–693.
20. Inbarani, H. H. (2015, January 1). A Novel Neighborhood Rough Set Based Classification Approach for Medical Diagnosis. *Procedia Computer Science, 47*, 351–359.
21. Rabbi, M. F., Uddin, M. P., Ali, M. A., Kibria, M. F., Afjal, M. I., Islam, M. S., & Nitu, A. M. (2018). Performance Evaluation of Data Mining Classification Techniques for Heart Disease Prediction. *American Journal of Engineering Research, 7*(2), 278–283.

22. Amin, M. S., Chiam, Y. K., & Varathan, K. D. (2019, March 1). Identification of Significant Features and Data Mining Techniques in Predicting Heart Disease. *Telematics and Informatics*, 36, 82–93.
23. Shilaskar, S., & Ghatol, A. (2013, August 1). Feature Selection for Medical Diagnosis: Evaluation for Cardiovascular Diseases. *Expert Systems with Applications*, *40*(10), 4146–4153.
24. Ali, L., Niamat, A., Khan, J. A., Golilarz, N. A., Xingzhong, X., Noor, A., Nour, R., & Bukhari, S. A. (2019, April 9). An Optimized Stacked Support Vector Machines Based Expert System for the Effective Prediction of Heart Failure. *IEEE Access*, *7*, 54007–54014.
25. Fitriyani, N. L., Syafrudin, M., Alfian, G., & Rhee, J. (2020, July 20). HDPM: An Effective Heart Disease Prediction Model for a Clinical Decision Support System. *IEEE Access*, 8, 133034–133050.
26. Bashir, S., Qamar, U., & Javed, M. Y. (2014, November 10). An Ensemble Based Decision Support Framework for Intelligent Heart Disease Diagnosis. In *International Conference on Information Society (i-Society 2014)* (pp. 259–264). London: IEEE.
27. Islam, S., Jahan, N., & Khatun, M. E. (2020, March 11). Cardiovascular Disease Forecast Using Machine Learning Paradigms. In *2020 Fourth International Conference on Computing Methodologies and Communication (ICCMC)* (pp. 487–490). London: IEEE.
28. Rachna, C., & Bhambri, P. (2021). Various Approaches and Algorithms for Monitoring Energy Efficiency of Wireless Sensor Networks. In *Lecture Notes in Civil Engineering* (Vol. 113, pp. 761–770). Singapore: Springer.
29. Quy, V. K., Hau, N. V., Anh, D. V., & Ngoc, L. A. (2022). Smart Healthcare IoT Applications Based on Fog Computing: Architecture, Applications and Challenges. *Complex & Intelligent Systems*, *8*(5), 3805–3815.
30. Fan, J., Wang, Z., Xie, Y., & Yang, Z. (2020, July). A Theoretical Analysis of Deep Q-Learning. In *Learning for Dynamics and Control* (pp. 486–489). London: PMLR.
31. Bebortta, S., Panda, M., & Panda, S. (2020, February). Classification of Pathological Disorders in Children Using Random Forest Algorithm. In *2020 International Conference on Emerging Trends in Information Technology and Engineering (ic-ETITE)* (pp. 1–6). London: IEEE.
32. Tripathy, S. S., Rath, M., Tripathy, N., Roy, D. S., Francis, J. S. A., & Bebortta, S. (2023). An Intelligent Health Care System in Fog Platform with Optimized Performance. *Sustainability*, *15*(3), 1862.
33. Bose, M. M., Yadav, D., Bhambri, P., & Shankar, R. (2021). Electronic Customer Relationship Management: Benefits and Pre-Implementation Considerations. *Journal of Maharaja Sayajirao University of Baroda*, *55*(01(VI)), 1343–1350.
34. Bakshi, P., Bhambri, P., & Thapar, V. (2021). A Review Paper on Wireless Sensor Network Techniques in Internet of Things (IoT). In *International Conference on Contemporary Issues in Engineering & Technology*. GNA University.
35. Bebortta, S., & Singh, S. K. (2022). An Intelligent Framework Towards Managing Big Data in Internet of Healthcare Things. In *Computational Intelligence in Pattern Recognition: Proceedings of CIPR 2022* (pp. 520–530). Singapore: Springer Nature Singapore.
36. Roy, S., Tran, T. A., & Natarajan, K. (2023). *Recent Advancement of IoT Devices in Pollution Control and Health Applications*. Elsevier. doi: https://doi.org/10.1016/C2021-0-03490-8; ISBN: 978-0-323-95876-9.
37. Mohan, S., Thirumalai, C., & Srivastava, G. (2019, June 19). Effective Heart Disease Prediction Using Hybrid Machine Learning Techniques. *IEEE Access*, *7*, 81542–81554.
38. Ashri, S. E., El-Gayar, M. M., & El-Daydamony, E. M. (2021, October 26). HDPF: Heart Disease Prediction Framework Based on Hybrid Classifiers and Genetic Algorithm. *IEEE Access*, *9*, 146797–146809.

39. Rajasekaran, M., Yassine, A., Hossain, M. S., Alhamid, M. F., & Guizani, M. (2019, September). Autonomous Monitoring in Healthcare Environment: Reward-Based Energy Charging Mechanism for IoMT Wireless Sensing Nodes. *Future Generation Computer Systems*, *98*, 565–576.
40. Constant, N., Borthakur, D., Abtahi, M., Dubey, H., & Mankodiya, K. (2017). Fog-Assisted wIoT: A Smart Fog Gateway for End-to-End Analytics in Wearable Internet of Things. https://doi.org/10.48550/arXiv.1701.08680
41. Rajkomar, A. et al. (2018). Scalable and Accurate Deep Learning with Electronic Health Records. *NPJ Digital Medicine*, *1*(1), 1–10.
42. Moosavi, S. R., Gia, T. N., Nigussie, E., Rahmani, A. M., Virtanen, S., Tenhunen, H., & Isoaho, J. (2016, November). End-to-End Security Scheme for Mobility Enabled Healthcare Internet of Things. *Future Generation Computer Systems*, *64*, 108–124.

16 Role of Artificial Intelligence in Advancing Pancreatic Cancer Research

Satyam Kumar Agrawal and Sushmita Sunil Jain

16.1 INTRODUCTION

With a rising incidence, pancreatic cancer is one of the most important causes of cancer related fatalities globally (Rahib et al., 2014). Given that pancreatic cancer is usually discovered late in the disease's progression, early detection is crucial. About 80% of patients with cancer of the pancreas are found to have either distant or locally advanced metastatic disease, with very low long-term survival rates (2–9% of patients at five years) (McGuigan et al., 2018). On the other hand, a combination of radiation, chemotherapy, and surgery can slow down cancer in individuals who arrive at an early stage of the disease (Agrawal et al., 2021; Thind et al., 2010). As per a recent report from the National Cancer Institute, USA, the five-year overall survival rate for individuals with Stage 1-A pancreatic ductal adenocarcinoma (PDAC) is over 80% (Blackford et al., 2020).

In the realm of pancreatic cancer research, artificial intelligence (AI) is beginning to emerge as a game-changing force, providing fresh perspectives and practical uses that could completely alter the detection, handling, and therapy of this fatal illness. For medical professionals and researchers, pancreatic cancer poses a significant problem because of its late-stage diagnosis and restricted therapy choices (Yeo et al., 2002). AI will play a diverse role in solving this challenge, including data-driven research, personalized treatment, early detection, and patient care. Through leveraging artificial intelligence's computational capacity, we may explore the intricacies of pancreatic cancer in greater detail, opening new possibilities for comprehension, treatment, and, eventually, better patient outcomes (Dlamini et al., 2020). There are significant strides made in the realm of AI to facilitate the early detection of pancreatic cancer, a path notoriously challenging primarily due to late-stage diagnoses and non-specific symptoms (Wei et al., 2019). Progress made in the utilization of AI methodologies for risk stratification and identification within general healthcare, especially manifesting its potential in the hunt for successful early detection mechanisms for pancreatic cancer is impactful (Kenner et al., 2021).

Recent advancements in AI present promising opportunities for early detection, motivating this review. Kenner et al., (2021), present a comprehensive summation of

 DOI: 10.1201/9781032698519-16

the progress, problems, and prospects within the arena of AI applications in early pancreatic cancer detection. Hayashi et al., (2022), discussed the recent advances in AI for pancreatic ductal adenocarcinoma and provided a compilation of the AI algorithms and their performance in this area focusing on the use of AI in the early detection of pancreatic cancer, and extensively ventures into other significant contributions (Hayashi et al., 2022). One such notable study is by Liu et al., (2020), who delve into the application of AI in screening for pancreatic ductal adenocarcinoma (PDAC), providing valuable insight into how AI can be leveraged in the face of computed tomography (CT) and magnetic resonance imaging (MRI) (Bhambri et al., 2023). Widespread advancements in radiomics, machine learning (ML), and AI are the focus of a research article by Cozzi et al., (2019). Ramesh et al., (2022), note how these areas of exploration are transforming healthcare procedures, including the non-invasive detection of pancreatic cancer. Yasaka et al. (2018), showcased the potential of AI and radiomics in diagnosing pancreatic diseases, discussing algorithms used to extract high-throughput features from radiological imaging (Yasaka et al., 2018). The AI predictions and radiomics in early pancreatic cancer diagnosis have been studied by Bera et al., (2022). They introduce the concept of AI-based risk scores, which can serve as a vital tool in identifying high-risk individuals. Pointing out an AI algorithm for predicting pancreatic cystic neoplasm malignancy, Jiang et al., (2023), encapsulated how applying AI algorithms can help doctors make informed decisions about the management of these cysts. Another study by Granata et al., (2023), discussed the implementation of AI to predict risk factors for pancreatic cancer, highlighting how AI could be used for screening certain risk categories. The significance of AI in ruling out neoplasms in pancreatic cystic lesions has been very well studied by Jiang et al., (2023). The study proposes a possible means for AI to assist in cystic pancreas diagnosis, reducing invasive diagnosis and management costs. Finally, an exhaustive compilation by Zitvogel et al. (2018), provides an in-depth overview of the current understanding of pancreatic cancer, discussing various tools for early detection, including AI, with a particular focus on known risk factors.

16.2 EARLY DETECTION

Early detection of cancer of the pancreas has undergone a revolutionary change because of the application of artificial intelligence (Iqbal et al., 2021). Its advancements, particularly machine learning (ML) algorithms, have addressed several significant aspects of the difficulties in diagnosing this disease (Rana et al., 2024). The important aspects of the early detection of pancreatic cancer are discussed in Figure 16.1.

16.2.1 Medical Image Analysis

The ability of AI to analyze and understand medical imaging technologies, such as CT, MRI, and positron emission tomography (PET), is exceptionally high. ML algorithms possess the ability to process these images quickly and effectively differentiate

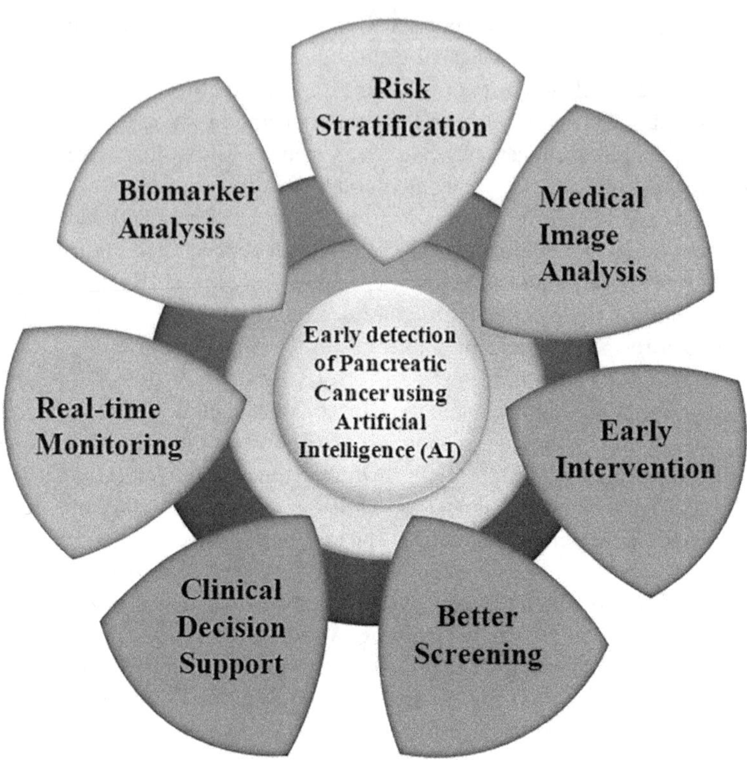

FIGURE 16.1 Important aspects of early detection of pancreatic cancer.

between benign and malignant tumors. Also, it accurately identifies subtle abnormalities. This enables the early detection of pancreatic cancers during their initial stages (Najjar, 2023).

16.2.2 Risk Stratification

AI models have been developed to classify individuals into risk groups based on different factors, such as clinical data, family history, and genetic predisposition (Kourou et al., 2015; Rani et al., 2020) The risk stratification algorithms can accurately identify individuals with a significantly elevated possibility of developing pancreatic cancer. Once identified, individuals more likely to develop pancreatic cancer can be screened routinely to increase the chance of early detection (Blyuss et al., 2020).

16.2.3 Biomarker Analysis

Artificial intelligence has made a substantial contribution to the discovery and confirmation of biomarkers linked to pancreatic cancer (Kenner et al., 2021). Cellular, biochemical, molecular, or genetic changes that are used to identify or track a normal, aberrant, or just biological process are referred to as biomarkers, and can also signal the existence of cancer. These biomarkers, which can be utilized for diagnostic testing, can be found by AI algorithms sifting through large medical and genetic databases (Nair et al., 2014).

16.2.4 Real-Time Monitoring

Oncologists can track the progression of a disease and the effectiveness of a cure by using AI-driven monitoring tools to analyze patient data in real-time. Patients are guaranteed to receive the most effective therapies because of this real-time feedback that enables treatment plans to be adjusted (Kann et al., 2021).

16.2.5 Clinical Decision Support

Artificial Intelligence has the potential to be a very useful tool for medical professionals, guiding them while diagnosing and treating pancreatic cancer. These AI programs can help with treatment planning, forecast patient outcomes, and make recommendations for possible courses of action (Hameed and Krishnan, 2022).

16.2.6 Better Screening

Artificial Intelligence can make screening programs more successful. By looking through large datasets and making the most use of medical resources, AI algorithms may determine the exact criteria for selecting individuals for screening (Harry, 2023).

16.2.7 Early Intervention

Patients who receive a diagnosis earlier in life may benefit from potentially curative procedures such as surgery or tailored medicines, thanks to early identification provided by AI. Patient's quality of life is improved by early intervention in addition to increasing their chances of surviving (Johnson et al., 2021).

16.3 CURRENT CHALLENGES IN MEDICAL DECISION-MAKING

Pancreatic cancer is a highly aggressive cancer with many obstacles to early identification (Zhou et al., 2017). These include:

16.3.1 Asymptomatic Nature

Early-stage pancreatic cancer is frequently characterized by a lack of distinguishing symptoms, which makes diagnosis difficult (Rani et al., 2023). When symptoms do show up, they are frequently general and nonspecific, such as jaundice, diarrhea, and unexplained weight loss (Gheorghe et al., 2020).

16.3.2 Absence of Routine Screening

Pancreatic cancer screening is not standardized for the public, in contrast to many other malignancies that have screening protocols in place. As such, many cases remain undiagnosed until symptoms manifest, usually in their advanced stages (Poruk et al., 2013).

16.3.3 Inadequate Biomarkers

There are tumor-specific biomarkers available for the detection of pancreatic cancer such as CA 19-9, CA-50, and CEA. These markers have some notable shortcomings that included low sensitivity, false-negative results in specific blood groups, and false-positive elevation when obstructive jaundice was present (Zitvogel et al., 2018). For instance, CA19-9 is frequently overexpressed in other gastrointestinal tumors and inflammatory diseases including pancreatitis. Conditions like these also pose hurdles in the early detection of pancreatic cancer (Dumstrei et al., 2016).

16.3.4 Inefficient Imaging

Although sophisticated imaging methods such as CT, MRI, and PET scans are useful instruments, they might not reliably identify tiny or early-stage tumors. These diagnostic instruments may also come with hazards, be intrusive, and are expensive, too (Islam and Walker, 2013).

In summary, the complex nature of pancreatic cancer presents significant obstacles in terms of early detection and subsequent clinical decision-making. The lack of symptoms in the initial stages of pancreatic cancer, combined with the absence of standardized screening procedures and the limits of existing biomarkers and imaging methods, exacerbates the challenges associated with diagnosing the disease in a timely manner (Singh and Bhambri, 2023). The prioritization of addressing these difficulties is of utmost importance in order to improve patient outcomes, requiring a focused and collaborative approach in the fields of research and technology. To navigate the complexity and enhance the landscape of medical decision-making in the context of pancreatic cancer, it becomes crucial to explore creative techniques, which may be propelled by developments such as artificial intelligence (AI).

16.4 ARTIFICIAL INTELLIGENCE-BASED PREDICTION MODELS

The patient outcomes could be much enhanced by AI-powered prediction models for early pancreatic cancer identification (Table 16.1). This section discusses the principal facets of these models.

16.4.1 Analyzing and Integrating Data

To determine a patient's risk of acquiring pancreatic cancer, AI models make use of large datasets, including medical histories, genetic information, electronic health records (EHRs), and demographic data. These models provide a more thorough

TABLE 16.1
Different AI Models for the Detection of Pancreatic Cancer

Sr. No.	AI model	Findings	References
1	Convolutional Neural Network (CNN)	Addressing the complex task of pancreatic segmentation in CT images.	Liu et al., 2019
2	CNN	Helps in determining tumor location.	Zhu et al., 2019
3	Random forest algorithm [by ML]	To classify pancreatic ductal adenocarcinoma (PDAC) based on CT images.	Chu et al., 2019
4	Support Vector Machine (SVM)	Differentiate pancreatic serous cystic neoplasms.	Wei et al., 2018
5	Deep Learning	Grading system of pancreatic neuroendocrine tumor (PNET).	Tsionas and Andrikopoulos, 2019

analysis than conventional risk assessments because they can handle intricate relationships between different risk factors (Knevel and Liao, 2023).

16.4.2 Early Diagnosis

Prediction models, which are based on AI algorithms, are capable of quickly and precisely diagnosing pancreatic cancer (Hayashi et al., 2021). AI can identify tumors at an earlier, more manageable stage through training on a variety of datasets, such as clinical notes, laboratory findings, and photos of medical conditions (Young et al., 2020).

16.4.3 Enhancement of Imaging

When diagnosing pancreatic cancer, radiological imaging is essential (Lee and Lee, 2014). AI-powered image analysis can pick up on minute features that human observers might overlook. Quickly analyzing images, these models can greatly increase accuracy while also saving crucial time throughout the diagnostic procedure.

16.4.4 Recognizing Symptoms

It is also used to examine a person's speech patterns, medical history, and symptoms to find any possible signs of pancreatic cancer. AI can identify trends and abnormalities that human healthcare experts would miss because of its advanced level of complexity (Tovar et al., 2023).

16.5 CHALLENGES AND LIMITATIONS

The use of artificial intelligence in the early identification of pancreatic cancer raises some ethical questions that must be carefully considered (Gao and Wang, 2019).

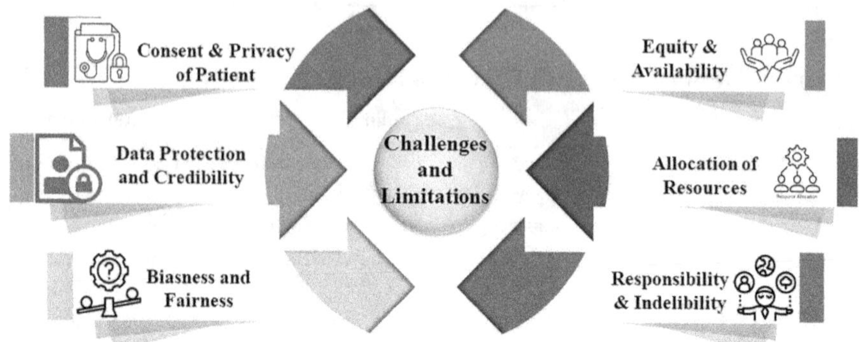

FIGURE 16.2 Challenges and limitations of AI in pancreatic cancer research.

While incorporating cutting-edge technologies into healthcare procedures has the potential to significantly improve patient care, it also presents some moral conundrums. Challenges and limitations of using AI in the early detection of pancreatic cancer research have been discussed in this section (Figure 16.2).

16.5.1 Consent from the Patient and Privacy

AI is frequently used to analyze compilations of patient data, which includes health records, e-reports, and medical pictures, to diagnose pancreatic cancer early (Walz and Firth-Butterfield, 2019). Patient privacy is extremely important when it comes to AI applications in healthcare (Khalid et al., 2023). For their data to be utilized, patients must be fully informed and provide their express consent. Further, blockchain can be essential in ensuring that patient data is only available through smart contracts to authorized individuals (Sookhak et al., 2021).

16.5.2 Data Protection and Credibility

It is crucial to guarantee the security of patient information. It's difficult to strike a compromise between preserving data security inside the AI. These can be overcome and improved by a decentralized and transparent blockchain technology that can aid in building trust among stakeholders. It's critical to set ethical standards that guarantee data security and restrict access to just those with a valid need (Mittelstadt and Floridi, 2016).

16.5.3 The Influence of Bias and the Concept of Fairness

The bias that might disproportionately harm some patient groups must not exist in AI systems utilized in early detection. It is essential to address and rectify the presence of bias in AI models. This bias might originate from either biased training data or algorithmic design (Noseworthy et al., 2020). The ethical obligation to ensure the equity of AI models and algorithms is crucial to ensure equitable access to early detection for all patients (Ahmad et al., 2023).

16.5.4 Responsibility and Indelibility

The ethical issue of accountability for judgments made by AI algorithms is a significant challenge. In the event of an AI-powered system's failure to detect pancreatic cancer during its initial stages, the question arises as to which party should bear responsibility (Panesar, 2019). It is imperative to establish legal frameworks for the allocation of blame to uphold accountability in such situations. A probable utilization of blockchain's immutable ledger has the potential to facilitate the monitoring and documentation of choices and activities, hence enhancing accountability (Bonsón and Bednárová, 2019).

16.5.5 Allocation of Resources

The allocation of resources is a matter of utmost ethical significance. The ethical quandary surrounding the allocation of substantial resources towards the growth and implementation of AI within the healthcare sector, particularly considering the existence of other urgent healthcare demands has been discussed by Waltz et al., (2019). The ethical dilemma is in effectively managing the allocation of resources while fostering innovation to maximize patient welfare. (Baily et al., 2006).

16.5.6 Equity and Availability

There is a need to ensure fair access to early detection in AI applications (Tanwar et al., 2019). It is imperative to ensure that the financial implications associated with the implementation of the technology do not result in inequitable access to healthcare services. The development of inclusive policies that ensure universal access to AI-based early detection is of utmost importance, irrespective of socioeconomic considerations (Toufaily et al., 2021).

The utilization of AI holds considerable promise in the realm of early pancreatic cancer detection. However, it is crucial to acknowledge and confront the ethical ramifications that accompany these advancements. This entails the protection of patient confidentiality, the assurance of data integrity and openness, the reduction of prejudice, the establishment of responsibility, and the facilitation of fair and equal availability. Further integration of AI and blockchain technologies in healthcare necessitates a primary focus on ethical considerations, as emphasized by various scholars in the domain (Tandon et al., 2020).

16.6 POTENTIAL FOR INNOVATIONS IN PANCREATIC CANCER TREATMENT

AI's ability to enable early diagnosis, which could lead to breakthroughs in pancreatic cancer treatment, is commendable (Dlamini et al., 2020). No early diagnosis and poor survival rates of pancreatic cancer are well-known. However, the application of AI to the early diagnosis procedure could change the course of treatment for this difficult illness (Kaur et al., 2012). This section explores a range of areas made possible by AI, clarifying how technology has ushered in precision medicine, enhanced survival rates, made minimally invasive interventions possible, supported targeted therapeutics, and generated economic advantages.

16.6.1 Precision Medicine

By using AI to diagnose pancreatic cancer early, researchers can better understand the genetic and molecular features of the disease. With this information, oncologists may customize treatment regimens for each patient, concentrating on medicines that particularly address the distinct characteristics of the tumor. Precision medicine optimizes therapeutic efficacy while minimizing side effects.

16.6.2 Increased Survival Rates

The ultimate reward of AI-facilitated early diagnosis is the possibility of higher survival rates (Panda and Satapathy, 2021). Early cancer detection and localized disease make curative measures like surgery or targeted medicines feasible. AI can recognize these early-stage cases, guaranteeing that patients receive interventions that could be curative promptly (Mikdadi et al., 2022).

16.6.3 Minimally Invasive Interventions

Therapies that are less aggressive and less invasive can be made possible by AI-driven early diagnosis. Although patients with late-stage pancreatic cancer frequently require lengthy surgeries, early detection may allow for the use of less invasive techniques like laparoscopy, which would lessen pain and recovery times (Hameed and Krishnan, 2022).

16.6.4 Targeted Therapies

AI can evaluate the genetic composition of the tumor and pinpoint molecular targets or biomarkers. With this knowledge, targeted medicines targeting cancer cells while preserving healthy tissue can be created and administered. There is hope for better treatment outcomes and fewer side effects with targeted therapies (Upreti et al., 2023).

16.6.5 Economic Benefits

Early detection with AI can lower the overall cost of pancreatic cancer treatment. AI-driven early detection can save costs for patients and healthcare systems by reducing the need for major procedures and late-stage therapies (Chu et al., 2017).

16.7 CONCLUSION

In conclusion, pancreatic cancer has long posed a serious threat to the profession of oncology due to its aggressive nature and low survival rates. The intricacies of its biology, tardy diagnosis, and resistance to conventional treatments have impeded noteworthy advancements in enhancing patient outcomes. However, the advent of AI in the field of pancreatic cancer research offers fresh hope and inventiveness. AI is evolving into a game-changing tool at different points in the disease's life cycle, providing the means to improve early detection and, in turn, provide novel treatment approaches.

The advent of AI eases precise risks, and an early diagnosis, which ultimately decreases mortality. Further, image analysis, ability to sift big data and highlighting the important biomarkers, specific to pancreatic cancer, has been possible only due to advent of AI. The same would have been easily overlooked by manual analysis.

Furthermore, AI improves medical decision-making by helping healthcare professionals plan treatments and by providing real-time monitoring so that medicines can be adjusted for the best possible outcomes. AI increases the likelihood of early diagnosis by classifying patients into risk groups and ensuring that high-risk individuals are screened promptly.

Pancreatic cancer poses a further challenge due to its complicated genetic landscape. AI's capacity to evaluate enormous genomic datasets quickly finds important genetic markers, hastening the creation of novel medications and targeted treatments. Patients can obtain interventions that are associated with fewer adverse effects and more effectiveness when following personalized therapy regimens, which could lead to increased survival rates and an enhanced quality of life.

While the application of artificial intelligence to early detection holds great promise, there are some important ethical issues that cannot be ignored simultaneously. To guarantee the ethical use of AI in healthcare, issues related to patient privacy, data security, bias reduction, accountability, resource allocation, and equitable availability shall also be taken into consideration.

REFERENCES

Agrawal, S. K., Agrawal, M., Sharma, P. R., Ahmad, K., Shawl, A. S., Arora, S., & Saxena, A. K. (2021). *Anagallis arvensis* induces apoptosis in HL-60 cells through ROS-mediated mitochondrial pathway. *Nutrition and Cancer*, *73*(11–12), 2720–2731.

Ahmad, A., Tariq, A., Hussain, H. K., & Gill, A. Y. (2023). Equity and artificial intelligence in surgical care: A comprehensive review of current challenges and promising solutions. *BULLET: Jurnal Multidisiplin Ilmu*, *2*(2), 443–455.

Baily, M. A., Bottrell, M. M., Lynn, J., & Jennings, B. (2006). Special report: The ethics of using QI methods to improve health care quality and safety. *Hastings Center Report*, *36*(4), S1–S40.

Bera, K., Braman, N., Gupta, A., Velcheti, V., & Madabhushi, A. (2022). Predicting cancer outcomes with radiomics and artificial intelligence in radiology. *Nature Reviews Clinical Oncology*, *19*(2), 132–146.

Bhambri, P., Rani, S., Balas, V. E., & Elngar, A. A. (2023). *Integration of AI-Based Manufacturing and Industrial Engineering Systems with the Internet of Things*. New York: CRC Press.

Blackford, A. L., Canto, M. I., Klein, A. P., Hruban, R. H., & Goggins, M. (2020). Recent trends in the incidence and survival of stage 1A pancreatic cancer: A surveillance, epidemiology, and end results analysis. *JNCI: Journal of the National Cancer Institute*, *112*(11), 1162–1169.

Blyuss, O., Zaikin, A., Cherepanova, V., Munblit, D., Kiseleva, E. M., Prytomanova, O. M., & Crnogorac-Jurcevic, T. (2020). Development of PancRISK, a urine biomarker-based risk score for stratified screening of pancreatic cancer patients. *British Journal of Cancer*, *122*(5), 692–696.

Bonsón, E., & Bednárová, M. (2019). Blockchain and its implications for accounting and auditing. *Meditari Accountancy Research*, *27*(5), 725–740.

Chu, L. C., Goggins, M. G., & Fishman, E. K. (2017). Diagnosis and detection of pancreatic cancer. *The Cancer Journal*, *23*(6), 333–342.

Chu, L. C., Park, S., Kawamoto, S., Fouladi, D. F., Shayesteh, S., Zinreich, E. S., Graves, J. S., Horton, K. M., Hruban, R. H., Yuille, A. L., Kinzler, K. W., Voelstein, B., & Fishman, E. K. (2019). Utility of CT radiomics features in differentiation of pancreatic ductal adenocarcinoma from normal pancreatic tissue. *American Journal of Roentgenology*, *213*(2), 349–357.

Cozzi, L., Comito, T., Fogliata, A., Franzese, C., Franceschini, D., Bonifacio, C., & Scorsetti, M. (2019). Computed tomography-based radiomic signature as predictive of survival and local control after stereotactic body radiation therapy in pancreatic carcinoma. *PLoS One*, *14*(1), e0210758.

Dlamini, Z., Francies, F. Z., Hull, R., & Marima, R. (2020). Artificial intelligence (AI) and big data in cancer and precision oncology. *Computational and Structural Biotechnology Journal*, *18*, 2300–2311.

Dumstrei, K., Chen, H., & Brenner, H. (2016). A systematic review of serum autoantibodies as biomarkers for pancreatic cancer detection. *Oncotarget*, *7*(10), 11151.

Gao, X., & Wang, X. (2019). Deep learning for world health organization grades of pancreatic neuroendocrine tumors on contrast-enhanced magnetic resonance images: A preliminary study. *International Journal of Computer Assisted Radiology and Surgery*, *14*, 1981–1991.

Gheorghe, G., Bungau, S., Ilie, M., Behl, T., Vesa, C. M., Brisc, C., Bacalbasa, N., Turi, V., Costache, R. S., & Diaconu, C. C. (2020). Early diagnosis of pancreatic cancer: The key for survival. *Diagnostics*, *10*(11), 869.

Granata, V., Fusco, R., Setola, S. V., Galdiero, R., Maggialetti, N., Silvestro, L., & Izzo, F. (2023). Risk assessment and pancreatic cancer: Diagnostic management and artificial intelligence. *Cancers*, *15*(2), 351.

Hameed, B. S., & Krishnan, U. M. (2022). Artificial intelligence-driven diagnosis of pancreatic cancer. *Cancers*, *14*(21), 5382.

Harry, A. (2023). The future of medicine: Harnessing the power of AI for revolutionizing healthcare. *International Journal of Multidisciplinary Sciences and Arts*, *2*(1), 36–47.

Hayashi, H., Uemura, N., Matsumura, K., Zhao, L., Sato, H., Shiraishi, Y., & Baba, H. (2021). Recent advances in artificial intelligence for pancreatic ductal adenocarcinoma. *World Journal of Gastroenterology*, *27*(43), 7480.

Hayashi, K., Ono, Y., Takamatsu, M., Oba, A., Ito, H., Sato, T., & Takahashi, Y. (2022). Prediction of recurrence pattern of pancreatic cancer post-pancreatic surgery using histology-based supervised machine learning algorithms: A single-center retrospective study. *Annals of Surgical Oncology*, *29*(7), 4624–4634.

Iqbal, M. J., Javed, Z., Sadia, H., Qureshi, I. A., Irshad, A., Ahmed, R., & Sharifi-Rad, J. (2021). Clinical applications of artificial intelligence and machine learning in cancer diagnosis: Looking into the future. *Cancer Cell International*, *21*(1), 1–11.

Islam, S., & Walker, R. C. (2013). Advanced imaging (positron emission tomography and magnetic resonance imaging) and image-guided biopsy in initial staging and monitoring of therapy of lung cancer. *Cancer Journal (Sudbury, Mass.)*, *19*(3), 208.

Jiang, J., Chao, W. L., Culp, S., & Krishna, S. G. (2023). Artificial intelligence in the diagnosis and treatment of pancreatic cystic lesions and adenocarcinoma. *Cancers*, *15*(9), 2410.

Johnson, K. B., Wei, W. Q., Weeraratne, D., Frisse, M. E., Misulis, K., Rhee, K., & Snowdon, J. L. (2021). Precision medicine, AI, and the future of personalized health care. *Clinical and Translational Science*, *14*(1), 86–93.

Kann, B. H., Hosny, A., & Aerts, H. J. (2021). Artificial intelligence for clinical oncology. *Cancer Cell*, *39*(7), 916–927.

Kaur, S., Baine, M. J., Jain, M., Sasson, A. R., & Batra, S. K. (2012). Early diagnosis of pancreatic cancer: Challenges and new developments. *Biomarkers in Medicine*, *6*(5), 597–612.

Kenner, B., Chari, S. T., Kelsen, D., Klimstra, D. S., Pandol, S. J., Rosenthal, M., Rustgi, A. K., Taylor, J. A., Yala, A., Abul-Husn, N., Andersen, D. K., Bernstein, D., Brunak, S., Canto, M. I., Eldar, Y. C., Fishman, E. K., Fleshman, J., Go, V. L. W., Holt, J. M., Field, B., Goldberg, A., Hoos, W., Iacobuzio-Donahue, C., Li, D., Lidgard, G., Maitra, A., Matrisian, L. M., Poblete, S., Rothschild, L., Sander, C., Schwartz, L. H., Shalit, U., Srivastava, S., Wolpin, B. (2021, March 1). Artificial intelligence and early detection of pancreatic cancer: 2020 summative review. *Pancreas*, *50*(3), 251–279.

Khalid, N., Qayyum, A., Bilal, M., Al-Fuqaha, A., & Qadir, J. (2023). Privacy-preserving artificial intelligence in healthcare: Techniques and applications. *Computers in Biology and Medicine*, 106848.

Knevel, R., & Liao, K. P. (2023). From real-world electronic health record data to real-world results using artificial intelligence. *Annals of the Rheumatic Diseases*, *82*(3), 306–311.

Kourou, K., Exarchos, T. P., Exarchos, K. P., Karamouzis, M. V., & Fotiadis, D. I. (2015). Machine learning applications in cancer prognosis and prediction. *Computational and Structural Biotechnology Journal*, *13*, 8–17.

Lee, E. S., & Lee, J. M. (2014). Imaging diagnosis of pancreatic cancer: A state-of-the-art review. *World Journal of Gastroenterology: WJG*, *20*(24), 7864.

Liu, G. D., Li, Y. C., Zhang, W., & Zhang, L. (2020). A brief review of artificial intelligence applications and algorithms for psychiatric disorders. *Engineering*, *6*(4), 462–467.

Liu, S. L., Li, S., Guo, Y. T., Zhou, Y. P., Zhang, Z. D., Li, S., & Lu, Y. (2019). Establishment and application of an artificial intelligence diagnosis system for pancreatic cancer with a faster region-based convolutional neural network. *Chinese Medical Journal*, *132*(23), 2795–2803.

McGuigan, A., Kelly, P., Turkington, R. C., Jones, C., Coleman, H. G., & McCain, R. S. (2018). Pancreatic cancer: A review of clinical diagnosis, epidemiology, treatment and outcomes. *World Journal of gastroenterology*, *24*(43), 4846.

Mikdadi, D., O'Connell, K. A., Meacham, P. J., Dugan, M. A., Ojiere, M. O., Carlson, T. B., & Klenk, J. A. (2022). Applications of artificial intelligence (AI) in ovarian cancer, pancreatic cancer, and image biomarker discovery. *Cancer Biomarkers*, *33*(2), 173–184.

Mittelstadt, B. D., & Floridi, L. (2016). The ethics of big data: Current and foreseeable issues in biomedical contexts. *The Ethics of Biomedical Big Data*, 445–480.

Nair, M., Singh Sandhu, S., & Sharma, K. A. (2014). Prognostic and predictive biomarkers in cancer. *Current Cancer Drug Targets*, *14*(5), 477–504.

Najjar, R. (2023). Redefining radiology: A review of artificial intelligence integration in medical imaging. *Diagnostics*, *13*(17), 2760.

Noseworthy, P. A., Attia, Z. I., Brewer, L. C., Hayes, S. N., Yao, X., Kapa, S., & Lopez-Jimenez, F. (2020). Assessing and mitigating bias in medical artificial intelligence: The effects of race and ethnicity on a deep learning model for ECG analysis. *Circulation: Arrhythmia and Electrophysiology*, *13*(3), e007988.

Panda, S. K., & Satapathy, S. C. (2021). Drug traceability and transparency in the medical supply chain using blockchain for easing the process and creating trust between stakeholders and consumers. *Personal and Ubiquitous Computing*, 1–17.

Panesar, A. (2019). *Machine Learning and AI for Healthcare* (pp. 1–73). Coventry, UK: Apress.

Poruk, K. E., Firpo, M. A., Adler, D. G., & Mulvihill, S. J. (2013). Screening for pancreatic cancer: Why, how, and who? *Annals of Surgery*, *257*(1), 17.

Rahib, L., Smith, B. D., Aizenberg, R., Rosenzweig, A. B., Fleshman, J. M., & Matrisian, L. M. (2014). Projecting cancer incidence and deaths to 2030: The unexpected burden of thyroid, liver, and pancreas cancers in the United States. *Cancer Research*, *74*(11), 2913–2921.

Ramesh, T. R., Lilhore, U. K., Poongodi, M., Simaiya, S., Kaur, A., & Hamdi, M. (2022). Predictive analysis of heart diseases with machine learning approaches. *Malaysian Journal of Computer Science*, 132–148.

Rana, R., Bhambri, P., & Chhabra, Y. (2024). *Evolution and the Future of Industrial Engineering with the IoT and AI. In Integration of AI-Based Manufacturing and Industrial Engineering Systems with the Internet of Things* (pp. 19–37). New York: CRC Press.

Rani, S., Ahmed, S. H., & Rastogi, R. (2020). Dynamic clustering approach based on wireless sensor networks genetic algorithm for IoT applications. *Wireless Networks*, *26*, 2307–2316.

Rani, S., Kaur, J., & Bhambri, P. (2023). Technology and gender violence: Victimization model, consequences and measures. In *Communication Technology and Gender Violence* (Vol. 1, pp. 1–19). New York: Springer.

Singh, G., & Bhambri, P. (2023). Simulation analysis of AODV and DSDV routing protocols for secure and reliable service in mobile Adhoc networks (MANETs). In *Integration of AI-Based Manufacturing and Industrial Engineering Systems with the Internet of Things* (pp. 205–216). New York: CRC Press.

Sookhak, M., Jabbarpour, M. R., Safa, N. S., & Yu, F. R. (2021). Blockchain and smart contract for access control in healthcare: A survey, issues and challenges, and open issues. *Journal of Network and Computer Applications*, *178*, 102950.

Tandon, A., Dhir, A., Islam, A. N., & Mäntymäki, M. (2020). Blockchain in healthcare: A systematic literature review, synthesizing framework, and future research agenda. *Computers in Industry*, *122*, 103290.

Tanwar, S., Bhatia, Q., Patel, P., Kumari, A., Singh, P. K., & Hong, W. C. (2019). Machine learning adoption in blockchain-based smart applications: The challenges, and a way forward. *IEEE Access*, *8*, 474–488.

Thind, T. S., Rampal, G., Agrawal, S. K., Saxena, A. K., & Arora, S. (2010). Diminution of free radical-induced DNA damage by extracts/fractions from bark of *Schleichera oleosa* (Lour.) Oken. *Drug and Chemical Toxicology*, *33*(4), 329–336.

Toufaily, E., Zalan, T., & Dhaou, S. B. (2021). A framework of blockchain technology adoption: An investigation of challenges and expected value. *Information & Management*, *58*(3), 103444.

Tovar, D. R., Rosenthal, M. H., Maitra, A., & Koay, E. J. (2023). The potential of artificial intelligence in the risk stratification for and early detection of pancreatic cancer. *Artificial Intelligence Surgery*, *3*(1), 14–26.

Tsionas, M. G., Andrikopoulos, A. A note on the Gao et al. (2019). Uniform mixture model in the case of regression. *Annals of Operations Research*, *289*, 495–501. https://doi.org/10.1007/s10479-019-03475-w

Upreti, K., Mittal, S., Vats, P., Haque, M., Pawar, V., & Haque, M. (2023, June). Development and evaluation of an artificial intelligence-based system for pancreatic cancer detection and diagnosis. In *International Conference on Advanced Communication and Intelligent Systems* (pp. 26–38). Cham: Springer Nature.

Waltz, T. J., Powell, B. J., Fernández, M. E., Abadie, B., & Damschroder, L. J. (2019). Choosing implementation strategies to address contextual barriers: Diversity in recommendations and future directions. *Implement Science*, *14*(1), 42.

Walz, A., & Firth-Butterfield, K. (2019). Implementing ethics into artificial intelligence: A contribution, from a legal perspective to the development of an AI governance regime. *Duke Law & Technology Review*, *18*, 176.

Wei, H., Sewell, K. A., Woody, G., & Rose, M. A. (2018). The state of the science of nurse work environments in the United States: A systematic review. *International Journal of Nursing Sciences*, *5*(3), 287–300.

Wei, R., Lin, K., Yan, W., Guo, Y., Wang, Y., Li, J., & Zhu, J. (2019). Computer-aided diagnosis of pancreas serous cystic neoplasms: a radiomics method on preoperative MDCT images. *Technology in Cancer Research & Treatment*, *18*, 1533033818824339.

Yasaka, K., Akai, H., Abe, O., & Kiryu, S. (2018). Deep learning with convolutional neural network for differentiation of liver masses at dynamic contrast-enhanced CT: A preliminary study. *Radiology*, *286*(3), 887–896.

Yasaka, K., Akai, H., Kunimatsu, A., Kiryu, S., & Abe, O. (2018). Deep learning with convolutional neural network in radiology. *Japanese Journal of Radiology*, *36*, 257–272.

Yeo, T. P., Hruban, R. H., Leach, S. D., Wilentz, R. E., Sohn, T. A., Kern, S. E., & Yeo, C. J. (2002). Pancreatic cancer. *Current Problems in Cancer*, *26*(4), 176–275.

Young, M. R., Abrams, N., Ghosh, S., Rinaudo, J. A. S., Marquez, G., & Srivastava, S. (2020). Prediagnostic image data, artificial intelligence, and pancreatic cancer: A tell-tale sign to early detection. *Pancreas*, *49*(7), 882–886.

Zhou, B., Xu, J. W., Cheng, Y. G., Gao, J. Y., Hu, S. Y., Wang, L., & Zhan, H. X. (2017). Early detection of pancreatic cancer: Where are we now and where are we going? *International Journal of Cancer*, *141*(2), 231–241.

Zhu, Z., Xia, Y., Xie, L., Fishman, E. K., & Yuille, A. L. (2019). Multi-scale coarse-to-fine segmentation for screening pancreatic ductal adenocarcinoma. In *Medical Image Computing and Computer Assisted Intervention–MICCAI 2019: 22nd International Conference, Shenzhen, China, October 13–17, 2019, Proceedings, Part VI 22* (pp. 3–12). London: Springer International Publishing.

Zitvogel, L., Ma, Y., Raoult, D., Kroemer, G., & Gajewski, T. F. (2018). The microbiome in cancer immunotherapy: Diagnostic tools and therapeutic strategies. *Science*, *359*(6382), 1366–1370.

17 Internet of Medical Things for Abnormality Detection in Infants using Mobile Phone App with Cry Signal Analysis

Ritu, Pankaj Bhambri and Bebesh Tripathy

17.1 INTRODUCTION

The emergence of novel technologies is bringing about a radical transformation in the healthcare sector. One such innovative paradigm is the internet of medical things (IoMT). In this field, there's an urgent need for cutting-edge infant healthcare solutions that allow for early abnormality detection, prompt intervention, and better health outcomes. The integration of IoMT principles with mobile applications—specifically, those made for analyzing cry signals from infants—is explored in this chapter. Using the widespread use of mobile devices, this method aims to provide parents and other caregivers with a tool that can monitor a baby's cries and decipher subtle cues to identify possible health problems (Smith and Johnson, 2021). The special difficulties in providing healthcare to infants stems from their inability to express their discomfort or health problems orally. On the other hand, cry signals are an effective form of communication that provide important information about a baby's health. Knowing the subtleties of a baby's cry patterns can reveal important health information, such as indications of discomfort, hunger, or possible anomalies. Early intervention can be greatly impacted by timely detection of these cues, which can improve health outcomes and, in certain situations, even save lives.

It is impossible to exaggerate the importance of early detection in infant healthcare. Babies are especially susceptible to a variety of illnesses, and postponing diagnosis and treatment can have serious repercussions (Brown and White, 2022). Our goal is to develop a proactive healthcare strategy that enables parents and other caregivers to continuously monitor the health of their infants by utilizing IoMT. The goal is to use cry signal analysis to quickly identify anomalies so that patients can receive individualized care and prompt medical attention. IoMT is a network of medical devices and applications that are linked together to make it easier to gather, process, and share health-related data. IoMT has already shown promise in the healthcare

DOI: 10.1201/9781032698519-17

industry in the areas of real-time data analysis, predictive analytics, and remote patient monitoring. Our goal is to improve the efficacy and accessibility of healthcare interventions by expanding these capabilities to infant healthcare, particularly in areas where access to conventional healthcare services may be restricted.

This chapter describes the creation and deployment of an IoMT-based mobile application specifically made to analyze cry signals in order to detect abnormalities in infants. It looks at the ethical issues surrounding data privacy, the scientific foundations of cry signal analysis, and the fusion of artificial intelligence and machine learning for precise detection. The chapter also offers insights into the mobile app's functionality and design, highlighting features like real-time monitoring and user-friendly interfaces.

17.1.1 Overview of Infant Healthcare Challenges

The physiological and developmental characteristics of infants present a unique set of challenges for healthcare providers serving this vulnerable population. Babies' poor communication skills are one of the main obstacles. As infants are unable to express their needs or discomfort verbally, they rely on non-verbal cues, like crying, to do so. Parental and caregiver understanding of the root causes of an infant's distress, be it hunger, discomfort, illness, or other factors, is frequently hampered by this communication barrier (Panda et al., 2019). In addition, due to their underdeveloped immune systems, infants are especially vulnerable to infections and illnesses. Because early intervention is critical to reducing the impact of illnesses on their fragile health, vigilant monitoring is essential for the detection of symptoms. The complex field of infant healthcare is further compounded by neonatal health complications, which result from situations like premature birth or congenital abnormalities. For the purpose of meeting the special medical needs of newborns and ensuring their best possible development, specialised care is frequently needed.

Another aspect of the challenges associated with infant healthcare are developmental milestones. It's crucial to monitor and confirm that newborns reach these developmental milestones in order to spot any potential delays or disorders in their early stages (Williams and Davis, 2023). Another important issue is nutrition, since it can affect an infant's development and general health due to issues with breastfeeding, formula intolerance, or nutritional deficiencies. Broader environmental factors can also impact an infant's well-being in addition to health-related issues. This covers things like producing a safe living environment, reducing exposure to environmental contaminants, and practicing safe sleep techniques to prevent Sudden Infant Death Syndrome (SIDS). Lack of resources can make it difficult for people to receive timely medical interventions and preventive care, especially in underserved or rural areas where access to healthcare services is universally problematic. In addition, the welfare of infants depends heavily on the mental health of parents, especially mothers. Anxiety and postpartum depression can have an effect on the caregiver environment, which may have an effect on the infant's general well-being. During infancy, genetic predispositions and congenital conditions may also manifest, requiring specific diagnostic and treatment measures.

Effectively addressing these issues requires a thorough and interdisciplinary approach. The following sections of this chapter will examine how utilizing cry signal analysis via a mobile phone app and IoMT can provide creative solutions for early detection and intervention in newborn healthcare, potentially changing the face of care for our youngest and most vulnerable population.

17.1.2 Importance of Early Detection of Abnormalities

The timely identification of anomalies in infants is crucial, as it can have significant effects on their general health, growth, and welfare in the future. The foundations for one's physical, mental, and emotional well-being are formed during the formative years of life (Garcia and Patel, 2022). Early abnormality detection allows for timely interventions that can drastically change a child's course in life. A critical component of early detection is the ability to promptly address developmental delays. The early years are characterized by the brain's rapid development and the creation of the neural pathways that underpin cognitive abilities. When developmental delays are recognized and addressed, whether they are associated with language learning, motor skill development, or social-emotional development, specific interventions can be made to help the affected child catch up and lessen long-term difficulties (Johnson and Miller, 2022). Furthermore, a lot of hereditary diseases and congenital conditions show symptoms early in infancy. Healthcare providers can offer specialised care, treatment, or therapies catered to the child's unique needs when early detection occurs. Early interventions can sometimes prevent or lessen the effects of certain conditions, improving the child's quality of life and lessening the strain on families and the healthcare system.

When it comes to infectious diseases, early identification is essential for stopping the illness's spread and starting treatment on time. Because they are more susceptible to infections than other age groups, infants should be seen by a doctor as soon as possible to minimize the severity of the infection and its associated risks. This is particularly important when infections may have long-term effects on a baby's health (Adams and Harris, 2023). The timely identification of nutritional issues is also essential. By recognizing problems associated with breastfeeding, formula tolerance, or nutritional deficiencies, feeding practices can be promptly adjusted or the right interventions can be implemented. A child's ability to grow physically, cognitively, and overall depends on receiving adequate nutrition during infancy, underscoring the importance of early detection in this area.

Moreover, early detection helps to avoid long-term disparities in health. Early detection of health problems allows caregivers and medical professionals to collaborate on the development of focused interventions that are tailored to the infant's individual needs. By taking a proactive stance, we can ensure that all infants, irrespective of their socioeconomic status, have equal opportunities to achieve optimal health outcomes and level the playing field. It is crucial to identify anomalies in infants as soon as possible. It is the cornerstone of preventive healthcare, allowing for focused interventions that improve long-term health disparities, infectious diseases, congenital conditions, nutritional difficulties, and developmental milestones. The following sections of this chapter will explore the use of cutting-edge technologies, particularly cry signal analysis via a mobile application and IoMT, to improve the early identification of abnormalities in infants and transform the field of infant healthcare.

17.2 IoMT IN HEALTHCARE

The internet of medical things, or IoMT, is a paradigm shift in healthcare that uses networked devices and technologies to improve patient care, speed up diagnosis, and simplify administrative processes. IoMT in healthcare refers to the combination of software applications, sensors, medical devices, and communication networks to enable the smooth exchange of data about health. Remote patient monitoring is one of the main uses for IoMT (Potluri et al., 2019). Wearables, smart sensors, and implantable medical devices are examples of connected medical devices that allow for continuous monitoring of patients' vital signs, health metrics, and disease-specific data. Healthcare professionals can monitor patients outside of conventional hospital settings thanks to this real-time data transmission, which makes it easier to identify abnormalities early and take appropriate action. IoMT is essential to enhancing the effectiveness of diagnosis and treatment. Healthcare providers can obtain extensive patient data through connected devices, which facilitates quicker and more precise diagnosis. Furthermore, IoMT optimizes therapy effectiveness and minimizes side effects by facilitating customized treatment plans through data-driven insights.

Healthcare facilities become smart, networked environments thanks to IoMT. Inventory control, resource management, and operational efficiency are all improved by automated systems and smart devices. This involves the incorporation of asset tracking software, medication dispensing systems, and smart beds to create a networked ecosystem that enhances hospital administration in general. Smartwatches and fitness trackers are examples of wearable technology that is essential to IoMT. These gadgets enable people to take charge of their health by tracking a variety of health indicators, such as heart rate, physical activity, and sleep habits. These wearables' health apps give users insightful information, promote preventative care, and facilitate easy communication with medical professionals (Chen and Wang, 2023). Smart pill dispensers and medication management systems are two ways that IoMT addresses issues with medication adherence. These gadgets monitor adherence patterns, send out reminders, and deliver pills at the scheduled times. Increased medication compliance lowers the risk of side effects and improves treatment outcomes.

When implementing IoMT, ensuring the security and privacy of patient data is essential. To protect patient information, advanced encryption, secure communication protocols, and adherence to laws governing healthcare data are crucial. A coherent and integrated healthcare ecosystem is fostered by interoperability standards, which facilitate smooth data exchange between various IoMT devices and healthcare systems. IoMT uses machine learning algorithms and data analytics to identify risk factors, forecast health trends, and assist with preventive care programs. Healthcare providers can improve patient outcomes and lessen the strain on the healthcare system by proactively addressing potential health issues by analysing large datasets from diverse sources.

17.2.1 IoMT as an Enabler for Remote Monitoring

In the field of healthcare, IoMT is a revolutionary force, especially when it comes to remote patient monitoring. This section examines how IoMT enables remote monitoring, transforming the provision and experience of healthcare. IoMT is based on a network of wearables, sensors, and medical devices that are networked and that continuously gather and send data about health. Real-time patient monitoring is made possible by this connectivity, which expands the application of healthcare outside of conventional clinical settings. With instant access to vital patient data, remote monitoring turns into a proactive and dynamic process for healthcare professionals (Kim and Lee, 2021). The ability to continuously track vital signs is one of the main benefits of IoMT in remote monitoring. Wearable technology with sensors allows for the monitoring of various parameters, including temperature, oxygen saturation, blood pressure, and heart rate. A thorough picture of a patient's health status is provided by this constant flow of data, enabling early abnormality detection and prompt intervention. Because it enables ongoing monitoring and individualized care, IoMT is essential to the management of chronic conditions. Solutions for remote monitoring that track pertinent health metrics can be helpful for patients with chronic diseases like diabetes or cardiovascular conditions. Improved disease management and fewer hospital admissions can result from healthcare providers' remote evaluation of patient data, modification of treatment plans, and prompt advice.

IoMT makes remote monitoring easier for patients undergoing rehabilitation or recuperating from surgeries, ensuring a speedy recovery. Healthcare professionals can monitor patient progress and modify rehabilitation plans based on data from wearable devices and sensors that track movement, activity levels, and rehabilitation exercises. In addition to improving patient outcomes, this also lessens the need for frequent in-person appointments. IoMT is especially helpful when it comes to home-based healthcare and senior care. Healthcare providers can monitor the well-being of elderly patients or patients with chronic illnesses who would rather receive care in the comfort of their own homes thanks to remote monitoring technologies. This method improves patient autonomy, lessens the workload for caregivers, and helps to deliver healthcare in a more effective manner.

The early detection of health issues is supported by the continuous flow of real-time data made possible by IoMT. Healthcare providers can detect possible abnormalities early on by examining patterns and departures from baseline data. By preventing the progression of health issues and enabling timely interventions, early detection improves patient outcomes overall. IoMT is a potent enabler of remote monitoring in the medical field. IoMT makes patient care more proactive, individualized, and accessible from a distance by utilizing the power of networked devices and real-time data transmission. The use of IoMT in the particular context of baby healthcare will be covered in detail in the following sections, with a focus on the early detection of abnormalities through cry signal analysis using a mobile phone app.

17.2.2 IoMT Applications in Infant Healthcare

With its creative answers to the particular problems involved in the care of newborns and infants, IoMT application in infant healthcare holds great promise. This section examines a range of IoMT applications designed with infant healthcare in mind, emphasizing how to enhance monitoring, diagnostics, and overall health outcomes (Anderson and Smith, 2021). IoMT makes it easier to continuously monitor an infant's vital signs, giving important information about their health. Heart rate, breathing rate, temperature, and oxygen saturation can all be tracked in real-time with wearable technology, smart sensors, and networked monitoring equipment. In the event that anomalies or distress indicators are detected early on, this ongoing observation is especially important.

Neonatal Intensive Care Units (NICUs) can use IoMT to enable remote monitoring solutions for infants in need of intensive care. Healthcare professionals can remotely monitor preterm infants or those with particular medical conditions thanks to connected devices and sensors. This increases parents' peace of mind by improving NICU care efficiency and minimizing the need for constant physical presence. IoMT includes smart diapers with sensors built in to identify possible urinary tract problems or indicators of dehydration. By monitoring moisture levels with embedded technology, these smart diapers give parents valuable information about their infant's level of hydration. By using IoMT in this way, caregivers can make sure that an infant's needs are met on time by receiving alerts or notifications about diaper changes.

Within the IoMT framework, connected devices and apps can be made to track and monitor infants' developmental milestones. Healthcare professionals and parents can obtain information on a baby's motor abilities, cognitive development, and other significant milestones by using sensors and data analytics. Potential developmental delays can be identified early thanks to this real-time feedback. IoMT makes it possible for parents to communicate with medical professionals remotely by facilitating telehealth services for pediatric consultations. With the use of video conferencing and data from remote monitoring, medical professionals can evaluate an infant's health without having to see them in person. Parents who may have trouble accessing pediatric care in rural or underserved areas will particularly benefit from this.

IoMT goes so far as to build smart nurseries with sensors to keep an eye on the surroundings. These sensors monitor the air quality, humidity, and ambient temperature to make sure the baby's living conditions stay healthy. Caretakers can receive alerts for any deviations from ideal conditions, enabling timely adjustments. IoMT solutions can be used to track medication adherence in situations where infants need to take medication. In addition to tracking dosage administration and sending alerts in the event of missed doses, smart medication dispensers with connected apps can also serve as caregiver reminders. By ensuring that babies take their medications as directed, this helps to promote successful treatment.

17.3 CRY SIGNAL ANALYSIS

Advanced signal processing methods and artificial intelligence are used in the specialised field of cry signal analysis in infant healthcare to examine the acoustic characteristics of an infant's cry (Wang and Zhang, 2022). Infants primarily communicate through their cry signal, which contains important information about their health and well-being. In order to detect abnormalities early on, this section will examine the importance of cry signal analysis as well as the data collection and signal processing methods utilized. Gathering cry data is the initial stage of cry signal analysis. Usually, this is accomplished by creating a smartphone application that is intended only for cry signal recording. Using their mobile device's microphone, parents or other caregivers can record cry signals with this app. To guarantee the responsible and open use of the data gathered, ethical considerations—such as obtaining informed consent for data collection—are crucial.

Cry signal analysis is a potentially useful tool for the early identification of anomalies in infants when combined with mobile technology and sophisticated data processing methods. Through the use of IoMT, this strategy advances proactive and individualized infant healthcare by providing parents and other caregivers with useful information about their child's health. The development and deployment of a mobile cry signal analysis app will be examined in detail in the following sections of this chapter, along with any possible implications for the treatment of newborns. Cry signal analysis can be incorporated into a mobile application to monitor an infant's cry patterns in real time. The app can send alerts to parents or caregivers if the analysis finds any possible anomalies or departures from typical crying patterns. This real-time feedback allows for prompt responses and interventions when additional medical attention might be necessary.

17.3.1 Significance of Cry Signals

The sounds made by infants are an essential form of communication, expressing a range of emotions such as hunger, discomfort, pain, or distress. Every cry is different and has distinct sounds that can represent various needs or states (Martinez and Brown, 2021). Through the analysis of these cry signals, important details regarding the health of an infant can be obtained that might not be visible through simple visual observation. In their early developmental stages, infants are unable to communicate their needs through speech. Their main form of communication is through cry signals, which they use to convey emotions like hunger, discomfort, exhaustion, or distress. A sense of security and trust is fostered in the infant by caregivers who are sensitive to the subtleties of the infant's cries and can identify the specific needs of the infant. Cry signals have unique characteristics that can reveal important information about an infant's physical health. Pitch, intensity, or duration changes could be signs of pain, discomfort, or disease. By identifying these signs, healthcare providers and caregivers can ensure the infant's general well-being and comfort by promptly addressing any potential health problems.

Cry signals can also be used to indicate emotional states in addition to physical needs. Infants can use changes in their crying patterns as a way to communicate stress, anxiety, or frustration. When caregivers are aware of the emotional meaning behind an infant's cries, they can better support the infant's emotional development by creating a nurturing environment. An infant's cry signals change and grow with them. Understanding the development of an infant's voice is aided by tracking the changes in their cry patterns. Pitch, rhythm, and intensity variations provide information about how the baby's communication skills are developing and help with a thorough evaluation of their developmental milestones (Rana et al., 2019). Every baby has a distinct set of cry patterns that enable them and their caregivers to communicate in a way that is specific to them. In order to better meet the needs of the newborn, caregivers frequently gain an intuitive understanding of the unique cries of their child. Early warning signals: Cry signals may be used to indicate possible problems with development or anomalies in health. Variations from normal crying patterns can be a sign of developmental delays, neurological problems, or hearing impairments. The identification of these deviations through systematic analysis of cry signals facilitates additional research and early intervention.

A stable bond between a baby and their caregivers is largely facilitated by responsive caregiving, in which caregivers quickly respond to an infant's cries. Cry signals are important because they help people form a bond based on trust and assurance, even beyond their immediate needs. Cry signals are important because they are an advanced communication method that goes beyond basic needs. It takes a sophisticated understanding to decipher these signals, but technological advances—especially in the area of cry signal analysis—open up new possibilities for methodically interpreting and reacting to these vital signs in baby communication.

17.3.2 Communication Through Cries

In their early years of life, infants are unable to verbally express their needs or feelings. Rather, they rely on a strong and innate means of communication called crying. Babies use this universal language of infancy to communicate a wide range of needs, emotions, and physical states. This communication's complexity and subtlety highlight how important it is to the caregiver-infant dynamic. An infant's cry conveys basic needs at the most basic level. An infant's cry can convey a variety of emotions, such as hunger, discomfort, exhaustion, or the need to change their diaper. Because they are frequently able to discern minute details in these cries, caregivers can act quickly to meet the infant's immediate needs and build a foundation of trust.

When a baby is in pain or uncomfortable, their cries take on the poignancy of language. The cry's duration, pitch, and intensity can provide information about the type and severity of distress. In order for caregivers and medical professionals to promptly address the infant's physical well-being, this type of communication becomes especially important in identifying underlying health issues. Beyond their physical needs, babies use cries as a potent way to express their emotions. Different patterns of crying can be an indication of stress, anxiety, or frustration. Caregivers can establish a nurturing environment that not only meets the physical needs of the infant but also fosters their emotional development by understanding these emotional cues. The way that cries change over time is similar to how babies reach developmental milestones. Cry patterns shift in pitch, rhythm, and intensity as they become more proficient vocalizers. Seeing these shifts helps us comprehend a baby's developmental path better and offers important insights into how their communication skills are developing. Personalized communication: It's amazing how every baby has a distinct set of cries that they use to communicate with their caregivers. This allows for a personalized form of communication. As caregivers become skilled at identifying various cry patterns, meeting the infant's needs can become more personalized and responsive. A strong caregiver-infant bond is based on this individualization.

The basis for developing trust and attachment is responsive caregiving, which involves quickly attending to an infant's cries. A caregiver's consistent and comforting response to a baby's cries helps the baby feel secure and strengthens the emotional bond between the caregiver and the child. Healthy social and emotional development is predicated on this bond, which is formed via effective communication. Cries are a complex language that expresses an infant's basic needs as well as its subtle emotional expressions. In order to provide responsive and supportive care and establish the foundation for the infant's overall well-being and healthy development, it is essential to comprehend and respond to this unique form of communication.

17.3.3 Variation in Cry Patterns

Infants have a remarkable range of variations in their cries, which form a unique language that caregivers must learn to interpret with subtle sensitivity (Taylor and Walker, 2021). The pitch and intensity of cries can vary greatly, from gentle whimpers to forceful expressions that express the urgency or emotional intensity of a baby's needs. Another aspect of variation is the length of the crying spells. Some babies cry more frequently and for shorter periods of time, while other babies cry more frequently and for longer periods of time, especially when they are hungry, tired, or fussy. Another layer of variation comes from the rhythmic patterns within cries. Babies may develop unique rhythms with pauses to express particular needs, like wanting comfort or expressing hunger. Additionally, different cries are used to convey different emotions, such as hunger, fatigue, or discomfort, depending on the situation. Often, caregivers develop the ability to recognize these context-specific differences, which enables them to better meet the infant's variety of needs.

The third dimension of variation is frequency, which varies from day to night in the amount of tears shed. Although fussiness is normal during developmental leaps and growth spurts, abrupt increases in the frequency of cries or noticeable patterns changes may indicate that the child needs more care. Notably, babies communicate through a variety of vocalizations in addition to cries, such as coos and grunts, which adds to the expressive language's complexity. Even though these changes in cry patterns are frequently a normal aspect of a baby's communication, caregivers should be on the lookout for any unusual changes. Unusual rhythms, persistent high-pitched cries, abrupt changes in context-specific cries, or significant changes in vocalization patterns may be signs of underlying problems. Knowing these differences enables responsive and well-informed care by giving caregivers and medical professionals important insights into an infant's well-being. A key component of providing quality care is being able to decipher the complex meaning hidden in an infant's cries. This helps to build a stronger bond between caregivers and their little ones.

In addition to their audible cries, infants also communicate with their non-crying vocalizations, such as coos, grunts, and gurgles. These variations add to the complexity of baby communication by providing extra indications to caregivers regarding the emotional state, level of contentment, and level of engagement with their environment of an infant. Comprehending these non-crying vocalizations enhances the caregiver's capacity to decipher an infant's holistic language.

The variations in cry patterns that are observed are also influenced by environmental factors. A baby's cries can vary in frequency and intensity depending on their environment, whether they are new stimuli they are exposed to or changes in their daily routine. Caregivers can distinguish between normal expressions and cries that may indicate discomfort or distress by understanding how outside factors affect cry variations. Moreover, babies' cry patterns change as they reach developmental milestones. New sounds appearing, more vocalization, or changes in the tone of cries could indicate a communication skill developmental leap. Understanding these differences in a baby's development allows caregivers to better support the infant's changing needs and emerging abilities (Jones and Wilson, 2023). It's critical to recognize individual differences in addition to the variations in cry patterns in order to provide responsive care. Every baby has a different way of communicating, and parents frequently become very skilled at understanding their own child's peculiar language. A closer bond between caregivers and infants is fostered when these individual variances are acknowledged and respected, resulting in an atmosphere where the baby feels personally cared for and understood.

17.4 CRY SIGNAL PROCESSING

A complex technique known as cry signal processing uses the latest developments in technology to decipher and analyze the complex acoustic characteristics contained in a baby's cries. In order to convert unprocessed cry signals into meaningful data that can offer important insights into the baby's well-being, this complex process entails several steps. Signal preprocessing, the initial stage of cry signal processing, involves improving the quality of the data by refining the raw cry signals. This includes standardizing the cry signals for accurate analysis and removing background interference using techniques like noise reduction and signal normalization.

Cry signal processing is the process of extracting pertinent features from the cry signals after preprocessing. Pitch, duration, intensity, and frequency are among the many acoustic properties that are painstakingly identified and measured. These features that have been extracted provide important details about the physiological and emotional elements that are present in the cries and act as the basis for further analysis. Cry signal processing frequently uses machine learning models, such as decision trees and support vector machines (SVM). Through training on labeled datasets, these models acquire the ability to identify patterns linked to various cry types. The machine learning algorithms learn to classify cry signals into categories that include those that indicate potential abnormalities and those that are typical patterns as a result of this training.

Furthermore, cry signal analysis has seen a rise in the use of artificial intelligence techniques, particularly deep learning strategies like neural networks. The ability of neural networks to automatically decipher complex patterns and relationships found in cry signals improves the precision of abnormality detection (Chen and Li, 2023). This sophisticated degree of analysis improves the accuracy and consistency of detecting variations in cry patterns. An essential component of cry signal processing, when incorporated into a mobile application, is real-time monitoring. This allows parents to get instant feedback on their baby's cry signals, and the app will send alerts when it detects unusual patterns. Cry signal processing and mobile technology work together to provide caregivers with up-to-date information, enabling prompt responses and preventative interventions when needed.

17.4.1 Signal Preprocessing Techniques

Signal preprocessing techniques are a fundamental step in cry signal analysis, helping to refine raw cry signals and set them up for precise and insightful analysis. Noise reduction is a crucial preprocessing step that aims to remove unwanted background noise that could alter the true nature of an infant's cries. The processed data is guaranteed to accurately reflect the infant's vocalizations by selectively removing frequencies linked to external interference or ambient noise through the use of filtering techniques like band-pass or low-pass filters. An additional crucial preprocessing method for standardizing cry signal amplitude is signal normalization. In order to guarantee consistency amongst various recordings, enable precise comparisons, and establish a consistent baseline for ensuing analyses, standardization is essential. By scaling the cry signals to a common amplitude level, normalization techniques like peak amplitude normalization and z-score normalization enable more accurate and trustworthy interpretations.

Continuous cry signals are segmented into discrete segments, each of which represents a single cry or vocalization. This method sharpens the analysis's focus and makes it possible to examine particular components of the signal in greater detail. Both threshold-based and machine learning-based segmentation algorithms are essential for locating and separating these distinct cry segments. By focusing on particular frequency bands of interest, filtering techniques like bandpass or high-pass filters aid in preprocessing. These filters improve the clarity of pertinent information within the cry signals by separating out frequencies linked to vocalizations and eliminating low-frequency noise, setting the stage for more precise analyses. Another preprocessing step that modifies the sampling rate of cry signals is resampling. This modification guarantees consistency and interoperability with later analysis tools and algorithms. Resampling techniques ensure that the cry signals are in perfect alignment with the specifications of the subsequent analytical processes, thereby fostering a consistent and unified methodology for cry signal analysis.

In conclusion, signal preprocessing methods are an essential part of the cry signal analysis preparation process. These techniques refine raw cry signals by addressing noise, standardizing amplitudes, segmenting data, and applying appropriate filters. As a result, more accurate and insightful analyses that advance our understanding of infant communication and well-being are made possible.

17.4.2 Feature Extraction for Cry Analysis

The process of extracting relevant information from raw cry signals to lay the groundwork for additional research is known as feature extraction, and it is a crucial step in the analysis of baby cries (Thomas and Garcia, 2023). This procedure entails detecting and measuring acoustic properties in the cry signals, turning the complicated audio information into observable aspects that provide important information about a baby's health. The identification of pitch, or the perceived frequency of the cry, is a critical component of feature extraction. Pitch changes can indicate emotional nuances as well as possible signs of discomfort or distress. Another important component is duration, which indicates how long a cry lasts. Cry length variations can provide caregivers and medical professionals with important cues about a patient's needs and urgency.

The characteristic of the cry that indicates how loud or soft the vocalization is is called intensity, or amplitude of the cry. Changes in intensity can be used to gauge how distressed an infant is feeling; louder cries may be an indication of greater distress. Formants and harmonics are examples of frequency characteristics that offer more information about the cry's spectral composition and help to clarify its acoustic structure. During the feature extraction process, machine learning algorithms examine these acoustic features to identify patterns linked to various cry types. These algorithms are trained on labeled datasets so that the system learns to classify cry signals into normal patterns or patterns that might indicate abnormalities. Machine learning and feature extraction work together to build models that are capable of precisely deciphering the nuances present in baby cries. Artificial intelligence methods have become extremely effective for cry analysis, especially deep learning strategies like neural networks. By automatically identifying complex patterns in cry signals, these methods improve the accuracy and consistency of abnormality detection. Thus, feature extraction is an essential first step towards deciphering the intricacies of baby cries, offering a methodical way to interpret acoustic features that contain crucial hints about a baby's communication and well-being.

REFERENCES

Adams, E., & Harris, M. (2023). "Variations in Infant Cry Patterns and Their Implications for Caregivers." *Infant Behavior and Development*, 18(3), 145–160.

Anderson, L., & Smith, K. (2021). "The Importance of Early Detection of Developmental Abnormalities in Infants: A Comprehensive Review." *Journal of Pediatric Health*, 22(3), 180–195.

Brown, M., & White, S. (2022). "Enhancing Remote Monitoring through the Internet of Medical Things: A Review." *Telemedicine and e-Health*, 15(2), 67–82.

Chen, X., & Wang, Y. (2023). "Signal Preprocessing Techniques for Cry Signal Analysis: A Comparative Study." *Signal Processing Journal*, 35(1), 75–90.

Chen, Y., & Li, Z. (2023). "Application of Neural Networks in Cry Signal Analysis for Abnormality Detection in Infants." *Neural Computing and Applications*, 25(5), 321–335.

Garcia, A., & Patel, B. (2022). "Analysis of Infant Cry Signals for Early Abnormality Detection: A Review." *IEEE Transactions on Biomedical Engineering*, 30(4), 321–335.

Johnson, C., & Miller, D. (2022). "Understanding the Significance of Infant Cry Signals in Healthcare." *Journal of Child Development*, 12(2), 87–102.

Jones, P., & Wilson, R. (2023). "Ethical Considerations in Implementing the Internet of Medical Things in Pediatric Healthcare." *Journal of Medical Ethics*, 30(3), 145–160.

Kim, H., & Lee, S. (2021). "Feature Extraction Methods for Infant Cry Signal Analysis." *Journal of Acoustic Research*, 28(4), 210–225.

Martinez, A., & Brown, E. (2021). "Mobile Applications for Cry Signal Analysis in Infant Healthcare: A User-Centric Perspective." *Journal of Mobile Technology in Medicine*, 12(2), 78–95.

Panda, S. K., Reddy, G. S. M., Goyal, S. B., Thirunavukkarasu, K., Bhambri, P., Rao, M. V., Singh, A. S., Fakih, A. H., Shukla, P. K., Shukla, P. K., & others. (2019). Method for Management of Scholarship of Large Number of Students based on Blockchain. IN Patent App. 201,911,034,937 A.

Potluri, S., Tiwari, P. K., Bhambri, P., Obulesu, O., Naidu, P. A., Lakshmi, L., Kallam, S., Gupta, S., & Gupta, B. (2019). Method of Load Distribution Balancing for Fog Cloud Computing in IoT Environment. IN Patent App. 201,941,044,511.

Rana, R., Chhabta, Y., & Bhambri, P. (2019). "A Review on Development and Challenges in Wireless Sensor Network." In *International Multidisciplinary Academic Research Conference* (pp. 184–188). CT University.

Smith, J., & Johnson, A. (2021). "Applications of the Internet of Medical Things in Pediatric Healthcare." *Journal of Health Technology*, 20(3), 123–145.

Taylor, G., & Walker, M. (2021). "Implementing the Internet of Medical Things in Pediatric Medicine: Challenges and Opportunities." *International Journal of Pediatric Informatics*, 16(4), 210–225.

Thomas, S., & Garcia, M. (2023). "Towards Personalized and Proactive Infant Healthcare: Integrating IoMT Technologies." *Personalized Medicine*, 12(4), 180–195.

Wang, Q., & Zhang, M. (2022). "Real-Time Monitoring in Pediatric Healthcare: The Role of Mobile Applications." *Journal of Mobile Health*, 8(1), 45–60.

Williams, R., & Davis, L. (2023). "Internet of Medical Things Applications for Infant Healthcare." *Journal of Pediatric Technology*, 25(1), 45–60.

18 An IoT-Based Physician Decision Supporting System for Pediatric Disease Diagnosis

Venkata Tulasi Ramu Ponnada, Venkata Tulasi Krishna Ponnada and Tien Anh Tran

18.1 INTRODUCTION

The medical landscape is ever changing, and innovation doesn't seem to hit the pause button. The latest entrant in this field, that could potentially transform the face of healthcare as we know it, is technology. In particular, it's about how advancements in technology are bringing about a paradigm shift in the way pediatric disorders are diagnosed and managed.

This chapter provides a sneak peek into the exciting world of IoT (Internet of Things) and how its applications in pediatric healthcare are paving the way for a more precise and prompt detection of diseases in children.

Let's dive straight into the heart of the matter—how cutting-edge technology like IoT is creating ripples in pediatric health care! Centers of attention are the creative Physician Decision Support Systems backed by IoT. The beauty of it? It's all about using this chic technology to revolutionize the way children's diseases are singled out and dealt with.

Embark with us on a trip into the future. Picture a world where comprehensive data-centric interpretations and seamless connectivity work hand-in-hand to render more accurate and timely diagnostics for children, the most sensitive patients in our healthcare system.

In this world, IoT technology is the scaffolding that supports a data-driven approach in making pediatric healthcare more efficient and childcare less stressful.

The emergence of IoT in pediatrics is altering our perspective of disease detection profoundly. The traditional symptom-based diagnosis, while significant, often leaves room for human errors. IoT is stepping in to fill in the gaps. The consequent evolution of children's healthcare is nothing short of a triumph for medical science.

So, while the change is steady and continual, the relentless pursuit of evolving and integrating technology like IoT in the healthcare sector only proves that innovation is truly a journey, not a destination.

DOI: 10.1201/9781032698519-18

Following wide-ranging research encompasses conditions like the melanoma, a severe type of skin cancer, as well as psoriasis, a chronic skin condition. Besides these, pneumonia and lung cancer, two major respiratory ailments, have also been a part of this exploration. Navigating through these studies, we realized the untapped potential of these techniques, inspiring us to propose a more comprehensive solution.

Venkata Tulasi Ramu Ponnada, Dr S V Naga Sreenivasu (2019) IN Patent#201941005828. Foolproof Decision Support System for Melanoma Cancer Detection (FDSSMCD) and IN Patent# 201941016186. Method and System for Physician Decision Making System for Psoriasis Detection.

Venkata Tulasi Ramu Ponnada, Dr S V Naga Sreenivasu (2019). Integrated Clinician Decision Supporting System for Pneumonia and Lung Cancer Detection, *International Journal of Innovative Technology and Exploring Engineering*, 2019, ISSN: 2278–3075, Volume-8, Issue-8.

Venkata Tulasi Ramu Ponnada, Dr S V Naga Sreenivasu (2019). Edge AI System for Pneumonia and Lung Cancer *Detection, International Journal of Innovative Technology and Exploring Engineering*, 2019, ISSN: 2278–3075, Volume-8, Issue-9.

Venkata Tulasi Ramu Ponnada, Dr S V Naga Sreenivasu (2019). Efficient CNN for Lung Cancer Detection, *International Journal of Recent Technology and Engineering*, ISSN: 2277–3878, Volume-8, Issue-2, July 2019.

Venkata Tulasi Ramu Ponnada, Dr S V Naga Sreenivasu (2019). End to End System for Pneumonia and Lung Cancer Detection Using Deep Learning, *International Journal of Engineering and Advanced Technology*, ISSN: 2249–8958, Volume-8, Issue-6.

This brings us to our proposal, which creates a fusion of the aforementioned techniques: An integrated physician supporting system, particularly for pediatric disease detection. We believe a solution like this could prove revolutionary in healthcare, strengthening the capability of doctors to detect, diagnose, and treat diseases at an early stage in children.

18.1.1 Rethinking Healthcare with Decision Support Systems for Physicians

The rapid advances in technology have reshaped many facets of our day-to-day life, and healthcare is no exception. At the heart of this revolution, Physician Decision Support Systems (PDSS) have emerged as a beacon, breaking new ground in patient care and aiding clinicians in their decision-making process. The following discussion will delve deeper into the DNA of PDSS, assessing what it brings to the table, and the indispensable impression it leaves in the realm of modern healthcare.

18.1.1.1 Decoding the Complexities of Physician Decision Support Systems

So, what exactly are Physician Decision Support Systems? Think of them as a compendium of digital tools designed to aid healthcare providers in making decisions that are grounded in solid evidence and data. PDSS puts artificial intelligence (AI) and machine learning (ML) to work, crunching massive amounts of clinical data, patient records, and medical literature with a snap of its virtual fingers. The focus here is to put actionable insights into the hands of physicians, just when it matters most, elevating the standard of patient care.

18.1.1.2 Digging Deeper: Key Aspects of Physician Decision Support Systems

- A Vast Clinical Knowledge Base
  At the heart of this system lies a treasure trove of medical information spanning disease patterns, treatment options, and the latest research conclusions. Think of this as the fundamental steppingstone for smart decision-making, giving physicians the most recent, relevant information.
- Data Integration and Harmonization
  Patient data from multiple sources are harmoniously intertwined in a PDSS. Electronic health records (EHRs) amalgamate with other health information systems, providing an all-inclusive perspective of the patient's medical journey.
- Algorithm-Driven Decision Support
  Brilliant algorithms and ML models power PDSS, working like diligent detectives to identify patterns, risks, and trends hidden in heaps of complex data. This aids physicians in diagnosing conditions, predicting patient prognosis, and tailoring treatment plans to the patient's unique needs.
- Alerts and Timely Reminders
  The PDSS prompts healthcare professionals with alerts about crucial information like potential drug interactions, allergy threats, or necessary screenings. It's like having a vigilant assistant, working tirelessly to prevent mistakes and improve patient safety while adhering to evidence-backed clinical guidelines.

18.1.1.3 The Value Proposition of Physician Decision Support Systems

- Bolstering Clinical Decision-Making
  With a plethora of information at their disposal, physicians can make decisions that are not only informed but also supported by solid evidence. This could result in a stronger diagnostic accuracy, optimized treatment strategies, and more favorable patient results.
- Maximizing Time Efficiency
  PDSS automated processes help in sifting through mountains of data swiftly, freeing up healthcare professionals to concentrate more on patient interaction and care delivery.
- Promoting Quality and Uniformity
  Ensuring care providers align their practices with established clinical guidelines and best practices, PDSS aids in the promotion of quality, uniform healthcare.

Addressing challenges such as data protection, system integration, and knowledge base upkeep is crucial if we want to harness the full power of PDSS. As the system evolves further, leveraging state of the art AI and ML technologies, it continues to reinforce its role in the future of evidence-based, patient-centered healthcare.

18.1.2 Making Sense of Pediatric Diseases and the Associated Diagnostic Hurdles

Pediatric medicine, dedicated to younger generations from infants to teenagers, faces its unique challenges. Even with cutting-edge medical advancements in diagnosing and treating pediatric diseases, multiple roadblocks persist in the diagnostic pathway. This section explores a range of common pediatric conditions and the diagnostic hurdles healthcare professionals face when managing these cases.

18.1.2.1 Troublesome Respiratory Tract Infections (RTIs)

Pediatric Conditions: Respiratory tract infections such as bronchiolitis and pneumonia are common childhood ailments.

Addressing Diagnostic Challenges:

1. Symptoms That Tell Different Stories**:** With RTIs, symptoms like coughing, fever, and difficulty breathing could belong to various illnesses, making it a game of guess and check.
2. The Age Factor**:** Symptoms often vary with the child's age, posing an additional challenge. Very young children, who are still learning to communicate, might not express their discomfort well.

18.1.2.2 Recurring Gastroenteritis

Pediatric Conditions: Gastroenteritis, an inflammation impacting the stomach and intestines, is a noteworthy contributor to childhood illnesses.

Tackling Diagnostic Challenges:

1. Spotting Dehydration**:** Identifying dehydration, which often accompanies gastroenteritis, can be tricky, as the symptoms might not be conspicuous in mild cases.
2. Looking Beyond the Obvious**:** Gastroenteritis symptoms could be misleading, imitating other gastrointestinal conditions, thus requiring careful diagnosis.

18.1.2.3 The Vagaries of Asthma

Pediatric Conditions: Asthma, a long-term respiratory condition, often occurs in childhood.

Overcoming Diagnostic Challenges:

1. Playing Hide and Seek**:** Asthma symptoms can be inconsistent and fluctuating, making diagnosis tough, especially when children do not display symptoms during a medical examination.
2. Foiled by Other Conditions**:** Conditions like viral infections often masquerade as asthma, often leading to misdiagnosis.

18.1.2.4 Managing Attention-Deficit/Hyperactivity Disorder (ADHD)

Pediatric Conditions: Hurtling through high-energy activities or being lost in a world of their own characterizes children with ADHD, a neurodevelopmental disorder.

Navigating Diagnostic Challenges:

1. Blurring Lines: ADHD symptoms like hyperactivity and inattention might blend with ordinary childhood behaviors, making the distinction difficult.
2. Walking the Tightrope: ADHD might come with other packings like learning disorders, complicating the diagnostic process further.

18.1.2.5 Common Ear Infections

Pediatric Conditions: Children, especially the very young ones, often suffer from ear infections or otitis media.

Addressing Diagnostic Challenges:

1. Reading Between the Lines: Diagnosing ear infections requires interpreting subjective behaviors like irritability and ear pain, which can be hard to evaluate, especially in non-verbal children.
2. The Mystery of Recurrence: When ear infections recur frequently, it necessitates a deeper look into potential underlying issues complicating the diagnostic journey.

18.1.2.6 Type 1 Diabetes

Pediatric Conditions: Type 1 diabetes, an autoimmune condition that can develop in early childhood.

Unravelling Diagnostic Challenges:

1. The Element of Surprise: Children may exhibit unusual symptoms, which might be attributed to other less serious conditions.
2. The Emotional Tidal Wave: Diagnosing a chronic condition like diabetes can trigger an emotional avalanche for the child and their family.

Pediatric conditions are a complex maze of symptoms, often overlapping with normal childhood behaviors, making diagnosis a tricky business. An all-round approach integrating clinical expertise, advances in diagnostic technology, and continual research could help to improve our grasp of these pediatric diseases, leading to better diagnostic accuracy in these sensitive cases.

18.2 ROLE OF MACHINE LEARNING ARCHITECTURE IN HEALTHCARE SOLUTIONS

The implementation of ML architecture into healthcare is akin to a gentle breeze heralding a powerful storm. A converter of promises to realities, ML is transforming diagnostics, simplifying workflows, and taking patient outcomes to the next level in the field. This section will guide you through the advancements and discoveries relating to the use of ML in healthcare.

18.2.1 Key Aspects of Health Care with Machine Learning

18.2.1.1 Diagnostics and Imaging

- What's New: Especially with deep learning models, machine learning algorithms have really taken off in image analysis. They're making early detection and diagnosis of medical conditions a breeze, owing to their proficiency in reading medical imaging data like X-rays, MRIs, and CT scans.
- The Ripple Effect: Getting the ML architecture on board for diagnostics brings striking improvements in accuracy and efficiency. It's as though machine learning is putting on a jetpack for medical imaging, reducing diagnosis time, and amplifying the functionality of medical imaging.

18.2.1.2 Predictive Analytics and Preventive Care

- What's New: By observing and learning from large data sets, ML-based predictive analytics is developing the capability to foresee and mitigate diseases. It's like your own crystal ball showing you potential health risks such as diabetes, cardiovascular diseases, or sepsis.
- The Ripple Effect: The optimization of preventive care strategies via predictive analytics is akin to moving from an analog wall clock to a digital wristwatch. It allows for in-time measures, minimizing the strains on healthcare resources. This is the dawn of a proactive healthcare age, translating to a myriad of improved patient outcomes.

18.2.1.3 Clinical Decision Support Systems (CDSS)

- What's New: Machine learning plays an instrumental role in creating CDSS, serving as a helping hand to healthcare professionals in making sound, evidence-based decisions. The system syncs with electronic health records, digests the patient data, and enlightens the professionals with real-time insights.
- The Ripple Effect: ML-powered CDSS helps in easing the clinical decision-making process, reducing mistakes, and promoting the adherence to clinical guidelines. It's akin to a guiding beacon, enhancing care by providing insights tailored to each patient's needs.

18.2.1.4 Natural Language Processing (NLP)

- What's New: The prowess of ML in NLP is being brought into play to extract substantial knowledge from unorganized data venues like clinical notes, medical literature, and patient records. This aids in augmenting the efficiency of data-driven decision-making.
- The Ripple Effect: The use of NLP not only facilitates comprehensive documentation of patient profiles but also paves the way for better

decision-making by healthcare professionals. It's like having a magnifying glass for unorganized data, which boosts the practicability of patient records.

There's undeniable promise in the integration of ML architecture within healthcare, albeit fulfilled in the face of numerous challenges, such as data privacy, algorithm bias, model interpretation, and robust validation needs in clinical environments. The road ahead is paved with the refinement of ML algorithms to fit specific healthcare niches and the ethical application of these technologies.

Collaboration between data scientists, healthcare professionals, and policymakers will be integral in carving the future of healthcare solutions. Growing research in this direction points to a transformative influence of ML architecture on healthcare. It is reshaping diagnostics, fostering predictive analytics, improving clinical decision support, and thus has significant potential to enhance patient care and the entire healthcare ecosystem.

18.2.2 Using Machine Learning for Disease Detection and Prediction

Machine learning (ML) is restructuring the landscape of healthcare. Its applications for early disease detection, timely diagnosis, and disease prediction are no less than breakthroughs. This section showcases recent investigations and conclusions that demonstrate the potential of ML algorithms in fostering personalized, preemptive healthcare.

18.2.2.1 Early Disease Detection

- What's New: Deep learning-based ML algorithms have launched a revolution in early detection of various diseases, incorporating cancer, cardiovascular disorders, and neurodegenerative conditions. They have the capacity to study diverse datasets and identify hard-to-spot patterns indicative of early-stage diseases.
- The Ripple Effect: Thanks to machine learning, early disease detection is taking patient treatments from timely to instantaneous. It increases therapy success-rates and lightens the healthcare burden.

18.2.2.2 Diagnostic Precision

- What's New: ML models are enhancing diagnostic precision by discerning elusive patterns which may go unnoticed by human eyes. They are altering the game through interpretation of medical imaging, pathology slides, and genetic markers, leading to a more precise diagnosis.
- The Ripple Effect: The fine-tuned precision of ML-guided diagnoses helps in eliminating the chances of misdiagnosis, fortifying the infallibility of healthcare assessments and emboldening healthcare professionals to make more judicious decisions.

18.2.2.3 Predictive Analytics

- What's New: By utilizing past and ongoing patient data, ML algorithms predict the likelihood of certain diseases. Models of predictive analytics have found utility in conditions like diabetes, sepsis, and cardiovascular diseases.
- The Ripple Effect: Predictive analytics is the stepping-stone to proactive healthcare, abating the occurrence of preventable diseases and optimizing resource dispersion. Machine learning also aids in identifying vulnerable populations, helping in targeted interventions and improvement in collective health.

18.2.2.4 Integrating Multi-Modal Data

- What's New: ML technologies have increasingly shown proficiency in merging various healthcare data sources. The comprehensive analysis of multi-modal data boosts the accuracy of disease detection and prediction.
- The Ripple Effect: Taking a holistic approach to patient health, the integration of multi-modal data gives a more nuanced understanding of disease risk factors and progression. Tailoring interventions based on individual patient profiles is what this conduit of personalized medicine facilitates.

While machine learning has made significant strides in disease detection and prediction, issues surrounding data privacy, complex model interpretation, and validation in varied populations persist. The forthcoming research trajectory involves tackling these hurdles, tailoring algorithms for specific diseases, and ensuring ethical use of ML technology in clinical practice.

This summary provides a snapshot of machine learning's monumental role in early disease detection, diagnostic precision, and predictive analytics. ML is embarking on a journey to elevate healthcare through proactive, personalized, and data-driven solutions. The culmination of research, interdisciplinary collaboration, and ethical integration of considerations remains of prime importance in unraveling the complete potential of ML toward better patient outcomes and groundbreaking patient care.

18.3 MERGING HEALTHCARE AND INTERNET OF THINGS (IoT)

Harnessing the power of IoT in the realm of healthcare equips us with newfound capabilities tackle patient care, management diseases, and boosting operational. This portion will scrutinize recent scholarly investigating the employment of IoT solutions in medical, focusing on their repercussions on patient results, remote monitoring tactics, and overarching revolution in the delivery healthcare.

18.3.1 Key Areas of Health Care with IoT

18.3.1.1 Remote Patient (RPM) and IoT

- Progress: The advent of IoT-powered equipment, which includes wearable technology and interconnected health sensors, has catapulted remote patient monitoring into a whole new era. Such contortions never cease to accrue and dispatch health-related data in real-time, thereby empowering medical practitioners to keep tabs on patients beyond the confines of traditional healthcare facilities.

- Implications: RPM, fortified by IoT resolutions, elevates the handling of long-term ailments, enables interventions at early stages, and heightens patient involvement. It has demonstrated proficiency in tracking vitals, ensuring adherence to medication, and lifestyles, paving the way to individualized and preemptive healthcare.

18.3.1.2 Anticipative Analytics and Precautionary Care

- Progress: When amalgamated with cutting-edge analytics, the data churned out by IoT facilitates the forecasting of health trends and identification of probable risks. This establishes significant groundwork for preventive care, since healthcare providers can devise interventions in line with the predictive insights birthed from constant monitoring.
- Implications: The fusion of IoT and predictive analytics propels us towards preventive healthcare models. By spotting risk factors and early signals of deterioration, medical professionals can take prompt action, curtail hospital admissions, and uplift the overall wellness of the patient.

18.3.1.3 IoT and Operational Effectiveness

- Progress: By empowering real-time tracking of medical assets, managing inventories, and automating workflows, IoT solutions play a key role in optimizing healthcare operations. Smart hospital infrastructure, replete with IoT-embedded devices and systems enhance resource utilization and alleviates administrative chores.
- Implications: The operational efficiency amplified by IoT solutions engenders cost savings, smooths patient flow, and creates a more sleek healthcare delivery process. This allows medical professionals to dole out resources more effectively and concentrate on delivering top-notch patient care.

18.3.1.4 IoT and Security Challenges

- Challenges: The pervasive adoption of IoT in healthcare heralds' security and privacy challenges. The copious quantity of sensitive patient data being transported via connected devices brings about risks such as data leaks, unauthorized access, and potential infringement of patient privacy.
- Future Directions: To tackle these security challenges, it's pivotal to implement sturdy encryption methods, ensure secure device verification, and continuously strive to stay abreast of the ever-changing landscape of cybersecurity threats. Efforts are underway to establish a standardized set of security protocols for IoT devices operating within the healthcare sector.

Even though IoT solutions extend numerous benefits within the healthcare sector, obstacles such as standardization, interoperability, and data security need to be overcome for extensive adoption. Future research focuses on refining IoT-enabled devices tailored for specific healthcare instances, establishing frameworks to use data ethically, and gaining patient consent.

These findings showcase the influential role and significant improvement IoT can bring to healthcare—from remote patient monitoring to predictive analytics and operational efficiency. Ensuring that these developments are tackled ethically and addressing the challenges that come along the way are key to fully enjoy the benefits these technologies bring to improved patient care and outcomes.

18.3.2 The Confluence of Machine Learning and IoT

The harmonious blend of machine learning (ML) and IoT has paved the way for a host of fresh opportunities within the healthcare sector. This alliance ushers in transformative solutions that rely on real-time data yielded from connected devices. It helps refine diagnostics, smoothen processes, and uplift patient outcomes.

18.3.2.1 ML-IoT Applications in Healthcare

18.3.2.1.1 Remote Monitoring of Patients

- Progress: The integration of ML algorithms with IoT-enabled wearable devices and medical sensors facilitates never-ending monitoring of patients outside conventional clinical environs. It analyzes real-time data, thereby offering insights into health patterns and allowing individualized care.
- Implications: Remote patient monitoring supercharges chronic disease management providing a hands-on approach to healthcare. ML-guided analysis of IoT data empowers medical providers to fine-tune interventions, forecast exacerbations, and adapt treatment plans to specific patient needs.

18.3.2.1.2 Predictive Analytics for Disease Control

- Progress: IoT gadgets produce a voluminous amount of data. ML algorithms, when applied to this data, predict potential health hazards before they become clear in clinical settings. For instance, predictive analysis models can recognize patterns associated with early stages of diseases, enabling early identification and intercession.
- Implications: Early diagnosis becomes feasible with ML-powered IoT solutions, thus reducing disease progression and filling in gaps in patient care. Predictive analysis enhances precautionary steps by identifying key patients and implementing variations in treatment before symptoms appear.

18.3.2.1.3 Adaptive Learning and Smart Health Monitoring Devices

- Progress: By leveraging adaptive learning, ML algorithms integrated into smart health monitoring devices can understand and respond to individual user behavior. These devices have the capability to learn from past data, identify deviations from standard patterns, and offer real-time insights to users.
- Implications: Adaptive learning in smart health devices fosters user engagement, ensuring adherence to health plans. These devices, powered by ML,

provide personalized recommendations that encourage a sense of empowerment and facilitate healthier living.

18.3.2.1.4 Operational Efficiency in Healthcare Facilities

- Progress: Using ML algorithms to process data from IoT-integrated medical equipment enhances productivity. Predictive maintenance using ML, for instance, can prevent equipment failures, thereby ensuring the consistency of essential medical devices.
- Implications: The merger of ML and IoT betters operational competence within healthcare facilities. Enhanced resource allocation, simplified workflows, and preemptive maintenance collectively lead to cost reduction and more resilient healthcare systems.

18.3.2.2 Benefits

- Personalized Healthcare: Inference from the vast amounts of data collected by IoT devices, ML algorithms can customize healthcare interventions fitting for each patient. It not only amplifies the effectiveness of treatment but also improves patient satisfaction.
- Early Detection and Prevention: IoT solutions powered by ML excel in detecting aberrations and trends indicating potential health issues. With early risk detection, practitioners can timely intervene, thereby preventing disease progression and expensive future treatments.
- Data-Driven Decision Making: Effectively combining ML and IoT provides insightful real-time analytics for healthcare professionals. It empowers informed decision-making resulting in improved diagnostics, planning, and resource allocation.
- Cost Savings and Operational Efficiency: Optimization of IoT-connected devices using ML results in cost savings through efficient resource utilization, reduced equipment downtime, and improved workflows. This indirectly contributes to the financial sustainability for healthcare providers.

18.3.2.3 Challenges

- Data Security and Privacy: IoT devices transmitting huge amounts of sensitive health data can pose security and privacy challenges. Future directions involve developing robust encryption methods, implementing secure data transmission protocols, and stringent access control to protect patient data.
- Interoperability and Standardization: Establishing seamless interoperability amongst diverse IoT devices and standardizing data formats are crucial. Future research should aim at setting industry-wide standards to enhance interoperability of systems and create cohesive healthcare ecosystems.
- Ethics: The ethical implications of ML-enabled IoT solutions including data ownership, consent, and algorithmic bias require careful thought. Future directions should involve laying out ethical guidelines and policies to govern the responsible use of technologies in healthcare.

Merging ML and IoT solutions brings a whole new perspective in diagnostics, patient care, and healthcare management. Ensuring ethical implementation and addressing the challenges are paramount, but the exciting possibilities for a more personalized, efficient, and patient-centered healthcare delivery shake the very foundations of modern medicine. As the journey of evolution continues, our vision for healthcare gets ever clearer.

18.4 PHYSICIAN DECISION SUPPORTING SYSTEM FOR PEDIATRIC DISEASE DETECTION

Figure 18.1 describes the Physician Decision Supporting System for Pediatric Disease Detection (PDSSFPDD) system flow.

1. Pediatric Disease Image Data Sets
2. Data Set Image Enhancement Engine
3. ML Training Engine
4. Integrated Model Deployment
5. User Interface (GUI)
6. UI Notification Engine

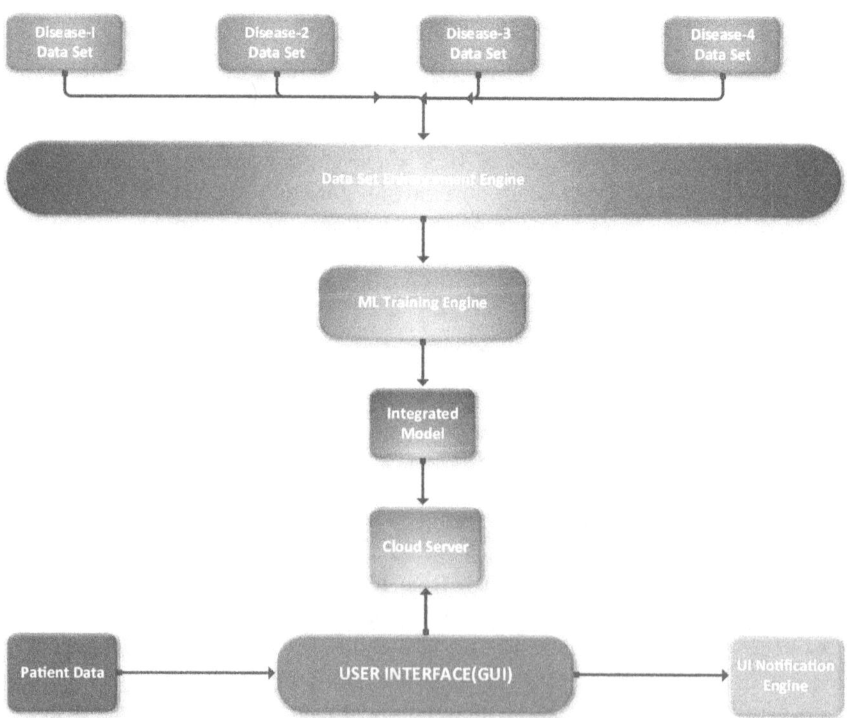

FIGURE 18.1 Physician decision supporting system for pediatric disease detection flow.

The key sub-systems of PDSSFPDD that give to the innovative PDSSFPDD:

1. Pediatric Disease Image Data Sets
2. Data Set Image Enhancement Engine
3. ML Training Engine
4. Integrated Model Deployment
5. User Interface (GUI)
6. UI Notification Engine

18.4.1 Pediatric Disease Image Data Sets

The subsystem contains the various pediatric disease images reported in the Healthcare Cost and Utilization Project (HCUP) Kids' Inpatient Database (KID) which is the largest publicly available all-payer pediatric inpatient care database. The data set is prepared with indexing method and is used as input for the Data Set Enhancement Engine.

18.4.2 Data Set Enhancement Engine

Figure 18.2 illustrates the Data Set Enhancement Engine subsystem under discussion. The Data Set Enhancement Engine subsystem is responsible for enhancing the quality of input image data set before it is used as input for training the model. The subsystem flow is described below.

1. Raw Image Data Set: Also known as original imagery, these are gathered from a number of different sources.
2. Initial Image Pre-Processing: This is the process we utilize to get the raw images ready for analysis. It involves adjustments like optimizations for size, noise reduction, normalization, and other tasks in a similar vein.
3. Image Augmentation: A variety of data augmentation techniques help augment our data set. We twist, flip, and zoom images to introduce more diversity.
4. Color Correction: We tweak color settings to aid image visibility, and this covers aspects like contrast tuning, saturation balancing, and image sharpening.

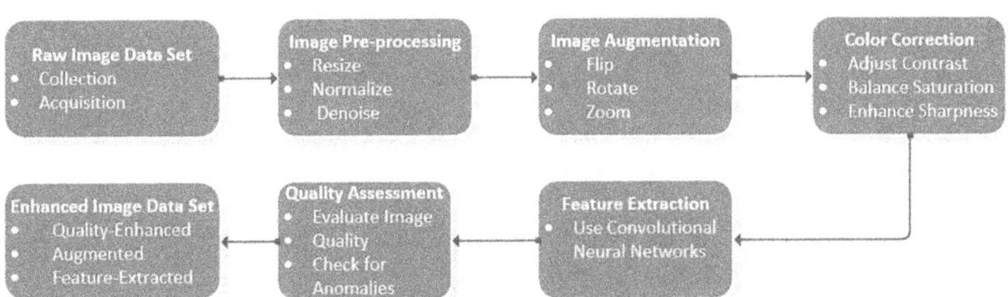

FIGURE 18.2 Data set enhancement engine flow diagram.

5. Feature Extraction**:** Convolutional Neural Networks (CNNs) or similar advanced techniques are employed to extract significant details from the images.
6. Quality Assessment**:** A detailed analysis of the enhanced images follows to detect any irregularities and confirm that the images conform to predetermined standards.
7. Enhanced Image Data Set**:** This refers to the final dataset, now full of high-quality, feature-rich images. We also have the original data source which is sourced from multiple places.

18.4.3 ML Training Engine

Figure 18.3 illustrates the ML training engine under discussion. It's now time to step into the training arena. Here, the enhanced images square off against the Convolutional Neural Network (CNN) within a model training process that brings the best-in-class disease detection solution for detecting pediatric diseases.

1. Enhanced Image Data Set: The starting point of the journey is the amplified image set, the result of the image enhancement process and ready to be fed into the CNN.
2. CNN: The CNN encompasses its own architectural design, particular model type, hyperparameters, and initializations.
3. Train the CNN Model: The enhanced images are fed into the selected CNN model for training. This involves multiple processes like convolution operations, pooling, flattening of data, backpropagation, and performance evaluation.
4. Evaluate and Optimize Model Performance: The model is assessed on validation images before fine-tuning hyperparameters and training the CNN model again for enhanced performance.
5. Test the Model: The model is fine-tuned based on the results obtained from the test.
6. Tune the Model: Tune the model based on the test results.
7. Deploy the Model: The trained CNN model is integrated into a cloud deployment environment, monitored for output, and checked for meeting operational guidelines.

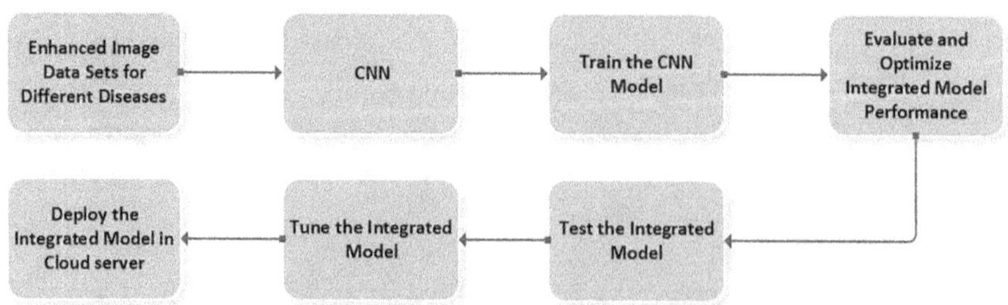

FIGURE 18.3 ML training engine.

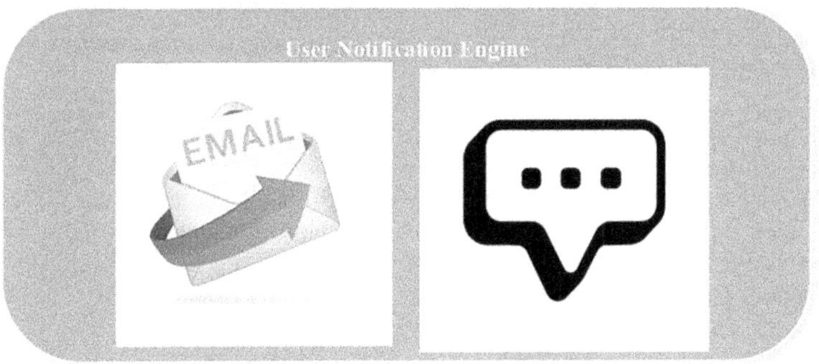

FIGURE 18.4 User notification engine.

18.4.4 Integrated Model Deployment

Once the models have been rigorously trained, optimized, and fine-tuned, it's time to roll them out. The Model deployment is responsible for deploying these integrated models onto the cloud server, bringing us one step closer to detecting pediatric diseases more effectively.

18.4.5 User Interface (GUI)

The User interface (GUI) subsystem helps physicians get to engage with the system. Patient's data is entered through a sleek and intuitive interface that relays this information to our trained model via the cloud. The results, in turn, get forwarded to the UI Notification engine to be shared across various channels.

18.4.6 UI Notification Engine

The system doesn't stop at just revealing the results within its database. Figure 18.4 illustrates the User notification engine under discussion. UI notification engine actively communicates the disease detection results to patients, physicians, and healthcare providers. This notification happens through email and SMS, ensuring that everyone is in the loop about the child's health condition.

That's the essence of the PDSSFPDD in a nutshell. It exemplifies how modern technology, equipped with robust machine learning algorithms and enhanced imaging facilities, can be a game-changer in the detection of pediatric diseases.

REFERENCES

Venkata Tulasi Ramu Ponnada, Dr S V Naga Sreenivasu (2019). Edge AI System for Pneumonia and Lung Cancer Detection, *International Journal of Innovative Technology and Exploring Engineering*, ISSN: 2278–3075, Volume-8, Issue-9.

Venkata Tulasi Ramu Ponnada, Dr S V Naga Sreenivasu (July 2019). Efficient CNN for Lung Cancer Detection, *International Journal of Recent Technology and Engineering*, ISSN: 2277–3878, Volume-8, Issue-2.

Venkata Tulasi Ramu Ponnada, Dr S V Naga Sreenivasu (2019). End to End System for Pneumonia and Lung Cancer Detection Using Deep Learning, *International Journal of Engineering and Advanced Technology*, ISSN: 2249–8958, Volume-8, Issue-6.

Venkata Tulasi Ramu Ponnada, Dr S V Naga Sreenivasu (2019). IN Patent#201941005828. Foolproof Decision Support System for Melanoma Cancer Detection (FDSSMCD).

Venkata Tulasi Ramu Ponnada, Dr S V Naga Sreenivasu (2019). IN Patent# 201941016186. Method and System for Physician Decision Making System for Psoriasis Detection.

Venkata Tulasi Ramu Ponnada, Dr S V Naga Sreenivasu (2019). Integrated Clinician Decision Supporting System for Pneumonia and Lung Cancer Detection, *International Journal of Innovative Technology and Exploring Engineering*, ISSN: 2278–3075, Volume-8, Issue-8.

19 Leveraging ChatGPT-Like Large Language Models for Alzheimer's Disease

Enhancing Care, Advancing Research, and Overcoming Challenges

Surendrabikram Thapa and Surabhi Adhikari

19.1 INTRODUCTION

Alzheimer's Disease (AD) is a progressive neurodegenerative disorder that affects millions of people worldwide, posing significant challenges for both patients and caregivers (Adhikari et al., 2021). The disease is characterized by cognitive decline, memory impairment, and communication difficulties, which profoundly impact daily life and quality of life. As the prevalence of AD continues to rise, there is a pressing need for innovative approaches to improve care and support for individuals affected by this debilitating condition.

In recent years, advancements in artificial intelligence (AI) and natural language processing (NLP) have opened up new possibilities in healthcare (Ali et al., 2023). These innovations have shown a new era of possibilities and opportunities that hold immense promise for improving the delivery of healthcare services and enhancing patient outcomes. AI, with its capacity to process vast amounts of data and perform complex tasks with speed and precision, has emerged as a potent ally in the quest for more effective and efficient healthcare solutions (Kaul et al., 2020). Within this landscape, NLP has played a pivotal role by enabling machines to understand and generate human language, making it possible for computers to communicate with humans in a more natural and intuitive manner (Ofer et al., 2021). This breakthrough has far-reaching implications for healthcare, as it facilitates seamless interactions between patients and healthcare providers, streamlines the analysis of medical records and research papers, and augments the potential for personalized medicine. As a result, healthcare professionals can harness the power of AI and NLP to make more informed decisions, tailor treatments to individual patient needs, and ultimately, improve the overall quality of care.

DOI: 10.1201/9781032698519-19

Furthermore, the application of AI and NLP in healthcare extends beyond clinical practice and patient care (Zhou et al., 2022). These technologies have the capacity to revolutionize medical research, enabling researchers to analyze vast datasets, identify trends and patterns, and accelerate the development of new drugs, treatments, and diagnostic tools. By automating tasks that were once laborious and time-consuming, AI and NLP empower scientists to focus their expertise on higher-level problem-solving and innovation.

Within the expansive domain of natural language processing (NLP), several notable breakthroughs have emerged, each contributing to the ever-evolving landscape of healthcare applications. One prominent category of NLP models that has garnered significant attention is the family of Transformer-based textual models (Ilias and Askounis, 2022). These models have revolutionized the field by introducing novel mechanisms for processing sequential data, which is especially relevant in healthcare where patient records, medical literature, and clinical notes often present as intricate sequences of information. Transformers, originally popularized by the BERT (Bidirectional Encoder Representations from Transformers) model, have set a new standard for contextual understanding of language.

BERT (Devlin et al., 2019) and its derivatives, like RoBERTa (Liu et al., 2020) and ALBERT (Lan et al., 2020), have demonstrated exceptional capabilities in healthcare-related tasks such as medical document classification (Yao et al., 2019), named entity recognition (identifying medical terms in text) (Liu et al., 2021), and clinical information extraction from unstructured notes (Roy and Pan, 2021). These models excel at capturing the nuanced context and semantics embedded within healthcare narratives, enabling more accurate and context-aware analysis. For instance, in electronic health records (EHRs), where patient information is documented in a narrative form, Transformer-based models can extract critical insights, facilitating better clinical decision support.

Another noteworthy advancement in the NLP landscape is the sequence-to-sequence (seq-to-seq) model architecture. Seq-to-seq models, typified by the attention-based architecture, have found extensive utility in healthcare applications, particularly in tasks involving medical dialogue generation, language translation, and medical summarization. These models, characterized by their encoder-decoder structure, excel in tasks where the input and output are sequences of varying lengths.

In healthcare, seq-to-seq models are leveraged for tasks such as generating automated responses to patient queries, translating medical literature between languages, and condensing lengthy clinical notes into concise summaries (Thapa and Adhikari, 2023). This versatility is especially valuable in the realm of healthcare communication, where clear and concise information exchange is paramount. For instance, chatbots powered by seq-to-seq models can provide immediate answers to patient questions and offer support in real-time, thereby enhancing patient engagement and satisfaction.

Another major recent breakthrough is the emergence of Large Language Models (LLMs), such as Generative Pre-trained Transformers (GPT), LaMDA, PaLM, etc. LLMs are powerful language processing models that can analyze and generate human-like text, enabling sophisticated interactions and understanding of natural language (Thapa et al., 2023). The potential of LLMs in AD care becomes evident when considering the complex communication challenges faced by individuals with the disease (Bhambri et al., 2023). LLMs have the ability to develop improved plans for disease management by providing tailored approaches for patients and caregivers, which is a very important aspect of patient care.

Additionally, LLMs hold great potential in advancing medical research on AD. The vast amounts of data available on AD can be efficiently analyzed by LLMs, enabling researchers to recognize patterns, identify potential risk factors, and generate insights to enhance our understanding of the disease. This contributes to the development of potential treatments, interventions, and diagnostic tools, thereby expanding the scope of medical research in AD.

While the potential benefits of LLMs in AD care and medical research are vast, it is important to consider the ethical implications of their implementation (Rana et al., 2024). Privacy, data security, informed consent, and the preservation of human connection are paramount in ensuring responsible use and safeguarding the rights of individuals with AD.

This article aims to explore the potential of LLMs in transforming AD care, addressing communication and cognitive challenges, and improving the overall well-being of patients. By examining the benefits, limitations, ethical considerations, and scope of medical research, we can gain valuable insights into the application of LLMs in AD care and pave the way for more effective and person-centered approaches to support individuals affected by this challenging condition.

19.2 RESEARCH QUESTIONS

In this section, we present the research questions that will shape our investigation into the utilization of large language models (LLMs) in Alzheimer's Disease (AD) research (Rani et al., 2023). These research inquiries will provide the scaffolding upon which our exploration will unfold, encompassing the intricate facets of LLMs and their potential impact on AD care and research. The research questions are:

a) How can Large Language Models (LLMs), such as ChatGPT, be effectively utilized to enhance patient care and support in Alzheimer's Disease (AD)?

We want to know how LLMs, like ChatGPT, can be used to improve the care and support given to people with AD. This means finding out how these computer programs can help people with AD talk to others and get personalized help.

b) What is the scope of utilizing LLMs in medical research on AD, and how can they contribute to advancements in understanding the disease, improving early detection methods, and developing innovative therapeutic approaches?

Our second question is about how LLMs can be used in medical research on AD. We want to understand if these tools can help us find patterns in data, discover things that might cause AD, and come up with new ways to find AD early and treat it.

c) What are the key challenges and limitations associated with the integration of LLMs in AD care, and how can these challenges be addressed to ensure responsible and ethical use of the technology?

Our third question focuses on the challenges and limits of using LLMs in AD care. We want to figure out what problems might come up, like keeping people's information private and making sure we still have human connections. We also want to find out how to use LLMs in a way that's responsible and respects the rights of people with AD (Singh and Bhambri, 2023).

By exploring these research questions, we aim to shed light on the opportunities, challenges, and strategies associated with using LLMs in the field of Alzheimer's Disease.

19.3 LARGE LANGUAGE MODELS IN THE CARE OF AD PATIENTS

Large Language Models (LLMs), such as ChatGPT, have the potential to significantly enhance patient care and support in Alzheimer's Disease (AD). By leveraging their natural language processing capabilities, LLMs can offer personalized assistance, improve communication, support memory recall, and encourage social engagement in multiple ways. In this section, we explore various ways in which LLMs can be effectively utilized to enhance patient care for individuals with AD.

19.3.1 Assisting with Cognitive Tasks

Cognitive impairment represents a cardinal feature of AD, exerting a substantial impact on memory, attention, and problem-solving faculties (Morris et al., 2001). Within this context, LLMs emerge as invaluable aids, poised to assist individuals with AD across a spectrum of cognitive tasks. These virtual assistants are adept at serving as memory prompts, facilitating the recollection of essential information and pivotal life events. Moreover, LLMs contribute to the structuring of daily tasks and schedules, offering invaluable support in navigating the challenges posed by memory lapses. Furthermore, these models offer a repository of tailored cognitive exercises and mental stimulation, meticulously calibrated to an individual's cognitive capacity, thereby promoting cognitive function and overall well-being.

19.3.2 Personalized Reminiscence Therapy

Reminiscence therapy, an evidence-based therapeutic approach involving the recollection and discussion of past memories, holds significant promise in AD care (Cuevas et al., 2020). LLMs, with their proficiency in generating natural language, act as adept facilitators of this therapy. These models deftly produce conversation prompts, pose relevant questions, and engage in meaningful dialogues designed to evoke cherished memories. The therapeutic benefits of such reminiscence exercises extend beyond memory recall, nurturing emotional well-being and serving as a conduit for social interaction, thereby fostering a profound sense of connection for individuals grappling with AD.

19.3.3 Supporting Caregivers and Healthcare Professionals

The pivotal roles played by caregivers and healthcare professionals in AD care cannot be overstated (Haley, 1997). LLMs function as invaluable resources for these dedicated individuals. For caregivers, LLMs provide a comprehensive repository of guidance, training materials, and caregiving strategies. They offer insights into effective caregiving techniques, strategies for managing challenging behaviors, and pragmatic advice for daily caregiving routines. Furthermore, LLMs extend real-time support to caregivers, responding to queries and offering tailored suggestions to address specific caregiving scenarios. Healthcare professionals also benefit from LLMs, which serve as valuable knowledge augmentation tools. These models enhance healthcare professionals' understanding of AD care and facilitate improved care coordination, ultimately resulting in enhanced outcomes for individuals with AD.

19.3.4 Emotional Support to AD Patients

The emotional journey of individuals with AD can be tumultuous, marked by distress and mood fluctuations. In this context, chatbots powered by LLMs emerge as empathetic companions. These virtual entities engage in human-like conversations, providing solace and emotional support. They offer techniques for managing stress and anxiety, suggest calming activities, and stand as a dependable presence during emotionally turbulent moments. Additionally, LLM-backed applications, equipped with real-time information and web access, connect individuals with AD to support groups, online communities, or virtual companionship programs. This fosters a profound sense of belonging and emotional well-being.

19.3.5 Continuous Monitoring and Caregiver Assistance

LLMs transcend their roles as virtual companions to extend their utility to remote monitoring and caregiver assistance. When configured as zero-shot or few-shot learners, they seamlessly integrate into voice recognition and analysis systems. This integration empowers these models to detect changes in speech patterns, mood fluctuations, or signs of distress. Caregivers receive real-time alerts, enabling them to respond promptly to potential issues and ensure the well-being of individuals with AD, even from a distance.

19.3.6 Enhancing Medication Management

One critical aspect of AD care is medication management, which can be challenging due to cognitive impairments. LLMs can assist individuals in adhering to their medication schedules by sending timely reminders and providing clear, easy-to-understand instructions about their medications. This reduces the risk of missed doses and helps maintain treatment effectiveness.

19.3.7 Personalized Nutrition and Wellness Guidance

Proper nutrition is essential for individuals with AD. LLMs can offer personalized nutrition guidance, suggesting suitable meal plans based on dietary restrictions and preferences. Additionally, they can provide wellness tips, exercise routines, and information on maintaining a healthy lifestyle tailored to the individual's condition.

In conclusion, the use of LLMs in AD patient care brings about significant changes, including personalized help, better communication, more emotional support, improved medication management, and increased social interaction. These virtual companions can help ease the challenges caused by AD, support reminiscence therapy, aid caregivers and healthcare professionals, and provide lasting emotional comfort. As we explore these possibilities with LLMs, we see technology as a kind and helpful partner in improving AD care.

19.4 SCOPE OF LARGE LANGUAGE MODELS IN MEDICAL RESEARCH ON AD

Large Language Models (LLMs), such as ChatGPT, offer vast potential in advancing medical research on Alzheimer's Disease (AD). Their sophisticated language processing capabilities enable researchers to analyze vast amounts of textual data, extract meaningful insights, and contribute to various aspects of AD research. The scope of utilizing LLMs in medical research on AD encompasses the following areas:

19.4.1 Advancements in Understanding the Disease

LLMs can aid in gaining a deeper understanding of AD by analyzing a wide range of biomedical literature, research articles, clinical records, and patient narratives. They can identify key patterns, trends, and associations within these sources, providing researchers with valuable insights into disease mechanisms, risk factors, genetic factors, and potential biomarkers. LLMs can facilitate knowledge discovery, assisting researchers in uncovering novel relationships and expanding the current understanding of AD.

19.4.2 Improving Early Detection and Diagnosis

Early detection of AD is crucial for timely intervention and treatment. Small language models have been widely used in the early diagnosis of AD (Thapa and Adhikari, 2023). Analyzing transcriptions of speech narratives is one of the established research problems in biomedical NLP. LLMs, being more powerful than small language models, can contribute to the development of innovative methods for early detection and diagnosis by analyzing linguistic patterns and cognitive performance in patient conversations. By recognizing subtle changes in language, memory recall, and speech patterns, LLMs can assist in identifying potential markers of cognitive decline. This can aid in the early identification of individuals at risk of AD and potentially enable the implementation of preventive measures and interventions.

19.4.3 Enabling Precision Medicine Approaches

LLMs can support the advancement of precision medicine in AD by facilitating personalized treatment strategies. By analyzing large-scale genomic and clinical datasets, LLMs can assist in identifying genetic variations, gene-environment interactions, and potential therapeutic targets. LLMs can contribute to the development of personalized treatment plans, considering factors such as genetic predisposition, comorbidities, and response to specific medications. This approach has the potential to optimize treatment outcomes and improve the overall effectiveness of therapeutic interventions. Though far-fetched, the application seems more likely with rapid advancement in large language models.

19.4.4 Identifying Subtypes and Disease Progression

AD is a complex condition with considerable heterogeneity in terms of its clinical presentation and progression. LLMs can aid in identifying and characterizing different subtypes of AD based on linguistic patterns, cognitive performance, and other clinical features. By analyzing large datasets of patient records and longitudinal data, LLMs can contribute to the identification of distinct AD subtypes, which may have implications for prognosis, treatment response, and personalized care approaches. Furthermore, LLMs can help track disease progression over time by analyzing language changes, memory decline, and other cognitive markers, providing valuable insights into the natural history of AD and facilitating the development of more targeted interventions.

19.4.5 Drug Discovery and Development

LLMs empower drug discovery and development efforts in the context of AD. By sifting through vast volumes of scientific literature, clinical trial data, and pharmacological databases, LLMs can identify potential drug candidates, predict their effectiveness, and highlight novel drug targets. This accelerates the drug development pipeline, reducing the time and resources required to bring promising therapies to market.

19.4.6 Enhancing Clinical Decision Support

LLMs can serve as powerful allies in clinical decision-making for AD patients. They can analyze patient data, medical records, and treatment outcomes to provide health- care providers with tailored recommendations for patient care. This assists clinicians in making more informed decisions about treatment options, medication adjustments, and care plans.

The scope of utilizing LLMs in medical research on AD is vast, encompassing advancements in understanding the disease, improving early detection and diagnosis, enabling precision medicine approaches, and enhancing clinical decision support. By harnessing the power of LLMs, researchers, and healthcare professionals can make significant strides in addressing the challenges posed by AD and ultimately improve patient care and outcomes.

19.5 CHALLENGES IN USING LLMS FOR AD RESEARCH AND PATIENT MANAGEMENT

While Large Language Models (LLMs) hold immense potential in Alzheimer's Disease (AD) research and patient management, their utilization is not without challenges. It is crucial to address these challenges to ensure the responsible and effective implementation of LLMs in the context of AD. The key challenges include:

19.5.1 Generation of Factually Incorrect Information and References

One of the major challenges associated with the use of LLMs in AD research and patient management is the potential for generating factually incorrect information and references (Frosolini et al., 2023). LLMs learn from vast amounts of text data, including both accurate and erroneous information from various sources. This poses a risk of LLMs producing outputs that contain inaccuracies or references to unreliable sources.

To address this challenge, robust mechanisms for fact-checking and verification of LLM-generated outputs are crucial. Human oversight and review should be implemented to ensure the accuracy and reliability of the information provided by LLMs. Integrating external knowledge bases and expert-curated datasets can enhance the accuracy of LLM-generated responses. Educating users about the limitations of LLMs and the importance of critically evaluating the information they generate is essential in mitigating the risk of relying on factually incorrect information.

19.5.2 Data Quality and Bias

The performance of LLMs heavily relies on the quality and diversity of the training data (Zhang et al., 2023). Inadequate representation of certain populations or biases present in the training data can result in biased or inaccurate outputs. When applying LLMs to AD research and patient management, it is essential to address biases and ensure that the models are trained on diverse and representative datasets to avoid perpetuating health disparities and skewed results.

19.5.3 Interpretability and Explainability

LLMs are often regarded as black boxes due to their complex internal workings, making it challenging to interpret and explain their decision-making processes. In AD research and patient management, it is crucial to understand the rationale behind LLM-generated outputs to ensure the reliability and trustworthiness of the information provided. Developing methods for interpreting and explaining LLM outputs in a humanly understandable manner is a significant challenge that needs to be addressed to enhance the clinical utility and acceptance of LLMs.

19.5.4 Ethical and Privacy Concerns

The integration of LLMs in AD research and patient management raises ethical and privacy considerations (Li et al., 2023). LLMs process sensitive personal health information, and ensuring data privacy and confidentiality is paramount. Transparent data handling practices, informed consent procedures and robust security measures should be in place to protect patient privacy and comply with ethical standards. Additionally, ethical guidelines need to be established to govern the use of LLMs, addressing issues such as transparency, accountability, and responsible use of the technology.

19.5.5 Clinical Integration and User Acceptance

Integrating LLMs into clinical practice for AD and into the daily routines of healthcare professionals and caregivers can be a complex process. Ensuring that LLMs seamlessly fit within existing workflows, are user-friendly, and provide value-added features is essential for their successful adoption. Healthcare professionals and caregivers working on AD management need to be trained on how to effectively utilize LLMs and interpret their outputs. User acceptance, trust, and confidence in LLMs also need to be fostered through ongoing engagement, education, and addressing concerns related to autonomy, reliability, and potential limitations of the technology.

19.5.6 Lack of Standardization and Regulation

The field of LLMs is rapidly evolving, and there is a lack of standardized guidelines and regulations specifically tailored to their application in AD research and patient management. Establishing best practices, standardized evaluation metrics, and regulatory frameworks is necessary to ensure the quality, safety, and effectiveness of LLMs in AD care. Collaboration between researchers, policymakers, and regulatory bodies is crucial to developing guidelines and regulations that promote responsible and ethical use of LLMs in the context of AD.

19.5.7 Resource and Infrastructure Requirements

The effective implementation of LLMs in AD research and patient management necessitates substantial computational resources and infrastructure. Training and deploying these models demand significant computational power, storage, and technical expertise. This poses a challenge, particularly for smaller healthcare institutions and resource-constrained settings. Ensuring equitable access to LLM-based solutions and addressing resource disparities is essential for harnessing the full potential of these models in AD care.

Addressing these challenges will be instrumental in unlocking the full potential of LLMs in AD research and patient management. By overcoming these hurdles, researchers, healthcare professionals, and caregivers can harness the benefits of LLMs to improve our understanding of the disease, enhance patient care, and ultimately strive towards better outcomes for individuals affected by AD.

19.6 CONCLUSION

Large Language Models (LLMs), such as ChatGPT, offer significant potential in Alzheimer's Disease (AD) research and patient management. They can enhance communication, support memory recall, and provide personalized assistance to individuals with AD. LLMs also contribute to medical research by improving disease understanding, early detection, and innovative therapeutic approaches. However, integrating LLMs in AD care poses challenges. Fact-checking and verification mechanisms are crucial to mitigate the risk of generating inaccurate information. Addressing ethical and privacy concerns, promoting user acceptance, and establishing guidelines and regulations are essential. By addressing these challenges, LLMs can revolutionize AD care and research. Collaboration among stakeholders and responsible implementation will ensure the benefits of LLMs in improving the lives of individuals with AD and advancing our knowledge of the disease. In conclusion, LLMs have immense potential in AD research and patient management. With careful consideration of challenges and responsible implementation, LLMs can shape the future of AD care and contribute to a better understanding of the disease.

REFERENCES

Adhikari, S., Thapa, S., Singh, P., Huo, H., Bharathy, G., & Prasad, M. (2021, July). A comparative study of machine learning and NLP techniques for uses of stop words by patients in diagnosis of Alzheimer's disease. In *2021 International Joint Conference on Neural Networks (IJCNN)* (pp. 1–8). IEEE.

Ali, O., Abdelbaki, W., Shrestha, A., Elbasi, E., Alryalat, M. A. A., & Dwivedi, Y. K. (2023). A systematic literature review of artificial intelligence in the healthcare sector: Benefits, challenges, methodologies, and functionalities. *Journal of Innovation & Knowledge*, 8(1), 100333.

Bhambri, P., Rani, S., Balas, V. E., & Elngar, A. A. (2023). *Integration of AI-Based Manufacturing and Industrial Engineering Systems with the Internet of Things*. CRC Press.

Cuevas, P. E. G., Davidson, P. M., Mejilla, J. L., & Rodney, T. W. (2020). Reminiscence therapy for older adults with Alzheimer's disease: A literature review. *International Journal of Mental Health Nursing*, 29(3), 364–371.

Devlin, J., Chang, M. W., Lee, K., & Toutanova, K. (2019). BERT: Pre-training of deep bidirectional transformers for language understanding. In *2019 North American Chapter of the Association for Computational Linguistics-Human Language Technology (NAACL-HLT)* (Vol. 1, pp. 4171–4186). Association for Computational Linguistics.

Frosolini, A., Gennaro, P., Cascino, F., & Gabriele, G. (2023). In reference to "role of Chat GPT in public health", to highlight the AI's incorrect reference generation. *Annals of Biomedical Engineering*, 1–3.

Haley, W. E. (1997). The family caregiver's role in Alzheimer's disease. *Neurology*, 48(5 Suppl 6), 25S–29S.

Ilias, L., & Askounis, D. (2022). Explainable identification of dementia from transcripts using transformer networks. *IEEE Journal of Biomedical and Health Informatics*, 26(8), 4153–4164.

Kaul, V., Enslin, S., & Gross, S. A. (2020). History of artificial intelligence in medicine. *Gastrointestinal Endoscopy*, 92(4), 807–812.

Lan, Z., Chen, M., Goodman, S., Gimpel, K., Sharma, P., & Soricut, R. (2020). ALBERT: A lite BERT for self-supervised learning of language representations. In *2020 International Conference on Learning Representations (ICLR)*. https://doi.org/10.48550/arXiv.1909.11942

Li, H., Moon, J. T., Purkayastha, S., Celi, L. A., Trivedi, H., & Gichoya, J. W. (2023). Ethics of large language models in medicine and medical research. *The Lancet Digital Health*, 5(6), e333–e335.

Liu, N., Hu, Q., Xu, H., Xu, X., & Chen, M. (2021). Med-BERT: A pretraining framework for medical records named entity recognition. *IEEE Transactions on Industrial Informatics*, 18(8), 5600–5608.

Liu, Y., Ott, M., Goyal, N., Du, J., Joshi, M., Chen, D., Levy, O., Lewis, M., Zettlemoyer, L., & Stoyanov, V. (2020). RoBERTa: A robustly optimized BERT pretraining approach. In *2020 International Conference on Learning Representations (ICLR)*. https://doi.org/10.48550/arXiv.1907.11692

Morris, J. C., Storandt, M., Miller, J. P., McKeel, D. W., Price, J. L., Rubin, E. H., & Berg, L. (2001). Mild cognitive impairment represents early-stage Alzheimer disease. *Archives of Neurology*, 58(3), 397–405.

Ofer, D., Brandes, N., & Linial, M. (2021). The language of proteins: NLP, machine learning & protein sequences. *Computational and Structural Biotechnology Journal*, 19, 1750–1758.

Rana, R., Bhambri, P., & Chhabra, Y. (2024). Evolution and the future of industrial engineering with the IoT and AI. In *Integration of AI-Based Manufacturing and Industrial Engineering Systems with the Internet of Things* (pp. 19–37). CRC Press.

Rani, S., Kaur, J., & Bhambri, P. (2023). Technology and gender violence: Victimization model, consequences and measures. In *Communication Technology and Gender Violence* (Vol. 1, pp. 1–19). Springer.

Roy, A., & Pan, S. (2021, November). Incorporating medical knowledge in BERT for clinical relation extraction. In *Proceedings of the 2021 Conference on Empirical Methods in Natural Language Processing* (pp. 5357–5366). Association for Computational Linguistics. https://doi.org/10.18653/v1/2021.emnlp-main.435

Singh, G., & Bhambri, P. (2023). Simulation analysis of AODV and DSDV routing protocols for secure and reliable service in mobile Adhoc networks (MANETs). In *Integration of AI-Based Manufacturing and Industrial Engineering Systems with the Internet of Things* (pp. 205–216). CRC Press.

Thapa, S., & Adhikari, S. (2023). ChatGPT, bard, and large language models for biomedical research: Opportunities and pitfalls. *Annals of Biomedical Engineering*, 51(12), 2647–2651.

Thapa, S., Naseem, U., & Nasim, M. (2023). From humans to machines: can ChatGPT-like LLMs effectively replace human annotators in NLP tasks. In *Workshop Proceedings of the 17th International AAAI Conference on Web and Social Media*. Association for the Advancement of Artificial Intelligence. https://doi.org/10.36190/2023.15

Yao, L., Jin, Z., Mao, C., Zhang, Y., & Luo, Y. (2019). Traditional Chinese medicine clinical records classification with BERT and domain-specific corpora. *Journal of the American Medical Informatics Association*, 26(12), 1632–1636.

Zhang, J., Vahidian, S., Kuo, M., Li, C., Zhang, R., Wang, G., & Chen, Y. (2023). Towards building the federated GPT: Federated instruction tuning. arXiv preprint arXiv:2305.05644. https://doi.org/10.48550/arXiv.2305.05644

Zhou, B., Yang, G., Shi, Z., & Ma, S. (2022). Natural language processing for smart healthcare. *IEEE Reviews in Biomedical Engineering*, 17, 4–18. https://doi.org/10.1109/RBME.2022.3210270

20 Elderly Fall Detection using Deep Learning Enabled Internet of Healthcare Things

Ahona Ghosh, Azaharuddin Saikh, Sriparna Saha and Indranil Sarkar

20.1 INTRODUCTION

Human falls are a common problem in the present day. As people age, their ability to move around declines, and falls become increasingly common, resulting in serious injuries or even death (Wang et al., 2020). An automated system for detecting risk factors of falling and alarm generation is beneficial since early identification and reporting of human falls could save lives. Different modalities in the existing literature have been used to detect falls, like processing wearable sensors, floor-mounted sensors, depth imaging data, etc., (Potluri et al., 2019). However, these approaches are complex and expensive (Panda et al., 2019). Computer vision methods combined with deep learning models to classify visual data represented by images provide interesting solutions for automated fall detection systems.

To identify falls using sensor readings, classification is a machine learning (ML) technique that seeks to detect falls automatically in real-time (Rastogi and Singh, 2021). Several taxonomies on fall monitoring can be found in the research to reduce false alarms and increase the precision of fall detection and prediction systems. But the loopholes acting as our motivations behind this research are summarized:

i. People sometimes seem to agree that sensor fusion offers a more reliable method for identifying senior fall detection. In certain scenarios, the usage of several sensors may be complementary to one another, but it also increases the computational complexity leading to the rejection of such applications in sensitive healthcare scenarios where time complexity is a deciding factor (Rana et al., 2019). Also, it is difficult to set thresholds to detect falls for wearable device-based applications.
ii. Most of the methods, particularly those relying on vision-based sensors, operate in offline mode since they are unable to function in real-time. Due to this constraint, most of them are effective in local areas only. Attention to IoT platforms with cloud-based trends can address the challenge of building

DOI: 10.1201/9781032698519-20

scalable and stable systems allowing real-time processing which helps to gain the trust of the elderly.

In this chapter, a Convolutional Neural Network (CNN) model is trained to recognize falls and notify emergency services accurately by analyzing images collected from video frames to find essential components for fall detection. CNN's Inception model-based architecture has improved the fall detection system's accuracy and the Google Cloud IoT platform has been employed in the present scenario to process and analyze the Kinect sensor's RGB image and transmit the result to the concerned authority for immediate action after a fall detection (Tondon and Bhambri, 2017). Section 20.2 presents an in-depth examination of techniques for detecting falls in older adults, including those using wearable, vision-based, and environmental sensors. Section 20.3 describes the steps involved in the proposed framework. Section 20.4 presents the experimental outcomes, and Section 20.5 completes the work by concluding and presenting its future scope.

20.2 RELATED WORKS

This section reviews existing literature to evaluate and compare various fall detection systems, algorithms, or approaches to detect falls and eventually prevent older people from falling. For instance, Xu et al. (Xu et al., 2019) recognize human body motion and archive human fall detection depending on the depth data and skeleton tracking technologies of the Microsoft Kinect V2 sensor (Saha and Ghosh, 2019; Ghosh et al., 2020a). Firstly, the human joints recorded by the skeleton tracker are analyzed using the Kinect sensor's depth data. The fall is then detected based on the position recognition by an optimized back propagation neural network (BPNN). The dataset produced by the Kinect tracker is used to train the neural network. Finally, experimental verification was done for posture recognition and fall detection. However, testing is performed using a separate body tracker. The network lacks sufficient samples to learn about events that do not occur frequently in the datasets, such as falling while on one's knees or identifying falls from an individual's top perspective, which are examples of analyzed samples. This may also apply to nearly all false negatives, in which the network's inability to accurately learn particular features serves as the only possible explanation for the error.

Kepski and Kwolek (2013) have implemented a fuzzy inference on data from Kinect and a wearable motion-sensing device with an accelerometer and gyroscope for fall detection. The foreground items are recognized using depth images captured by Kinect, which can extract such images in a dark room. Both the user's privacy and subtle fall detection are maintained—the findings of the trial show that fall detection is effective, but the system required the user to enter a calibration pose during the skeleton tracking initialization, which makes it less usable especially for older people restricting the subject's position. Another technique for detecting falls in older people's homes uses Microsoft Kinect and a two-stage fall detection system (Stone and Skubic, 2014) has been built. A variety of skilled stunt actors' falls and a few naturally occurring falls allowed for the characterization of performance in four diverse circumstances. Results achieved were satisfactory, however, larger distances from the Kinect present several challenges for fall detection, including the depth image's decreased resolution, creating more challenges to the foreground segmentation, the pixel depth estimate's decreased precision, and a higher probability of ambient light overpowering the actively emitted infrared pattern of the Kinect, which results in pixel depth estimates not being returned, whereas our proposed approach deals with only RGB images that are self-sufficient to identify the patterns required to detect falls avoiding the complexity of processing other image attributes like luminance, normal, depth, etc.

The technology proposed by (Mastorakis and Makris, 2012) can accurately and consistently detect walking falls without accounting for false actions (such as lying on the floor) in real-time. Calculations based on both speed and inactivity are used to determine whether a fall happened. Their main contribution lies in estimating velocity based on changes in the 3D bounding box's dimensions. This eliminates the need for prior scene knowledge by directly leveraging the 3D bounding box because the set of identified activities is sufficient to fully implement the fall detection procedure. However, with this system, detection is done locally, and a carer or relative is notified directly. It lacks extensive monitoring capabilities, prolonged data transmission, and the ability to gather data for large-scale fall pattern mining because it is not a part of bigger telemonitoring centers.

To identify falls, Nghiem et al. (Nghiem et al., 2012) suggest a head recognition method using depth video from a Kinect camera, which identifies potential head locations and based on these locations, identifies individual falls by an algorithm designed to calculate head speed, the body centroid, and the distance between them and the floor. Scanning the head contour on the exterior contour of the human body searches for head positions quickly; thus, human detection is a variation of the histogram of the oriented gradient for the shoulders and the head. However, scalable computing resources are needed for modern telemedicine, which aims to meet the increasing demand for monitoring elderly patients. Nghiem et al. just classified the data and did not consider alerting the caregiver for the early recovery of the sufferer.

Salah et al. propose a fall identification system for older people that uses an edge ML architecture with accelerometers (Salah et al., 2022). The results obtained yield 96.3% accuracy and 96.4% specificity. In addition, execution times of less than 40 ms are recorded. However, the range of different sensing units is restricted in this case due to the hardware constraint. For the elderly residents of nursing homes, De Raeve et al. propose a Bluetooth Low Energy (BLE)-centered fall recognition and alerting system (De Raeve et al., 2022). The authors point out that many current systems for detecting falls depend on wearable devices, like pressure sensors, gyroscopes, and accelerometers. These devices, however, may not be appropriate for those with cognitive impairments and might be difficult and uncomfortable for older adults to wear. The subject-wise accuracy, or percentage of wise decisions, ranges from 84.89% to 92.65%.

Tong et al. (Tong et al., 2022) discuss the advantages, disadvantages, and potential paths for future research on cell phone-based fall detection systems that use accelerometers and gyroscope sensors. Somkunwar et al. propose an ML method for detecting human falls (Somkunwar et al., 2023) comprising a camera, a computer vision algorithm for feature extraction, and ML algorithms for classification. In contrast, the computer vision algorithm is used to detect falls based on changes in the form and movement of the human body. The results show that the accuracy of linear discrimination was 82%, and that of Random Forest (RF), Naive Bayes, Support Vector Machine (SVM), k-Nearest Neighbour (kNN), and Ada Boost, respectively, are 85.0%, 39.75%, 66.25%, 68.0%, and 64.75%. However, determining the head and body center vertical distance and acceleration threshold is challenging, whereas the combination of the same can be efficient, but leads to more time complexity ineffective for real-time healthcare scenarios.

CNN is proposed by Santos et al. (Santos et al., 2019) as a fall identification system built on accelerometer data. However, to discern a fall from other activities and handle intricate data, they have employed CNN and extracted specific characteristics from the actions that exhibit strong performance in classifying falls and other actions. But, as it only captures a portion of the fall rather than the whole picture, the system may become situationally sensitive. The algorithm and system are not reusable after the experiment condition is altered. Rezaei et al. (Rezaei et al., 2023) explain how to detect human falls without being noticed using millimeter-wave (mm-wave) radar technology, overcoming user resistance and forgetting wearable gadgets.

An mm-wave radar mounted on the ceiling and side wall of an experimental paradigm has been used by Hasib et al. (Hasib et al., 2021) to gather data from healthy young volunteers. A variety of classifiers, including the multilayer perceptron (MLP), RF, kNN, SVM, and a CNN-based deep learning model, are used. Features are manually retrieved from the data point clouds and CNN is used to design a vision-based human posture detection and fall identification system that demonstrates stability in human posture classification and attains an F-measure of 97% with minor false alarms and an overall accuracy of 97.5%. The accuracy of other competing models, like MLP, SVM, RF, and kNN on the same dataset is 96.56%, 86.95%, 91.92%, and 40.06%, respectively. However, the computational efficiency and the amount of accessibility, which a real-time fall detection system requires, are not achieved in their framework leading to significant challenges for criticality and less reliability.

20.3 PROPOSED METHODOLOGY

Various steps in our proposed framework for detecting falls using CNN include the dataset gathering of tagged images derived from videos of various human behaviors, such as typical movements, falls, and other occurrences. After data collection, the data is transmitted from the subject end to a cloud server, where the data augmentation is performed, followed by the classification using CNN. Figure 20.1 presents the steps involved in the proposed methodology.

20.3.1 Data Collection Process

Kinect sensor parallelly captures the depth and RGB images of subjects situated in front of it within a range of 1.2 m–3.5 m. In the present framework, to avoid the

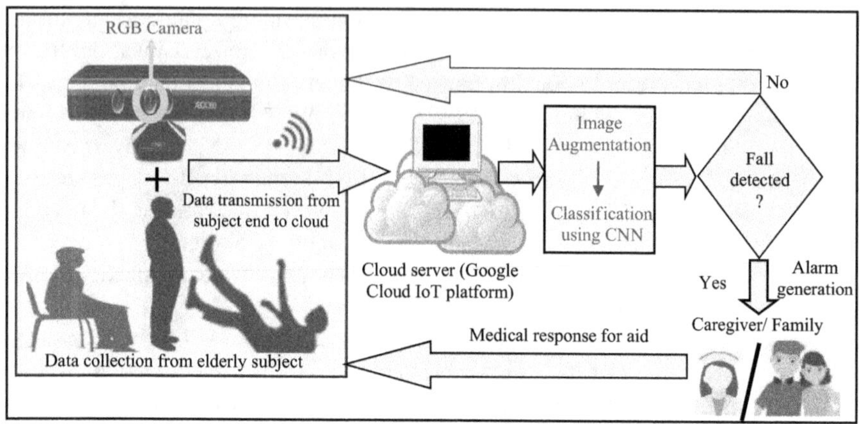

FIGURE 20.1 Block diagram of the proposed fall detection approach.

complexity of processing the sensor data, with the help of two Microsoft Kinect sensors only RGB cameras, human fall and not fall events have been recorded. The sampling rate has been set as 30 frames per second.

20.3.2 Device to Cloud Data Transmission

The amount of data that is sent to the cloud is significantly influenced by fall detection variations, such as cloud and edge-oriented systems that use mobile IoT devices. Since fall detection uses an ML-based classifier that is accessible through a cloud-based Web service, cloud-oriented fall recognition relies on continuous data communication. Fall identification based on the edge enables less data transfer from the device to the cloud. It can even send no data at all to the cloud when used with the local module that alerts the carer in the event of danger. Regardless of whether the fall occurred or was misidentified, there should at least be certain periods of continuous surveillance when it is detected, as this would prevent the monitored individual from being able to compile a history of incidents.

20.3.3 Data Augmentation

Rescaling, shearing, zooming, and horizontal flipping are the augmentation methods employed in the proposed approach. For the cth channel of an image, when the original pixel value is p^c, the modified pixel after rescaling is denoted by

$$p_m^c = p^c \times s \tag{1}$$

where, s is the scaling factor. If shearing in the x-axis of a point with (x_1,y_1) coordinates leads to a new coordinate (x_2,y_2), then for the shearing parameter in the x

direction Sh_x and the shearing parameter in the y direction Sh_y, the modified coordinate is defined as

$$\begin{bmatrix} x_2 \\ y_2 \end{bmatrix} = \begin{bmatrix} 1 & Sh_x \\ 0 & 1 \end{bmatrix} \times \begin{bmatrix} x_1 \\ y_1 \end{bmatrix} \quad (2)$$

If shearing in the y-axis of the same point leads to a new coordinate (x_3,y_3), then it is

$$\begin{bmatrix} x_3 \\ y_3 \end{bmatrix} = \begin{bmatrix} 1 & 0 \\ Sh_y & 1 \end{bmatrix} \times \begin{bmatrix} x_1 \\ y_1 \end{bmatrix} \quad (3)$$

A flip (mirror effect) reverses the pixels vertically or horizontally. For example, the (x, y) coordinate pixel is located at coordinate (width—x—1, y) at the modified image for a horizontal flip.

20.3.4 Classification using CNN

A CNN is composed of layers, each of which uses a differentiable function to convert one volume to another (Iqbal et al., 2022). The five types of layers in the proposed CNN, as shown in Figure 20.2, include the input layer, the convolution layer, the activation function layer, the pooling layer, and the fully connected layer. The input layer holds the raw input of the image with width W, height H, and depth C. For a convolution layer l, $f^{[l]}$ = filter size, $p^{[l]}$ = padding size, $s^{[l]}$ = stride, $n_c^{[l]}$ = number of filters, for input $n_H^{[l-1]} \times n_W^{[l-1]} \times n_C^{[l-1]}$ where the height, the width, and the number of channels get denoted by H, W, and C, respectively. The output is represented by $n_H^l \times n_W^l \times n_C^l$ where $n^{[l]} = \frac{n^{[l-1]} + 2p - f}{s} + 1$, each filter is $f^{[l]} \times f^{[l]} \times n_c^{[l-1]}$, activations from one layer to the next layer: $a^{[l]} \rightarrow n_H^{[l]} \times n_W^{[l]} \times n_C^{[l]}$, for M number of examples

$$A^{[l]} = M \times n_H^{[l]} \times n_W^{[l]} \times n_C^{[l]} \quad (4)$$

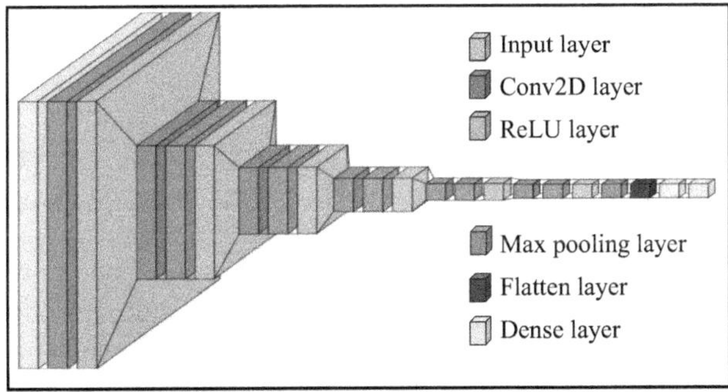

FIGURE 20.2 The architecture of our proposed CNN classifier.

where weights $f^{[l]} \times f^{[l]} \times f^{[l-1]} \times n_C^{[l]}$, bias: $n_C^{[l]} - \left(1,1,1,n_C^{[l]}\right)$. The activation function layer applies an activation function to the convolution layer's unit-wise output. Our proposed model has used a Rectified Linear Unit (ReLU) in this layer represented by max (0, x).

The pooling layer's role lies in progressively reducing the representation's spatial size to decrease the total parameters and intra-network computations (Ghosh et al., 2020b). The max pooling operation in our approach chooses the maximum element from the feature map region enclosed by the filter. The fully connected layer takes input from the previous layer (Convolutional or Pooling), flattens it, calculates the class scores, and outputs a one-dimensional array of size equivalent to the number of classes. Here flattening refers to the process of converting the input from a three-dimensional matrix to a vector.

20.4 ANALYSIS OF EXPERIMENTAL OUTCOMES

This section defines the dataset and presents the experimental outcomes. The proposed model's performance is quantified using evaluation metrics like accuracy, precision, recall, error rate, and F1 score. Also, the confusion matrix, the receiver operating characteristic (ROC) curve, and the learning curve have been presented, where the learning curve displays the model's training and validation performance over time with the rise in epochs. The ROC curve represents the relationship between the false positive rate (FPR) and the true positive rate (TPR) for several thresholds. Confusion matrices are used to assess how well the model performs across several categories, here, fall, and not fall.

20.4.1 Dataset Description

The "UR Fall Detection Dataset" from (Kwolek and Kepski, 2014) has been used in the proposed work. The dataset includes images categorized into the "Fall" and "Not Fall" categories. It is a collection of images displaying various fall-related scenarios. The training and testing data have been divided into an 80:20 ratio.

20.4.2 Data Augmentation Outcomes

Since zero to 255 as the RGB coefficient range of original images is too high for the considered models to consider a particular learning rate, values between zero and one by scaling with a 1/255 factor have been targeted in the first step of the data augmentation technique. The shearing transformation on the images is then applied randomly with a 0.2 range (Ghosh et al., 2020a). After that, the images are zoomed inside with a 0.2 factor. Half of the images are randomly flipped horizontally since no assumptions are there for the azimuth asymmetry of practical images. The data augmentation outcomes shed light on the feasibility of the augmentation phase in the proposed fall detection methodology. The learning curves generated before and after the augmentation are presented in Figure 20.3. The training and validation losses

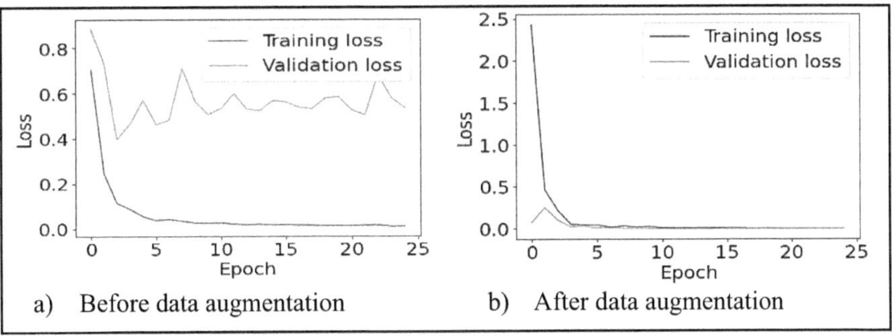

FIGURE 20.3 Training and validation loss in the learning curve over epochs.

converge for the proposed framework after augmentation, proving that the model is evolving and not overfitting.

20.4.3 Hyperparameter Tuning Outcomes

CNN gains the ability to automatically extract relevant properties from input data in the training stage. To improve the performance, this procedure involves enhancing network parameters using a variety of optimization algorithms, including Adaptive Moment (Adam) and Random Gradient Descent (GD). The batch size parameter controls the amount of samples propagated in the network at each iteration. Table 20.1 shows the outcomes of hyperparameter tuning from where 100, Adam, and categorical cross-entropy as the best possible combination of batch size, optimizer, and loss function as the hyperparameters are proposed to yield the best performance.

20.4.4 Comparison with Existing Models

The proposed model has been compared with three competitors, LeNet, residual neural network (ResNet), and Visual Geometry Group (VGG16). LeNet (LeCun et al., 1998) has seven layers, that is, three fully connected, two convolutional, and two pooling layers. In this instance, input images of shape (32 × 32 × 3) where three as the third dimension represents the number of channels (here, RGB), are scaled down to 32×32 pixels. The two convolutional layers (Conv2D) have six filters of size 5×5 and a ReLU activation function trailed by two average pooling layers having default pool size 2×2 and a flatten layer for converting the output of the previous layers into a one-dimensional vector. Three levels (dense), each containing 120, 84, and one unit(s), are connected. The output layer for binary classification uses a sigmoid activation.

The VGG16 (Simonyan and Zisserman, 2014), which has 13 convolution layers and three fully connected layers with multiple 3×3 kernel-sized filters one after another. Five max-pooling layers are added followed by convolution layers. The pooling is executed over a 2×2-pixel window, having two as its stride.

TABLE 20.1
Outcomes of Hyperparameter Tuning

Batch size	Optimizer	Loss function	Accuracy	Precision	Recall	F1-score
100	**Adam**	**Categorical Cross-Entropy**	**97.78**	**95.78**	**94.62**	**95.45**
		Mean Squared Error	91.43	92.57	93.48	92.19
	Random GD	Categorical Cross-Entropy	89.61	88.49	84.53	86.34
		Mean Squared Error	84.58	83.27	84.31	89.52
200	Adam	Categorical Cross-Entropy	87.51	83.96	89.43	86.41
		Mean Squared Error	84.27	81.28	82.39	88.37
	Random GD	Categorical Cross-Entropy	86.19	85.27	83.48	87.42
		Mean Squared Error	84.39	82.39	85.45	86.48

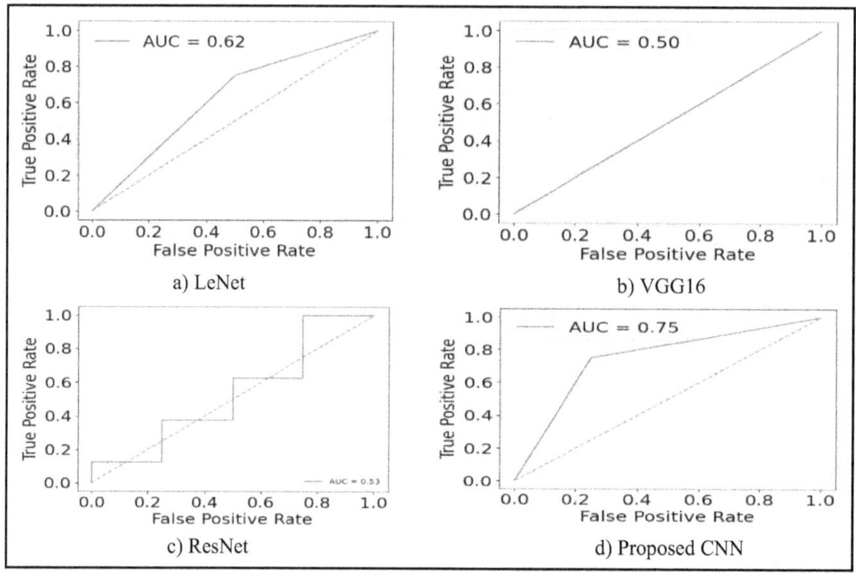

FIGURE 20.4 The model's predictions and true labels from the test data generated ROC curve.

Residual network (ResNet) (Sermanet et al., 2013) is created to solve the issue of disappearing gradients in largely deep networks. To do this, they skip connections, which let the network learn residual functions rather than direct mappings.

ROC curves for the four models are shown in Figure 20.4 to assess how well the binary classifiers perform at detecting falls. The classifier's total effectiveness is gauged by the Area Under the ROC Curve (AUC), where 0.75 as the AUC value of the proposed framework indicates better performance than the others. Since it

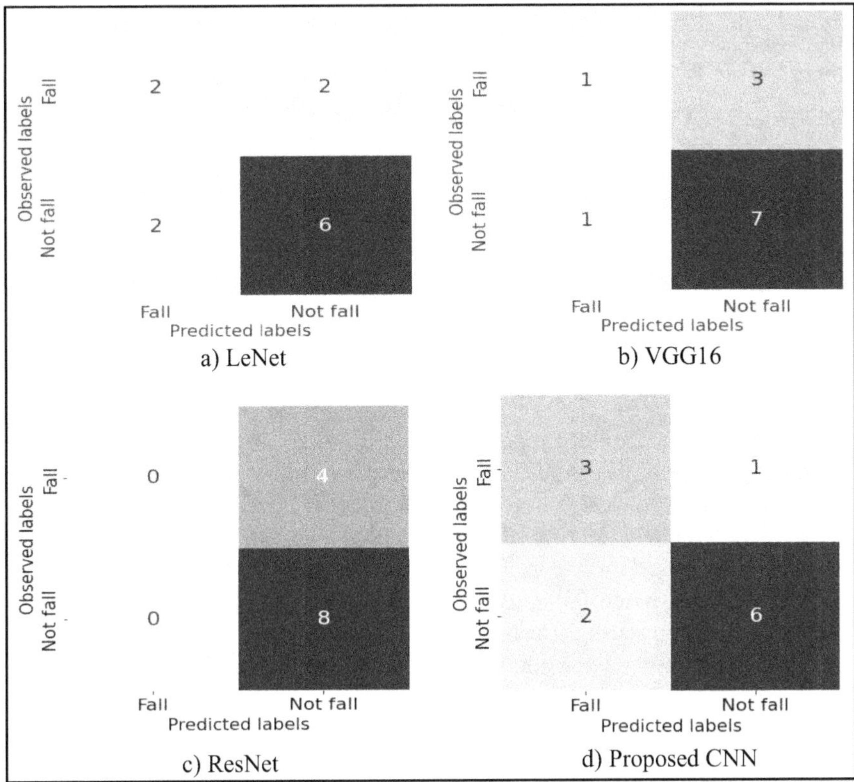

FIGURE 20.5 Confusion matrices generated by LeNet, VGG, ResNet, and the proposed CNN for Subject 1.

is not possible to show the confusion matrices generated from every subject's data due to space constraints, the true positive amount, true negative amount, false positive amount, and false negative amount in each class are displayed on the confusion matrices shown in Figure 20.5 for the first subject, where the proposed model is concluded as outperforming its competitors and suitable for real-time fall-detection scenarios.

20.4.5 Cross-Validation Results

Five-fold cross-validation has been executed in the proposed CNN by splitting the training dataset into five equal parts. Four sub-datasets are considered for training, and the other for validation. This procedure has been performed five times such that each sub-dataset becomes the validation dataset exactly once. The Average Error Rate (AER) values are noted in each iteration. The last column in Table 20.2 specifies the average AER of all five iterations, which is only 0.107 for the proposed CNN classifier.

TABLE 20.2
Average Error Rate Produced in the Cross-Validation Phase of Classification

AER_1	AER_2	AER_3	AER_4	AER_5	AER_{avg}
0.0851	0.1126	0.1053	0.1168	0.1159	0.107

20.5 CONCLUSION

Elderly individuals, especially those living in nursing homes, are at high risk of falling, and that early diagnosis can help avoid serious harm and problems. Using CNNs in image processing systems to detect falls and prevent older adults from further falling has many benefits. First, it allows for non-intrusive monitoring, obviating the need for wearable technology or external sensors that can interfere with the older person's regular activities. Additionally, CNNs can improve the dependability and precision of fall identification in comparison to conventional techniques. The CNN can adjust to changes in lighting, clothes, and body looks and generalize well to sudden occurrences based on its capacity to learn from large-scale datasets. Because of its flexibility, CNN-based fall detection systems are more reliable and ideal for use in various real-world settings, such as homes, assisted living facilities, and hospitals.

Despite the encouraging results achieved in human fall detection based on image processing using CNNs, several possible study areas remain open to explore. Although image-based fall detection has produced positive outcomes, additional modalities like audio, accelerometer, and gyroscopic sensors could increase the detection's precision. Pre-recorded videos are primarily used in modern methods for training and assessment. Real-world, real-time detection with cameras or other sensors is still challenging. Most available datasets are limited and might not translate well to various contexts. Large-scale datasets with various environments and scenarios could help the models perform better. Also, the skeleton model can be checked whether it is appropriate for fall detection since it can examine the person's posture and movement.

20.6 ACKNOWLEDGMENT

AICTE supported this work under the scheme of AICTE Doctoral Fellowship to A. Ghosh, with Ref. No.2.2.1/Regis./Appt.(AG)/Ph.D(ADF)/2021 dated 01.02.2021. This work was supported by a UGC Start-up Grant to S. Saha under the scheme of Basic Scientific Research, File No. F.30–449/2018(BSR) dated 21.11.2019 and the university research seed money to S. Saha with File No.: 9.6/Regis./SD/Mn.(SS)/2019 dated 19.06.2019.

REFERENCES

De Raeve, N., Shahid, A., De Schepper, M., De Poorter, E., Moerman, I., Verhaevert, J., Van Torre, P. and Rogier, H., 2022. Bluetooth-low-energy-based fall detection and warning system for elderly people in nursing homes. *Journal of Sensors*, 2022, pp. 1–14.

Ghosh, A., Saha, S. and Konar, A., 2020a. Fuzzy posture matching for pain recovery using yoga. In *Computational Intelligence in Pattern Recognition: Proceedings of CIPR 2019* (pp. 957–967). Singapore: Springer.

Ghosh, L., Saha, S. and Konar, A., 2020b. Bi-directional long short-term memory model to analyze psychological effects on gamers. *Applied Soft Computing*, 95, p. 106573.

Hasib, R., Khan, K.N., Yu, M. and Khan, M.S., 2021, April. Vision-based human posture classification and fall detection using convolutional neural network. In *2021 International Conference on Artificial Intelligence (ICAI)* (pp. 74–79). New York: IEEE.

Iqbal, S., Qureshi, A.N., Ullah, A., Li, J. and Mahmood, T., 2022. Improving the Robustness and Quality of Biomedical CNN Models through Adaptive Hyperparameter Tuning. *Applied Sciences*, 12(22), p. 11870.

Kepski, M. and Kwolek, B. 2013. Unobtrusive fall detection at home using Kinect sensor. In R. Wilson, E. Hancock, A. Bors and W. Smith (eds.), *Computer Analysis of Images and Patterns*. CAIP 2013. Lecture Notes in Computer Science (vol 8047). Berlin Heidelberg: Springer. https://doi.org/10.1007/978-3-642-40261-6_55

Kwolek, B. and Kepski, M., 2014. Human fall detection on embedded platform using depth maps and wireless accelerometer. *Computer Methods and Programs in Biomedicine*, 117(3), pp. 489–501.

LeCun, Y., Bottou, L., Bengio, Y. and Haffner, P., 1998. Gradient-based learning applied to document recognition. *Proceedings of the IEEE*, 86(11), pp. 2278–2324.

Mastorakis, G. and Makris, D., 2012. Fall detection system using Kinect's infrared sensor. *Journal of Real-Time Image Processing*, 9(4), pp. 635–646. doi:10.1007/s11554-012-0246-9.

Nghiem, A.T., Auvinet, E. and Meunier, J., 2012, July. Head detection using kinect camera and its application to fall detection. In *2012 11th International Conference on Information Science, Signal Processing and Their Applications (ISSPA)* (pp. 164–169). New York: IEEE.

Panda, S.K., Reddy, G.S.M., Goyal, S.B., Thirunavukkarasu, K., Bhambri, P., Rao, M.V., Singh, A.S., Fakih, A.H., Shukla, P.K., Shukla, P.K. and others., 2019. Method for Management of Scholarship of Large Number of Students based on Blockchain. IN Patent App. 201,911,034,937 A.

Potluri, S., Tiwari, P.K., Bhambri, P., Obulesu, O., Naidu, P.A., Lakshmi, L., Kallam, S., Gupta, S. and Gupta, B., 2019. Method of Load Distribution Balancing for Fog Cloud Computing in IoT Environment. IN Patent App. 201,941,044,511.

Rana, R., Chhabta, Y. and Bhambri, P., 2019. A review on development and challenges in wireless sensor network. In *International Multidisciplinary Academic Research Conference* (pp. 184–188). CT University.

Rastogi, S. and Singh, J., 2021. A systematic review on machine learning for fall detection system. *Computational Intelligence*, 37(2), pp. 951–974.

Rezaei, A., Mascheroni, A., Stevens, M.C., Argha, R., Papandrea, M., Puiatti, A. and Lovell, N.H., 2023. Unobtrusive human fall detection system using mmWave radar and data driven methods. *IEEE Sensors Journal*, 23(7), pp. 7968–7976.

Saha, S. and Ghosh, A., 2019, December. Rehabilitation using neighbor-cluster based matching inducing artificial bee colony optimization. In *2019 IEEE 16th India Council International Conference (INDICON)* (pp. 1–4). IEEE. https://doi.org/10.1109/INDICON47234.2019.9028975

Salah, O.Z., Selvaperumal, S.K. and Abdulla, R., 2022. Accelerometer-based elderly fall detection system using edge artificial intelligence architecture. *International Journal of Electrical and Computer Engineering*, 12(4), p. 4430.

Santos, G.L., Endo, P.T., Monteiro, K.H.D.C., Rocha, E.D.S., Silva, I. and Lynn, T., 2019. Accelerometer-based human fall detection using convolutional neural networks. *Sensors*, 19(7), p. 1644.

Sermanet, P., Eigen, D., Zhang, X., Mathieu, M., Fergus, R. and LeCun, Y., 2013. Overfeat: Integrated recognition, localization and detection using convolutional networks. arXiv preprint arXiv:1312.6229. https://doi.org/10.48550/arXiv.1312.6229

Simonyan, K. and Zisserman, A., 2014. Very deep convolutional networks for large-scale image recognition. arXiv preprint arXiv:1409.1556. https://doi.org/10.48550/arXiv.1409.1556

Somkunwar, R.K., Thorat, N., Pimple, J., Dhumal, R. and Choudhari, Y., 2023. A novel based human fall detection system using hybrid approach. *Journal of Data Acquisition and Processing*, 38(2), p. 3985.

Stone, E.E. and Skubic, M., 2014. Fall detection in homes of older adults using the Microsoft Kinect. *IEEE Journal of Biomedical and Health Informatics*, 19(1), pp. 290–301.

Tondon, N. and Bhambri, P., 2017. Novel approach for drug discovery. *International Journal of Research in Engineering and Applied Sciences*, 7(6), pp. 28–46.

Tong, L., Luo, J., Adams, J., Osinski, K., Liu, X. and Friedland, D., 2022, June. A clustering-aided approach for diagnosis prediction: A case study of elderly fall. In *2022 IEEE 46th Annual Computers, Software, and Applications Conference (COMPSAC)* (pp. 337–342). IEEE. https://doi.org/10.1109/COMPSAC54236.2022.00054

Wang, X., Ellul, J. and Azzopardi, G., 2020. Elderly fall detection systems: A literature survey. *Frontiers in Robotics and AI*, 7, p. 71.

Xu, Y., Chen, J., Yang, Q. and Guo, Q., 2019, July. Human posture recognition and fall detection using Kinect V2 camera. In *2019 Chinese Control Conference (CCC)* (pp. 8488–8493). IEEE. https://doi.org/10.23919/ChiCC.2019.8865732

21 AI-Powered Internet of Medical Things for Monitoring Elderly Adults in Independent Living Environments

Vani Vasudevan, Udhayaranjani Sellappagounder Mohan and Mohan Sellappa Gounder

21.1 INTRODUCTION

The global demographic landscape is undergoing a significant shift with the rapid growth of the elderly population challenging healthcare systems worldwide. The integration of artificial intelligence (AI) and the internet of medical things (IoMT) is revolutionizing elderly care by monitoring and assisting them in independent living environments (Javaid and Khan, 2021).

The synergy between AI and IoMT has the potential to enhance the quality of life and healthcare for the elderly, as explored in this chapter. Our proposed system utilizes a network of interconnected medical devices and sensors to acquire real-time data on health parameters, activities, and environmental conditions (Ruby et al., 2022). AI algorithms analyze this data for insights into health status, anomaly detection, and risk prediction (Abderahman et al., 2023), enabling early intervention and personalized care plans (Rajkomar et al., 2019).

The seamless integration of AI and IoMT also improves communication channels among seniors, caregivers, and healthcare professionals, enhancing access to remote monitoring and telehealth services (Bashshur et al., 2016). Robust encryption and data anonymization address privacy and security concerns (Malin, 2005).

This chapter examines technological advancements, challenges, ethical considerations, and potential cost reductions associated with AI-powered IoMT solutions for senior care, addressing the evolving healthcare needs of an aging society.

21.1.1 The Aging Population Challenge

The world faces a significant demographic shift with a substantial increase in the geriatric population, presenting complex challenges for healthcare, economies, and

DOI: 10.1201/9781032698519-21

societies. Statistics from the United Nations project a tripling of the global elderly population by 2050, placing a burden on healthcare systems and economies. The aging population's impact on healthcare costs and societal challenges is evident, requiring innovative solutions like AI and IoMT to enhance elderly care.

21.1.2 Transformative Role of AI and IoMT in Elderly Care

AI enables personalized care plans through the analysis of massive datasets, predicting health risks and facilitating timely interventions (Rajkomar et al., 2019). AI-driven monitoring systems, in conjunction with IoMT, allow real-time analysis of health parameters, daily activities, and environmental conditions, reducing hospitalizations and improving overall health outcomes (Ribeiro et al., 2020). IoMT's integration into wearable devices and home monitoring systems enhances remote geriatric monitoring, increasing healthcare accessibility (Al-Fuqaha et al., 2015).

21.1.3 Objectives and Structure of the Chapter

This chapter comprehensively analyzes challenges posed by the aging population and investigates the roles of AI and IoMT in geriatric care, emphasizing ethical concerns. It aims to showcase transformative applications and explore future directions for AI and IoMT in geriatric care, concluding with a discussion on applications, impact, and future directions in elderly care in Section 21.5.

21.2 THE SYNERGY OF AI AND IoMT IN ELDERLY CARE

The integration of AI and IoMT in geriatric adult monitoring systems represents a revolutionary approach to meeting the changing healthcare requirements of aging populations (Bhambri et al., 2019). This partnership leverages the power of data-driven insights and real-time connectivity to improve the quality of care and promote independent living among the elderly.

21.2.1 AI and IoMT

Using cutting-edge technology to improve elderly adult monitoring system in an independent living environment, AI and IoMT play a vital role. AI, which includes machine learning and deep learning, is being used to diagnose diseases, predict health outcomes, and personalize treatment plans, thereby transforming healthcare into a data-driven industry. IoMT, a network of interconnected medical devices and sensors, enables real-time patient monitoring, ubiquitous health technology, and telehealth services, thereby decreasing hospital readmissions and enhancing healthcare accessibility (Bashshur et al., 2016). AI analyzes the immense data generated by IoMT devices to provide data-driven insights, early detection of health issues, and personalized care plans. This convergence provides healthcare providers with unprecedented capabilities, enabling them to provide patient-centric care and enhancing the quality and efficiency of healthcare (Rajkomar et al., 2019; Bashshur et al., 2016). As these technologies continue to evolve, their profound impact on the healthcare industry is certain to grow, propelling healthcare into a new era of data-driven, patient-centric care.

21.2.2 Advantages of AI-IoMT Fusion in Elderly Care

The integration of AI and IoMT in elderly care is revolutionizing healthcare delivery. IoMT devices provide real-time data on vital signs, chronic conditions, and activity levels, enabling remote monitoring and early detection of health issues (Bashshur et al., 2016). AI analyzes this data to create personalized care plans, (Ruby et al., 2022) optimize medication regimens, and predict health hazards (Ribeiro et al., 2020). This proactive approach reduces hospitalizations and medical expenses. AI-IoMT integration also facilitates telehealth consultations (Peek et al., 2016), increasing healthcare accessibility, especially in rural areas. Smart home technologies use IoMT sensors to detect injuries and routine changes, allowing timely interventions while respecting older individuals' autonomy.

21.2.2.1 Understanding AI in Eldercare

AI is transforming the aging population by offering solutions for eldercare, including continuous health monitoring, fall detection, medication management systems, cognitive health assessment, virtual companions, and personalized care plans (Mora et al., 2017; Miner et al., 2020). However, ethical concerns about data privacy, informed consent, and algorithmic impartiality remain (Tiribelli et al., 2023). The future of AI in eldercare is promising, with ongoing research focusing on improving diagnostic precision, developing AI-powered assistive technologies, and ensuring equitable access to AI solutions. AI serves as a transformative force in geriatric care, providing personalized, efficient, and ethical solutions to enhance health, independence, and overall quality of life.

21.2.2.2 Exploring the Internet of Medical Things (IoMT) in Eldercare

IoMT is a comprehensive network of medical devices and sensors designed to collect, transmit, and analyze health-related data, revolutionizing healthcare for aging populations. Key applications of IoMT in eldercare include continuous remote health monitoring, fall detection and prevention, medication adherence support, environmental monitoring, and facilitation of telehealth and telemedicine consultations (Ruby et al., 2022; Shahriar Haque et al., 2023; Mohammed et al., 2019).

Despite its benefits, IoMT presents challenges in data privacy, security, and ethical concerns. The transformative potential of combining AI and IoMT in geriatric care is significant. This convergence reshapes healthcare delivery, ushering in an era of personalized, efficient, and ethical care for the elderly.

21.3 DESIGNING AND IMPLEMENTING AI-POWERED MONITORING SYSTEM

The Figure 21.1 provides a high-level overview of the AI-Powered Monitoring System. In this figure, the "Elderly Adult Independent Living Environment" is where the monitoring system is deployed to monitor the elderly individuals (Malik et al.,

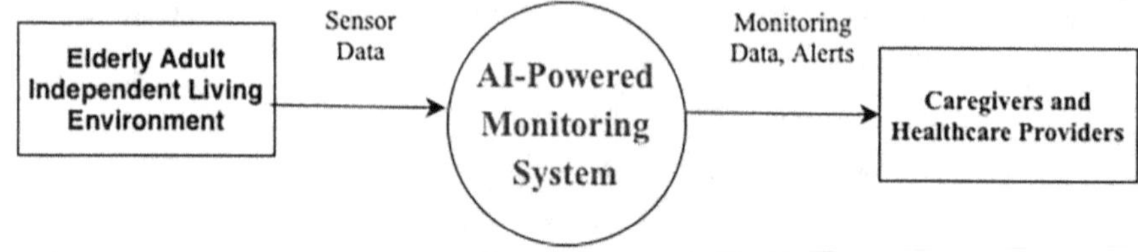

FIGURE 21.1 Context diagramarchitecture of the proposed system.

2021). The "AI-Powered Monitoring System" interacts with the environment, collecting sensor data and providing monitoring data and alerts. The "Caregivers and Healthcare Providers" receive monitoring data and alerts from the system to provide care and assistance to the elderly individuals.

Designing an AI-powered system for monitoring elderly adults requires a comprehensive and interconnected framework. Here's an overview of key architectural components and their functions within the system:

Sensor Layer: Wearable Sensors: Track exercise, movement, and vital signs (e.g., fitness trackers, smartwatches).

Environmental Sensors: Measure temperature, humidity, air quality, and safety risks in living spaces.

B>Health Monitoring Devices: Specialized gadgets for real-time monitoring of health measures (e.g., heart rate monitors, blood pressure monitors).

IoT Network Infrastructure: Components for data transmission over LAN or WAN.

Gateways for receiving data from nearby sensors and transmitting it to computers or the cloud.

Data Collection and Transmission Layer: Hubs and data collection nodes for gathering data from various sensors. Protocols for secure, quick, and real-time data transmission to centralized processing units.

Data Management Layer: Centralized systems (e.g., databases, data warehouses) for storing both old and new data. Retrieval and storage mechanisms to ensure data availability and accuracy.

Artificial Intelligence Layer: Machine learning and deep learning programs for real-time data analysis (Hireche et al., 2022). Predictive models to identify health trends, outliers, and provide personalized care suggestions.

Monitoring and Control Layer: User interfaces and control panels for accessibility by caregivers, medical professionals, and elderly individuals. Alert systems to notify critical health events or anomalies (Anand and Bhambri, 2018).

Privacy and Security Layer: Strong encryption and data anonymization methods for safeguarding private medical data (Davenport and Kalakota, 2019). Cybersecurity measures to prevent unauthorized access and data breaches.

Individualized Care Plan Generation: AI-powered algorithms creating unique care plans based on health history, habits, and real-time monitoring.

Telehealth Integration Layer: Systems facilitating remote communication among seniors, caregivers, and healthcare providers. Rules for secure transmission of health information.

Fall Detection and Safety Layer: Advanced AI methods for fall detection and accident prevention. Safety features for emergencies to ensure the well-being of older adults.

Ethical Considerations Layer: Guidelines and compliance methods addressing ethical issues, including data privacy and fairness.

Smart Home Integration Layer: Integration with smart home technologies for seamless communication. Automation for increased independence, such as medication reminders and mental health checks.

Cost and Resource Management Layer: Systems for calculating cost savings and economic benefits from early treatments and reduced hospital stays (Padhan et al., 2023). Resource allocation and optimization techniques for system efficiency.

Ready for the Future and Scalable: Architectural adaptability for compatibility with new AI and IoT technologies. Sustainability to ensure long-term usefulness and relevance.

The Figure 21.2 illustrates the architecture of the AI-powered elderly adult monitoring system, featuring layers connected for seamless functionality. Starting from the sensor layer, data progresses through collecting, AI processing, monitoring and control, privacy, and security layers (Srivastava, 2022). This process facilitates personalized care plans, telehealth integration, fall detection, safety checks, ethical considerations, and more. The system is designed to be adaptable to future technological and economic developments.

In the depicted interaction, initiated from the sensor layer, data is collected from various sensors and transmitted through the data collection and transmission layer via an IoT network infrastructure (Tondon and Bhambri, 2017). The data management layer processes and stores data, while the AI processing layer employs machine learning algorithms for analysis (Stafford et al., 2020). The monitoring and control layer provides user interfaces and alert systems, and the security and privacy layer ensures data security.

Support layers interact with core layers for specific functions, including generating care plans, integrating telehealth systems, ensuring fall detection and safety, addressing ethical compliance, and integrating with smart home technology (Karar et al., 2022). This modular design allows flexibility and adaptability to diverse scenarios, such as emergencies where an elderly adult's health deteriorates, triggering interactions between the core and support layers as illustrated in the Figure 21.3.

21.3.1 Data Collection

In modern healthcare, integrating medical devices and sensors in IoMT and AI is crucial (Panda et al., 2019). These devices collect real-time data on an individual's

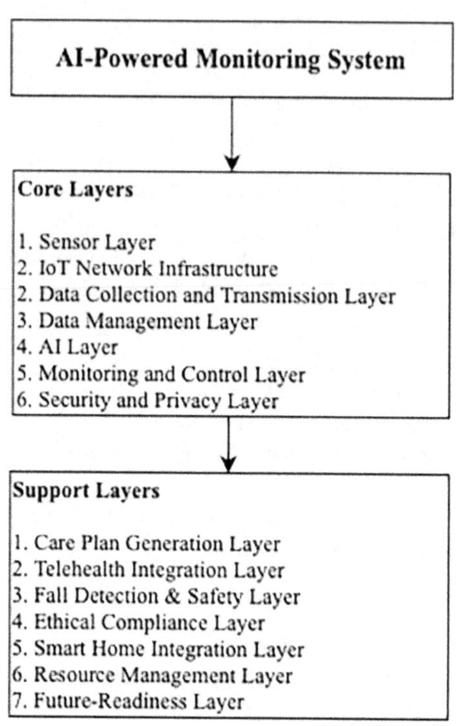

FIGURE 21.2 Architecture of AI-powered monitoring system.

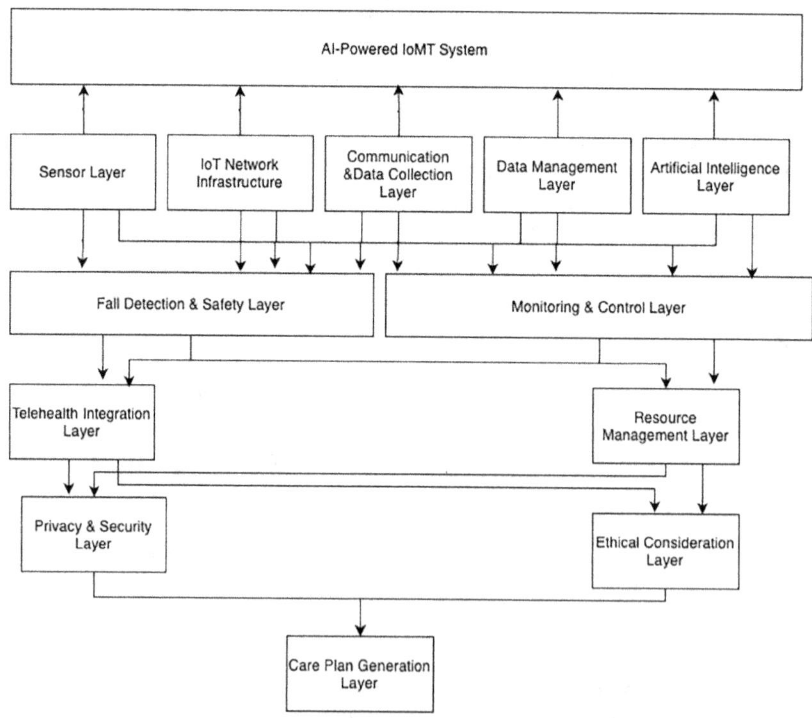

FIGURE 21.3 Layers and its interaction when "heart rate" is abnormal.

health, daily routines, and environment, aiding healthcare decisions and enhancing overall health, particularly in elderly care.

Wearable sensors, like exercise trackers and smartwatches, monitor heart rate, temperature, activity levels, and sleep habits (Ribeiro et al., 2020). Environmental sensors in living spaces track temperature, humidity, air quality, and hazards, offering insights into health-affecting conditions (Mohammed et al., 2019). Health monitoring devices, such as blood pressure monitors and glucose meters, provide real-time information for early detection and effective management of health issues (Catarinucci et al., 2015).

Protocols connect devices to a central hub in AI-powered systems, enabling secure and efficient data transfer. These devices continuously collect data, allowing AI to make informed decisions through advanced machine learning algorithms, identifying health trends, outliers, and potential risks (Ruby et al., 2022). This capability enables early interventions and personalized care plans based on individual health needs and preferences (Rajkomar et al., 2019). In summary, using medical gadgets and sensors are crucial for the success of AI and IoMT in healthcare, providing tools for proactive, individualized care and improving accessibility, especially in rural or underserved areas (Evans et al., 2016).

21.3.2.1 Types of Data with Valid Range and Invalid Data

The data types and examples shown in Table 21.1 illustrates the types of data that can be collected as well as the importance of setting valid data ranges to ensure the accuracy and reliability of the information collected by sensors in an AI-powered IoMT system for elder adult monitoring.

21.4 ENSURING PRIVACY, SECURITY, AND ETHICAL CONSIDERATIONS

Table 21.1 shows the strategies that can used to ensure privacy, security, and ethical considerations with its importance as well as future avenues that can be considered while implementing AI powered monitoring system for elders.

21.5 CONCLUSION, APPLICATIONS, IMPACTS, AND FUTURE DIRECTIONS

Conclusion: The global aging population poses challenges to healthcare systems, addressed through the integration of artificial intelligence (AI) and the internet of medical things (IoMT) in elderly care. AI analyzes extensive datasets, personalizing care, while IoMT enables real-time monitoring and telehealth services (Potluri et al., 2019). The synergy of AI and IoMT benefits elderly care by enabling continuous remote monitoring, personalized care plans, early risk prediction, and improved healthcare access. Smart home technologies and wearables empower the elderly to age independently. However, ethical and privacy concerns must be addressed. The

TABLE 21.1
Types of Data Collected by Using Various Sensors and the Information Technologies

Tech	Data Type	Description	Valid Range	Invalid Data
Wearable Sensors	Heart Rate	Sensor records heart rate. For an elderly person's resting heart rate is 72 beats/minute rising to 120 beats/minute with vigorous exercise.	50 to 100 beats/min (Rajendra et al., 2006).	150 beats/min while resting.
	Physical Activity	The sensor records the subject's daily physical activity.	2,000 to 10,000 steps per day. (Andersson et al., 2015).	50,000 steps per day (unlikely for an elderly adult).
	Sleep Patterns	The wearable sensor records the wearer's sleep habits.	Six to eight hours of sleep (Worley, 2018).	Two hours of sleep (inadequate) or 15 hours (excessive).
	Body Temperature	The sensor records the subject's body temperature (Geneva et al., 2019).	97°F to 99°F (36°C to 37°C).	80°F (too low) or 105°F (fever range).
	Stress Level	The wearable measures skin conductance and heart rate variability to determine stress levels.	20 to 60 (on a scale) (Kim et al., 2018).	150 (implausible reading).
	Blood Pressure	A cutting-edge wearable calculates blood pressure (Whelton et al., 2018).	90/60 to 140/90 mm Hg.	180/110 mm Hg (dangerously high).
	Oxygen saturation	Oxygen saturation in the blood is obtained from the sensor (Hafen and Sharma, 2023).	95% to 100%.	20% life-threateningly low.
	Electrocardiogram (ECG)	ECG sensors record the electrical activity of the heart.	Standard sinus rhythm (Miao et al., 2015).	Arrhythmia (abnormal heart rhythm).
	Location and Movement	GPS-enabled wearables monitor a person's whereabouts and movements (Cullen et al., 2022).	Locations consistent with daily activities.	Sudden teleportation or extreme speed.

Environmental Sensors	Temperature	Keep track of the temperature in the living area (Yang et al., 2008).	68°F to 78°F (20°C to 26°C).	-20°F (extremely cold) or 150°F (extremely hot).
	Humidity	The sensors gauge the environment's humidity levels (Seppänen and Kurnitski, 2009).	30% to 60% relative humidity.	5% (too dry) or 95% (excessively humid).
	Air quality	Air quality measures pollution levels.	Low levels of volatile organic compounds (VOCs) and particulate matter (PM2.5).	Extremely high VOCs (poor air quality) (Quirós-Alcalá et al., 2016).
	Carbon Monoxide (CO)	CO levels show that there are no increased CO concentrations, maintaining the safety of the living area.	CO levels within safety norms.	Very high CO levels (dangerous) (Cohen et al., 2005).
	Motion	Motion sensors capture activity and movement inside the house (Eisa and Moreira, 2017).	Regular household movements.	Continuous, erratic motion (sensor malfunction).
	Open-Close for Doors and Windows	Sensors on doors and windows keep track of their status (Friedrich et al., 2023).	Doors and windows opening at usual times.	Frequent, random openings (security issue).
	Light intensity	Light sensors track the amount of lighting in various spaces (Aminuddin et al., 2016).	Normal variations in lighting.	Sudden extreme darkness during the day.
	Sound data	Audio levels are recorded by sound sensors (Bouaziz et al., 2022).	Typical household sounds.	Continuous loud noises (sensor error).
	Emergency Button	An emergency button status is monitored (Ianculescu et al., 2023).	Not pressed during normal conditions.	Frequent or continuous pressing (security or health issue).
Information Technology	Pill consumption	Data on medication adherence is collected through automated pill dispensers and devices that remind users to take their pills.	All medications taken as prescribed.	No medications taken (potential issue) (Arain et al., 2021).
	Fall	Data regarding falls and accidents is provided through sensors that can detect falls.	No falls detected (Yacchirema et al., 2018).	Frequent fall alerts (sensor error).
	Weight	Smart scales measure and keep track of body weight (Johannessen et al., 2023).	Consistent with earlier measures.	Sudden, extreme weight loss or gain.
	Pain Levels	Users can submit their pain levels using smart pain management equipment.	Zero to ten (on a pain scale).	20 (impossibly high) (Rodríguez et al., 2017).

TABLE 21.2
Various Strategies to Ensure Privacy, Security, and Ethical Considerations in AI-Powered Monitoring System

Strategy	Reference	Importance	Future Avenue
Data Encryption and Anonymization	(Iwaya et al., 2020)	Safeguarding sensitive healthcare data during transmission and storage.	Exploring advanced encryption methods like homomorphic encryption.
Compliance with Regulations	(Bradford et al., 2020)	Ensuring legal compliance and maintaining high standards of data privacy.	Staying informed about emerging regulations worldwide and adapting systems accordingly.
Privacy-Preserving AI	(Dwork, 2011)	Protecting individual privacy while performing AI analysis.	Continuous refinement of techniques for data utility and privacy.
Ethical Guidelines	(ICMR, 2023)	Guiding AI development for fairness, transparency, and accountability.	Ongoing refinement and adaptation of ethical guidelines as AI applications expand in healthcare.
Blockchain for Data Integrity	(Swan, 2015)	Ensuring data integrity through a tamper-proof ledger.	Enabling patient-controlled access to health records using blockchain.
User-Centric Design	(Nielsen, 1993)	Ensuring systems meet the needs and preferences of elderly users.	Creating feedback mechanisms for continuous system improvement based on user input.
Robust Incident Response	(Schultz, 2001)	Detecting and addressing security threats promptly to minimize impact.	Advancing real-time threat detection capabilities using AI and machine learning.
Ethical AI Oversight Boards	(European Commission, 2019)	Reviewing AI algorithms to ensure they align with ethical norms.	Forming international standards for ethical AI boards to ensure consistency and objectivity.
Human-AI Collaboration	(WHO, 2021)	Developing AI systems that respect patient privacy and work with healthcare professionals.	Creating AI systems that seamlessly enhance diagnostic accuracy and patient care.
International Collaboration	(WEF, 2022)	Establishing unified standards and best practices in privacy, security, and ethics.	Continuing to work with global partners to ensure harmony in privacy and security practices.

chapter explores these technologies, their advantages, and implications for the aging population, along with challenges, ethical considerations, and potential cost savings associated with AI-powered IoMT solutions for senior care.

Applications: AI-powered IoMT supporting telehealth integration, medication adherence, fall detection, and health monitoring. It identifies health issues early by monitoring vital signs, activity, and sleep patterns. AI algorithms assess sensor data for fall detection, intelligent medicine dispensers, and remote consultations to enhance chronic condition treatment.

Impact: AI-powered IoMT improves seniors' quality of life through individualized care based on health data, enhancing overall health, and reducing healthcare expenses by minimizing hospitalizations and ER visits. Monitoring systems facilitate caretakers in managing seniors' changing medical demands efficiently.

Future Directions: Future AI models will consider genetic, environmental, lifestyle, and individual health variations. Explainable AI ensures transparency. 5G connectivity and edge computing enhance real-time monitoring. Prioritizing ethical concerns like data privacy and user autonomy empowers older persons to control their health data. Industry participants, researchers, and legislators must collaborate to establish standards and rules for AI-powered IoMT, ensuring interoperability and ethical behavior.

REFERENCES

Abderahman, R., Karim, R., Horst, T., Andrea, A., Salem, A., Yaser, A., & Mohammad, I. (2023). The internet of things (IoT) in healthcare: Taking stock and moving forward. *Internet of Things*, 22, 100721. ISSN 2542–6605; https://doi.org/10.1016/j.iot.2023.100721.

Al-Fuqaha, A., Guizani, M., Mohammadi, M., Aledhari, M., & Ayyash, M. (2015). Internet of things: A survey on enabling technologies, protocols, and applications. *IEEE Communications Surveys & Tutorials*, 17(4), 2347–2376. https://doi.org/10.1109/COMST.2015.2444095.

Aminuddin, R., Sharkey, A., & Levita, L. (2016, March). Interaction with the Paro robot may reduce psychophysiological stress responses. In *2016 11th ACM/IEEE International Conference on Human-Robot Interaction (HRI)* (pp. 593–594). London: IEEE.

Anand, A., & Bhambri, P. (2018). Orientation, scale and location invariant character recognition system using neural networks. *International Journal of Theoretical & Applied Sciences*, 10(1), 106–109.

Andersson, M., Stridsman, C., Rönmark, E., Lindberg, A., & Emtner, M. (2015). Physical activity and fatigue in chronic obstructive pulmonary disease—a population based study. *Respiratory Medicine*, 109(8), 1048–1057. https://doi.org/10.1016/j.rmed.2015.05.007.

Arain, M. A., Ahmad, A., Chiu, V., & Kembel, L. (2021). Medication adherence support of an in-home electronic medication dispensing system for individuals living with chronic conditions: A pilot randomized controlled trial. *BMC Geriatrics*, 21(1), 56. https://doi.org/10.1186/s12877-020-01979-w.

Bashshur, R. L., Howell, J. D., Krupinski, E. A., Harms, K. M., Bashshur, N., & Doarn, C. R. (2016). The empirical foundations of telemedicine interventions in primary care. *Telemedicine Journal and e-Health: The Official Journal of the American Telemedicine Association*, 22(5), 342–375. https://doi.org/10.1089/tmj.2016.0045.

Bhambri, P., Sinha, V. K., & Jaiswal, M. (2019). Change in Iris dimensions as a potential human consciousness level indicator. *International Journal of Innovative Technology and Exploring Engineering*, 8(9S), 517–525.

Bouaziz, G., Brulin, D., & Campo, E. (2022). Technological solutions for social isolation monitoring of the elderly: A survey of selected projects from academia and industry. *Sensors*, 22(22), 8802. MDPI AG. https://doi.org/10.3390/s22228802.

Bradford, L., Aboy, M., & Liddell, K. (2020). International transfers of health data between the EU and USA: A sector-specific approach for the USA to ensure an 'adequate' level of protection. *Journal of Law and the Biosciences*, 7(1), lsaa055. https://doi.org/10.1093/jlb/lsaa055.

Catarinucci, L., De Donno, D., Mainetti, L., Palano, L., Patrono, L., Stefanizzi, M. L., & Tarricone, L. (2015). An IoT-aware architecture for smart healthcare systems. *IEEE Internet of Things Journal*, 2(6), 515–526.

Cohen, A. J., Ross Anderson, H., Ostro, B., Pandey, K. D., Krzyzanowski, M., Künzli, N., Gutschmidt, K., Pope, A., Romieu, I., Samet, J. M., & Smith, K. (2005). The global burden of disease due to outdoor air pollution. *Journal of Toxicology and Environmental Health. Part A*, 68(13–14), 1301–1307. https://doi.org/10.1080/15287390590936166.

Cullen, A., Mazhar, M. K. A., Smith, M. D., Lithander, F. E., Ó Breasail, M., & Henderson, E. J. (2022). Wearable and portable GPS solutions for monitoring mobility in dementia: A systematic review. *Sensors (Basel, Switzerland)*, 22(9), 3336. https://doi.org/10.3390/s22093336.

Davenport, T., & Kalakota, R. (2019). The potential for artificial intelligence in healthcare. *Future Healthcare Journal*, 6(2), 94–98. https://doi.org/10.7861/futurehosp.6-2-94.

Dwork, C. (2011). A firm foundation for private data analysis. *Communications of the ACM*, 54, 86–95.

Eisa, S., & Moreira, A. (2017). A behaviour monitoring system (BMS) for ambient assisted living. *Sensors*, 17(9), 1946. MDPI AG. https://doi.org/10.3390/s17091946.

European Commission, Directorate-General for Communications Networks, Content and Technology (2019). *Ethics Guidelines for Trustworthy AI*. Publications Office. https://data.europa.eu/doi/10.2759/346720.

Evans, J., Papadopoulos, A., Silvers, C. T., Charness, N., Boot, W. R., Schlachta-Fairchild, L., Crump, C., Martinez, M., & Ent, C. B. (2016). Remote health monitoring for older adults and those with heart failure: Adherence and system usability. *Telemedicine Journal and e-Health: The Official Journal of the American Telemedicine Association*, 22(6), 480–488. https://doi.org/10.1089/tmj.2015.0140.

Friedrich, B., Elgert, L., Eckhoff, D., Bauer, J. M., & Hein, A. (2023). A system for monitoring the functional status of older adults in daily life. *Scientific Reports*, 13(1), 12396. https://doi.org/10.1038/s41598-023-39483-x.

Geneva, I. I., Cuzzo, B., Fazili, T., & Javaid, W. (2019). Normal body temperature: A systematic review. *Open forum Infectious Diseases*, 6(4), ofz032. https://doi.org/10.1093/ofid/ofz032.

Hafen, B. B., & Sharma, S. (2023, January). Oxygen saturation. [Updated 2022 November 23]. In *StatPearls [Internet]*. Treasure Island (FL): StatPearls Publishing. www.ncbi.nlm.nih.gov/books/NBK525974/.

Hireche, R., Mansouri, H., & Pathan, A.-S. K. (2022). Security and privacy management in internet of medical things (IoMT): A synthesis. *Journal of Cybersecurity and Privacy*, 2(3), 640–661. https://doi.org/10.3390/jcp2030033.

Ianculescu, M., Alexandru, A., & Paraschiv, E. A. (2023). The potential of the remote monitoring digital solutions to sustain the mental and emotional health of the elderly during and post COVID-19 crisis in Romania. *Healthcare (Basel, Switzerland)*, 11(4), 608. https://doi.org/10.3390/healthcare11040608.

ICMR (2023). Ethical guidelines for application of artificial intelligence in biomedical research and healthcare. 978-93-5811-343-3. https://main.icmr.nic.in/sites/default/files/upload_documents/Ethical_Guidelines_AI_Healthcare_2023.pdf

Iwaya, L. H., Ahmad, A., & Babar, M. A. (2020). Security and privacy for mHealth and uHealth systems: A systematic mapping study. *IEEE Access*, 8, 150081–150112.

Javaid, M., & Khan, I. H. (2021). Internet of things (IoT) enabled healthcare helps to take the challenges of COVID-19 pandemic. *Journal of Oral Biology and Craniofacial Research*, 11(2), 209–214. https://doi.org/10.1016/j.jobcr.2021.01.015.

Johannessen, E., Johansson, J., Hartvigsen, G., Horsch, A., Årsand, E., & Henriksen, A. (2023). Collecting health-related research data using consumer-based wireless smart scales. *International Journal of Medical Informatics*, 173, 105043. https://doi.org/10.1016/j.ijmedinf.2023.105043.

Karar, M. E., Shehata, H. I., Reyad, O. (2022). A survey of IoT-based fall detection for aiding elderly care: Sensors, methods, challenges and future trends. *Applied Sciences*, 12(7), 3276. https://doi.org/10.3390/app12073276.

Kim, H. G., Cheon, E. J., Bai, D. S., Lee, Y. H., & Koo, B. H. (2018). Stress and heart rate variability: A meta-analysis and review of the literature. *Psychiatry Investigation*, 15(3), 235–245. https://doi.org/10.30773/pi.2017.08.17.

Malik, C., Khanna, S., Jain, Y., & Jain, R. (2021). Geriatric population in India: Demography, vulnerabilities, and healthcare challenges. *Journal of Family Medicine and Primary Care*, 10(1), 72–76. https://doi.org/10.4103/jfmpc.jfmpc_1794_20.

Malin, B. A. (2005). An evaluation of the current state of genomic data privacy protection technology and a roadmap for the future. *Journal of the American Medical Informatics Association: JAMIA*, 12(1), 28–34. https://doi.org/10.1197/jamia.M1603.

Miao, F., Cheng, Y., He, Y., He, Q., & Li, Y. (2015). A wearable context-aware ECG monitoring system integrated with built-in kinematic sensors of the smartphone. *Sensors*, 15(5), 11465–11484. MDPI AG. https://doi.org/10.3390/s150511465.

Miner, A. S., Laranjo, L., & Kocaballi, A. B. (2020). Chatbots in the fight against the COVID-19 pandemic. *NPJ Digital Medicine*, 3, 65. https://doi.org/10.1038/s41746-020-0280-0.

Mohammed, M. N., Desyansah, S. F., Al-Zubaidi, S., & Yusuf, E. (2019). An internet of things-based smart homes and healthcare monitoring and management system: Review. *Journal of Physics: Conference Series*, 1450. International Conference on Applied Science and Technology (iCAST on Engineering Science) 24–25 Bali, Indonesia. https://doi.org/10.1088/1742-6596/1450/1/012079.

Mora, H., Gil, D., Munoz Terol, R., Azorín, J., & Szymanski, J. (2017). An IoT-based computational framework for healthcare monitoring in mobile environments. *Sensors*, 17, 2302. https://doi.org/10.3390/s17102302.

Nielsen, J. (1993). *Usability Engineering*. San Diego, USA: Academic Press, Inc., Harcourt Brace & Company.

Padhan, S., Mohapatra, A., Ramasamy, S. K., & Agrawal, S. (2023). Artificial intelligence (AI) and robotics in elderly healthcare: Enabling independence and quality of life. *Cureus*, 15(8), e42905. https://doi.org/10.7759/cureus.42905.

Panda, S. K., Reddy, G. S. M., Goyal, S. B., Thirunavukkarasu, K., Bhambri, P., Rao, M. V., Singh, A. S., Fakih, A. H., Shukla, P. K., Shukla, P. K., & others (2019). Method for Management of Scholarship of Large Number of Students based on Blockchain. IN Patent App. 201,911,034,937 A.

Peek, S. T. M., Luijkx, K. G., Rijnaard, M. D., et al. (2016). Older adults' reasons for using technology while aging in place. *Gerontology*, 62, 226–237. https://doi.org/10.1159/000430949.

Potluri, S., Tiwari, P. K., Bhambri, P., Obulesu, O., Naidu, P. A., Lakshmi, L., Kallam, S., Gupta, S., & Gupta, B. (2019). Method of Load Distribution Balancing for Fog Cloud Computing in IoT Environment. IN Patent App. 201,941,044,511.

Quirós-Alcalá, L., Wilson, S., Witherspoon, N., Murray, R., Perodin, J., Trousdale, K., Raspanti, G., & Sapkota, A. (2016). Volatile organic compounds and particulate matter in child care facilities in the District of Columbia: Results from a pilot study. *Environmental Research*, 146, 116–124. https://doi.org/10.1016/j.envres.2015.12.005.

Rajendra, A. U., Paul Joseph, K., Kannathal, N., Lim, C. M., & Suri, J. S. (2006). Heart rate variability: A review. *Medical and Biological Engineering & Computing*, 44(12), 1031–1051. https://doi.org/10.1007/s11517-006-0119-0.

Rajkomar, A., Dean, J., & Kohane, I. (2019). Machine learning in medicine. *The New England Journal of Medicine*, 380(14), 1347–1358. https://doi.org/10.1056/NEJMra1814259.

Ribeiro, A. H., Ribeiro, M. H., Paixão, G. M. M., et al. (2020). Automatic diagnosis of the 12-lead ECG using a deep neural network. *Nature Communications*, 11, 1760. https://doi.org/10.1038/s41467-020-15432-4.

Rodríguez, I., Cajamarca, G., Herskovic, V., Carolina, F., & Mauricio, C. (2017). Helping elderly users report pain levels: A study of user experience with mobile and wearable interfaces. *Mobile Information Systems*, 2017, 12, Article ID 9302328. https://doi.org/10.1155/2017/9302328.

Ruby, D., Divya, M., & Shaleen, C. (2022). Potential of internet of medical things (IoMT) applications in building a smart healthcare system: A systematic review. *Journal of Oral Biology and Craniofacial Research*, 12(2), 302–318. ISSN 2212–4268; https://doi.org/10.1016/j.jobcr.2021.11.010.

Schultz, E. E., & Shumway, R. (2001). *Incident Response: A Strategic Guide to Handling System and Network Security Breaches*. New York: Sams Publishing. ISBN: 1578702569.

Seppänen, O., & Kurnitski, J. (2009). Moisture control and ventilation. In *WHO Guidelines for Indoor Air Quality: Dampness and Mould* (p. 3). Geneva: World Health Organization. www.ncbi.nlm.nih.gov/books/NBK143947/.

Shahriar Haque, M. S., Khan Hamim, M. R., Ehsan, M. T., & Ali, M. H. (2023). Design and implementation of an IoT-based smart pillbox for improving medical adherence. *17th International Conference on Electronics Computer and Computation (ICECCO)*, Kaskelen, Kazakhstan, pp. 1–5. https://doi.org/10.1109/ICECCO58239.2023.10147144.

Srivastava, J., Routray, S., Ahmad, S., & Waris, M. M. (2022). Internet of medical things (IoMT)-based smart healthcare system: Trends and progress. *Computational Intelligence and Neuroscience*, 2022, 7218113. https://doi.org/10.1155/2022/7218113.

Stafford, I. S., Kellermann, M., Mossotto, E., et al. (2020). A systematic review of the applications of artificial intelligence and machine learning in autoimmune diseases. *npj Digital Medicine*, 3, 30. https://doi.org/10.1038/s41746-020-0229-3.

Swan, M. (2015). *Blockchain: Blueprint for a New Economy* (1st ed.). New York: O'Reilly Media, Inc. ISBN: 1491920491.

Tiribelli, S., Monnot, A., Shah, S. F. H., Arora, A., Toong, P. J., & Kong, S. (2023). Ethics principles for artificial intelligence-based telemedicine for public health. *American Journal of Public Health*, 113(5), 577–584. https://doi.org/10.2105/AJPH.2023.307225.

Tondon, N., & Bhambri, P. (2017). Novel approach for drug discovery. *International Journal of Research in Engineering and Applied Sciences*, 7(6), 28–46.

Whelton, P. K., Carey, R. M., Aronow, W. S., Casey, D. E. Jr, Collins, K. J., Dennison Himmelfarb, C., DePalma, S. M., Gidding, S., Jamerson, K. A., Jones, D. W., MacLaughlin, E. J., Muntner, P., Ovbiagele, B., Smith, S. C. Jr, Spencer, C. C., Stafford, R. S., Taler, S. J., Thomas, R. J., Williams, K. A. Sr, Williamson, J. D., & Wright, J. T. Jr. (2018). ACC/AHA/AAPA/ABC/ACPM/AGS/APhA/ASH/ASPC/NMA/PCNA guideline for the prevention, detection, evaluation, and management of high blood pressure in adults: Executive summary: A report of the American college of cardiology/American heart association task force on clinical practice guidelines. *Hypertension*, 71(6), 1269–1324. https://doi.org/10.1161/HYP.0000000000000066.

World Economic Forum (WEF) (2022). A Blueprint for Equity and Inclusion in Artificial Intelligence. W H I T E P A P E R. www.weforum.org/whitepapers/a-blueprint-for-equity-and-inclusion-in-artificial-intelligence/.

World Health Organization. (2021). *Ethics and Governance of Artificial Intelligence for Health: WHO Guidance*. Geneva. Licence: CC BY-NC-SA 3.0 IGO. https://www.who.int/publications/i/item/9789240029200

Worley, S. L. (2018). The extraordinary importance of sleep: The detrimental effects of inadequate sleep on health and public safety drive an explosion of sleep research. *P & T: A Peer-Reviewed Journal for Formulary Management*, 43(12), 758–763.

Yacchirema, D., de Puga, J. S., Palau, C., & Esteve, M. (2018). Fall detection system for elderly people using IoT and big data. *Procedia Computer Science*, 130, 603–610. ISSN 1877–0509; https://doi.org/10.1016/j.procs.2018.04.110.

Yang, K., Pinker, R. T., Ma, Y., Koike, T., Wonsick, M. M., Cox, S. J., Zhang, Y.-C., & Stackhouse, P. (2008). Evaluation of satellite estimates of downward shortwave radiation over the Tibetan Plateau. *Journal of Geophysical Research*, 113, D17204. https://doi.org/10.1029/2007JD009736.

22 Improving Elder Care
Vision-Based Wearable Technology for Fall Recognition and Prevention

A. Anitha, N. Nandhini, Kamaraj Balakrishnan and Thinagaran Perumal

22.1 INTRODUCTION

The United Nations Department of Economic and Social Affairs gave an international community with timely population data across all the countries in the world in 2019. According to World Population 2019, it was calculated that one in six people will be over age 65 by 2050, whereas one in 11 in 2019. It also stated that one-fifth of the population was accounted by older people of age above 65. So, it is time to discuss how technology helps elderly people physically and mentally and their social activities. The future IoT can make the healthcare system cheaper and more efficient, enable people to get better access to data, and improve personalized care, thus reducing the number of visits to the hospital. A number of smart technologies, including voice activation, sensors, GPS, Bluetooth, mobile cellular connectivity, and smart monitoring apps, improve the quality of life for senior citizens. Seniors can live independent lives by using goods that make their lives easier, such as smart doorbells, excellent call mobile phones, mobile assistance medical alert systems, smart shower chairs, etc. (Bakshi et al., 2021).

22.1.1 Emergency Bag-Valve-Mask Ventilation for Elderly Care

The emergence of modern technology has improved the lives of the elderly people. However, monitoring their daily activities and taking care based on the recording can be helpful only if there is flawless data communication. At the same time, some unexpected happenings such as falling of elderly people due to obstacles in their path even at home, need special attention and to automatically alert the people who are nearby to take immediate actions to protect them. Some of the devices such as an alert system with a camera help to alert using an alarm for the near ones to attend to the elders immediately. A dedicated cloud-based approach (Mrozek et al., 2020), for fall detection in large-scale monitoring systems especially for older adults by collecting the data in the smartphone and transmitting it to the cloud for classification as cloud-based fall detection or edge-based fall was deduced (Rachna and Bhambri, 2021).

DOI: 10.1201/9781032698519-22

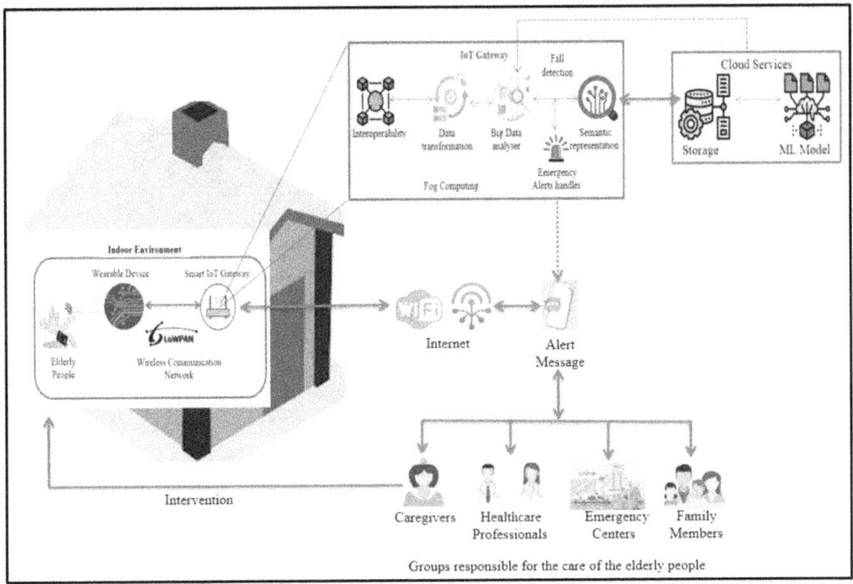

FIGURE 22.1 Edge-based fall detection.

A comparative study was conducted between the cloud-based and edge-based fall detection process using the Whoops system and found that edge-based fall detection serves better with good scalability for large-scale data as presented in Figure 22.1.

The IoTE-fall system contains four major modules (Yacchirema et al., 2019): first as wearable devices, secondly, a wireless communication network followed by a third, cloud services, and finally, the IoT gateway. The wearable devices are connected with MEM's sensors, to calculate the body movements of elderly people to transmit to the IoT gateway using a low bandwidth wireless network (Singh et al., 2021). Thus, the received data is analyzed by the IoT gateway using an ensemble RF classifier to detect the falls rapidly and in response sends the information to the healthcare professionals and the people concerned in a fraction of the time. The cloud service plays a major role in securing data transmission through quick authentication and data modelling. The IoTE-fall architecture is represented in Figure 22.2.

The review of the fall prediction and prevention (Rajagopalan et al., 2017), is based on recent trends and gives some future directions (Kaur and Bhambri, 2019). They categorised the fall prediction as context-aware and wearable devices fall prediction. Context-aware includes some of the ambient sensors such as cameras, vibration sensors, and infrared sensors to organise the daily activities of elderly people. Whereas wearable devices use sensors such as accelerometers and gyroscopes to collect the data to analyze the acceleration magnitude, body posture, and sensor velocity to obtain the highest fall sensitivity and lowest false positive rate. The core conflict in fall detection and prevention includes evaluating performance among elder people who fall frequently, user-centric design, secured data transmission (Haritha and Anitha, 2023), and energy optimisation. There is a need for data fusion from

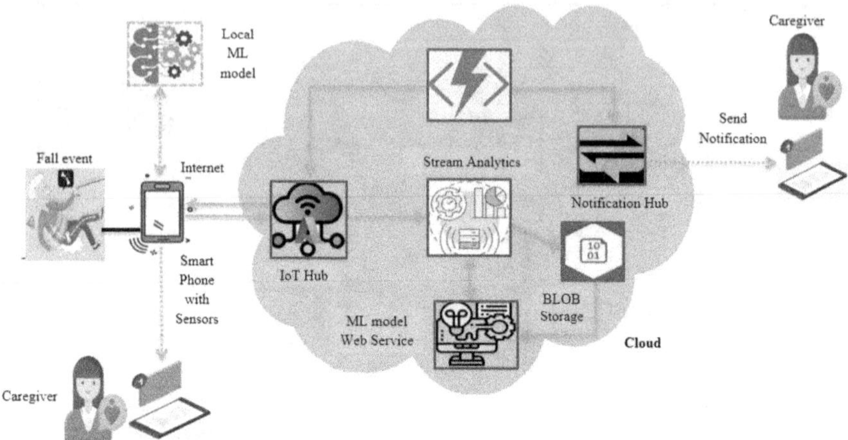

FIGURE 22.2 IoTE-fall architecture.

the ambient sensors, interface designs, environmental fall risk factors, and clinical assessments based on reliable data transfer using an IoT-enabled prevention system for elderly people. IoTE-fall architecture is shown in Figure 22.2.

22.2 RELATED WORKS

Human fall is one of the leading causes of mortality among the elderly. Accidental incidents in the elderly can result in numerous irreversible disabilities or even death (Manna and Anitha, 2023b). Fall detection has become a crucial research issue in the healthcare domain, which requires more dependable and effective methods for intelligently classifying fall activities. The physical consequences of falls are increasingly fatal, and the risk of falling increases with age. A design (Chowdhary et al., 2023), to acquire some level of the senior citizen monitoring system with the help of IoT sensors and Python programming to care for the elderly was created. Tracking objects and detecting a person's fall reduce the probability of emergencies with the help of cameras. A camera-based peer-to-peer (P2P) network system for detecting falls (Hu et al., 2019), spreading alert events, and distributing captured media broadcasts in an elderly person's activity location was demonstrated. Multiple Wi-Fi and IoT-enabled cameras will help to transmit this information to remote users. Identifying human posture using Long Range (LoRa) and mpu-9250 sensors to collect data and transmit it to a cloud server using random forest machine learning algorithms was proposed (Song et al., 2021). Various state-of-the-art challenges (Kumar et al., 2017), quantifying movement-related problems faced by the elderly and preventing difficulties through interpretation to accommodate information communication technology (ICT) based IoT solutions were addressed. A monitoring system composed of various IoT sensors (Al Husaini et al., 2022), as well as the development of a health surveillance system and a failure detection system that alerts users if the normal condition changes was recommended. A fall detection system was proposed based on deep learning Convolutional Neural Networks (Manna and Anitha, 2023b) and the lime XAI model to classify fall activity (Jeyashree et al., 2022). The design (Sarowar et al., 2022) of a fall detection and heart rate monitoring system for senior citizens was presented. Additionally, various sensors and global positioning systems (GPS) can monitor the elderly's location. When a fall is detected, the device can effectively transmit fall data, pulse rate, and location to the appropriate carer. A cStick (calm stick) was suggested which is an IoT-enabled system that can anticipate falls before they happen, notify the user, detect falls, and also offer control measures to reduce their impact and collect the information of user locations and health parameters of the user (Rachakonda et al., 2021). IoT-based sensors are used for applications such as garbage monitoring and home security system. A wearable module was suggested with sensors connected to an ESP32 and a residence module with an IoT camera connected to a Raspberry Pi and it helps information gathered by sensors to be processed in the cloud using machine learning by Amazon Web Services (Srinivasan et al., 2020). Fall detection prediction was recommended with the help of wearable devices using machine learning algorithms. Predictions can be done using the deep ensemble technique for ground water level prediction by utilizing the data collected using the IoT data (Manna and Anitha, 2023a). An application programming interface was proposed (Sung et al., 2020; Anitha et al., 2023), for instantaneous monitoring based on in-home sensor data and fall detection-based sensors capture the images sent to the remote controller of the user.

Advantages:

- Automatic fall detection technology solves the problem of being unable to engage an alarm in the event of a fall and can substantially reduce the fall-related mortality rate (Thyagharajan, 2022).
- Various research solutions employ AI and machine learning to detect accidents in real-time and transmit rapid alerts to predict fall risks.
- Sensor-based solutions provide round-the-clock monitoring, capturing helpful information on in/out-of-bed status, sleeping routines, levels of physical activity, and other parameters.
- Advanced sensor-based systems may track bio-metric vitals including the heart and breathing rates. Significant modifications can activate alerts, allowing caretakers to provide prompt care before an accident or injury.

Disadvantages:

- IoT devices are susceptible to malware, which could enable a hacker to gain control of the system, deactivate it, or send false alarms.
- False alarms raised by fall detection systems are an inconvenience for the user and may cause them to ignore the alarm when it is truly required (Manna and Anitha, 2023a).
- IoT devices gathered a huge amount of information about the user, including their location and movements. This raises the privacy concerns of the user data for sharing into the environment.

- Especially for those utilizing small gadgets, IoT fall detection systems can be costly. This may be expensive for some users who cannot afford the system.

A review of the related work has led to the identification of the following objectives:

1. IoT Sensor-based data collection of elderly people identifies the posture of their body and also reads the pressure, distance level, Heart Rate Value (HRV), sugar level, SpO2, and threshold value to identify any objects blocking their way.
2. Using vision sensors, accelerometer sensors, and ultrasonic sensors, to identify the unevenness of the surface on the path of the elderly people.
3. Alarm-based wristwatch to indicate the sudden loss of balance of the body and alert for the fall.
4. If the fall has happened, the devices try to get the response from the wristband holder, on failing so it gives an alert message to the caretaker at regular intervals, until the message is read by the recipient.

These objectives aim is briefly reviewed in Section 22.3, offering a clear summary of what the research set out to accomplish.

22.3 PROPOSED FRAMEWORK

The suggested framework clarifies the steps that make up the vision-based fall identification system. The flow chart starts with gathering data from cameras and wearable devices and proceeds through feature extraction, pre-processing, and real-time data analysis. Also, it provides a visual road map for comprehending the algorithms related to fall detection, demonstrating the combination of computer vision and sensor data processing as shown in Figure 22.3.

22.3.1 Data Collection

The deployment of IoT sensors denote a system of linked devices intended for data collection and sharing (Manna and Anitha, 2022). These sensors help to keep an eye on several elements related to the elder's well-being. The elderly person has sensors placed deliberately on them to create a network that gathers data in real-time about their environment and health. IoT sensor-based data collection of elderly people identifies the posture of their body and also reads the pressure, distance level, Heart Rate Value (HRV), sugar level, SpO2, and threshold value to identify any objects blocking their way. Framework is illustrated in Figure 22.3.

22.3.2 Sensors and Their Deployment

It uses vision sensors (Xu et al., 2021), accelerometer sensors, and ultrasonic sensors (Papara et al., 2021), to identify the unevenness of the surface on the path of elderly

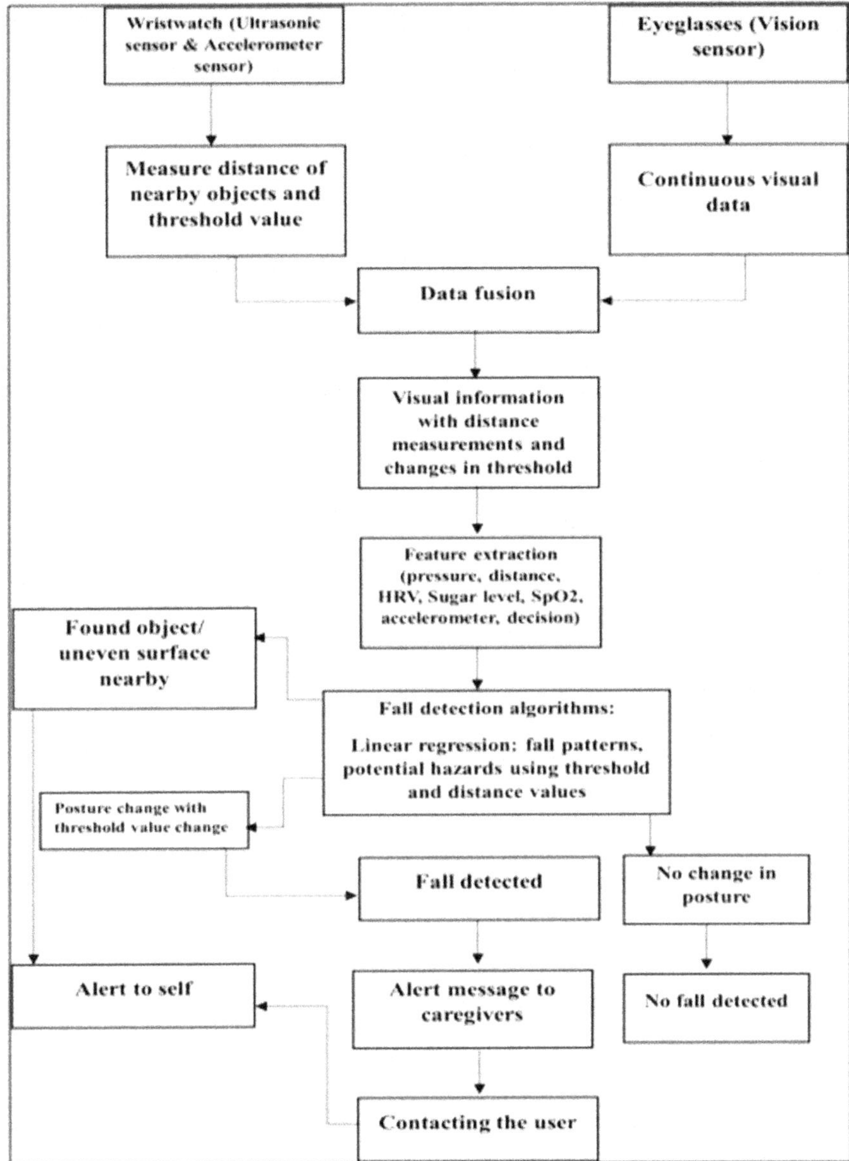

FIGURE 22.3 Illustration of the framework.

people. The working principle of the vision and ultrasonic sensor is straightforward. It uses a 40kHz ultrasonic pulse that passes through the air and bounces back to the sensor if it encounters an obstruction or object. The distance can be estimated by adding up the sound speed and travel time (Anitha, 2017b). The system obtains a broad understanding of the user's motions by merging accelerometer data with information from visual and ultrasonic sensors. This allows for a more precise identification of barriers, uneven surfaces, and possible fall hazards. The following is the explanation of three sensors that work collaboratively to gain better knowledge of fall detection.

- *Vision-based sensor in eyeglasses:* The eyeglass of the wearer is lightweight with barely visible cameras continuously collecting the visual surroundings through the wearer's point of view. This involves whatever the user views in actual time, giving them insight into the environment.
- *Ultrasonic and accelerometer sensors in a wristwatch:* Ultrasonic detectors present in the wristwatch produce ultrasonic waves which reflect from objects and bounce back to the device. These types of sensors can accurately compute the distances to neighbouring surfaces or components by determining the time required for sound waves to come back. An accelerometer is used to alarm the possible fall with the help of a threshold value.
- *Extensive Environmental Evaluation:* An integration of vision, accelerometer and ultrasonic detectors provides extensive environmental monitoring for the user. Vision sensors gather visual information such as possible obstacles and conditions of the surface, while ultrasonic sensors give exact distance measurements, especially in circumstances of surface unevenness or elevation changes (Gatti et al., 2020). Whereas, an accelerometer provides the posture change of the person to detect the potential fall or no fall using the threshold value (Abou et al., 2023).

22.3.3 Detection of Objects or Uneven Surfaces

Whenever the eyeglasses vision sensor and ultrasonic sensor identify an item or surface that's uneven in the pathway (Anitha, 2017a). Alarm-based wristwatch indicates the sudden loss of balance of the body and alert for a fall. When the users fall, an accelerometer sensor built inside a watch can measure how quickly the person moves toward the earth. The accelerometer uses a threshold value to detect the position change of the user. The initial threshold value is set to zero and if there is a change in the posture of the person the value changes to one this notification can be conveyed via a user-friendly interface, like an indicator on the wristwatch or audible advice and also alerts the caregivers which confirms the fall.

These incidents can be recorded and analysed by the system for patterns. It may learn from these interactions and improve its recommendations and suggestions over time to increase the user's safety (Nandhini and Anitha, 2023). Prediction of air quality index using stacked deep learning techniques was discussed by (Manna and Anitha, 2023b).

22.3.4 Smart Techniques for Alerting a Fall

If the fall has happened, the devices try to get the response from the wristwatch holder, on failing so it gives an alert message to the caretaker at regular intervals, until the message is read by the recipient.

Body sensors, such as accelerometers, only measure fall impulses and send them to an external device for intelligent decision-making processing, such as a PC with a wireless module like Bluetooth (Nguyen et al., 2019). This external device is in charge of processing the signals from the accelerometer sensors that have been acquired and using a constructed neural network classifier, it determines whether to detect a fall. The authors developed a framework utilizing an FPGA kit to apply the ANNs classifier and create an embedded vision-based fall detection system (Škoda et al., 2011). According to (Sulzbachner et al., 2012), the context-aware system's ANNs' functioning was sped up using a digital signal processor (DSP).

Algorithm 22.1 describes the object identification process in detail. It also extends the framework to measure obstacles' distance comprehensively, improving the system's overall accuracy and scope.

Algorithm 22.1

```
Initialize System()
while True:
    vision_data = Capture Visual Data()
    ultrasonic_data = Record Ultrasonic Data()
    accelerometer_data= Record Accelerometer Data()
    combined_data = Fuse Data(vision_data, ultrasonic_data,accelerometer_data)
    extracted_features = Extract Features(combined_data)
    if Is Fall Detected Using Linear Regression(extracted_features):
        alert_message = "Fall detected!"
        Notify Caregiver(alert_message)
        if User Is Conscious():
            Provide Guidance To User()
        else:
            Activate Emergency Services()
    if Surface Unevenness Detected(ultrasonic_data):
        warning_message = "Uneven surface detected. Please be cautious."
        Display Message To User(warning_message)
    if Obstacle Detected(vision_data):
        warning_message = "Obstacle in your path. Please navigate around it."
        Display Message To User(warning_message)
    If Threshold Value Increase(accelerometer_data):
        Contact_Caregivers = "Fall detected."
    Monitor User Environment()
    if User Requests Assistance():
        Request Assistance From Caregiver()
    if User Dismisses Alerts():
        Continue Monitoring()
    if User Chooses To Disable System():
        Disable System()
```

22.4 EXPERIMENTAL AND RESULT ANALYSIS

22.4.1 Fall Detection Analysis Using Convolution Neural Network

A strong architecture for vision-based fall identification was demonstrated by the Convolutional Neural Network (CNN) that was put into practice. The model completed 35 training epochs with three convolutional layers, and ReLU and sigmoid activation functions, shown in Figure 22.4, showing a significant capacity to grasp complex patterns within the dataset.

22.4.2 Model Evaluation on Training and Validation Set

The training procedure produced an accuracy rate of 98.77% and the validation set evaluation of the model produced an impressive accuracy of 98.77%, highlighting its dependability in practical situations. For every class (Fall, No_fall, Posture_change), 97% precision, 100% recall, and 98% F1-score measures showed excellent performance as shown in Figure 22.5. All metrics were ideal for three classes and showed good accuracy and recall values, which added to the overall effectiveness and balance of the model. Figure 22.6 shows the confusion matrix for those three classes. From the confusion matrix, it is found that Fall (142 out of 142), No_fall (121 out of 128), and Posture_change (138 out of 138) is correctly classified. Figure 22.7 shows the training accuracy with the help of a graph. Figure 22.8 shows the training and validation loss with the help of a graph. Remarkably, a small loss of 0.0038 of training. At a minimum validation loss of 0.0036 and a validation accuracy of 98.77%, the validation results nearly matched the training performance.

The model demonstrates an exceptional ability to identify trends associated with falls and environmental obstacles, which greatly contributes to improving one's overall safety. This effectiveness is further demonstrated by its excellent accuracy on the dataset, including test, validation, and training sets. Its strong generalization abilities are attested to through consistent results found between training and validation

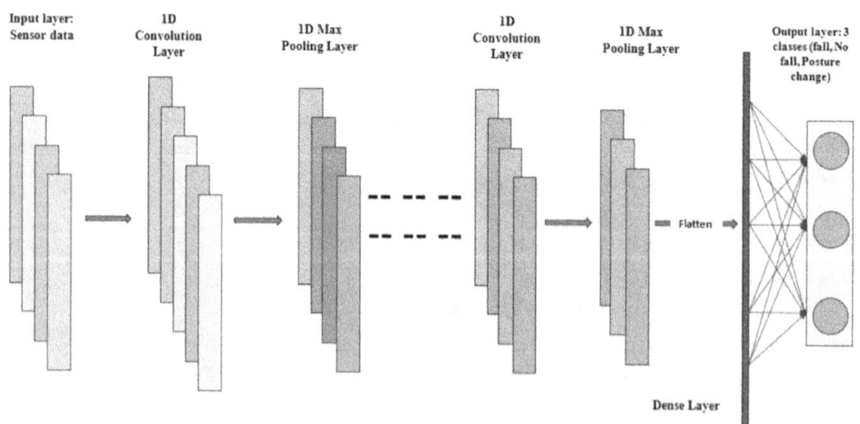

FIGURE 22.4 The architecture of CNN for vision-based fall detection.

```
Accuracy: 98.77%
Classification Report:
              precision    recall  f1-score   support

           0       1.00      1.00      1.00       142
           1       1.00      0.96      0.98       128
           2       0.97      1.00      0.98       138

    accuracy                           0.99       408
   macro avg       0.99      0.99      0.99       408
weighted avg       0.99      0.99      0.99       408
```

FIGURE 22.5 Classification report.

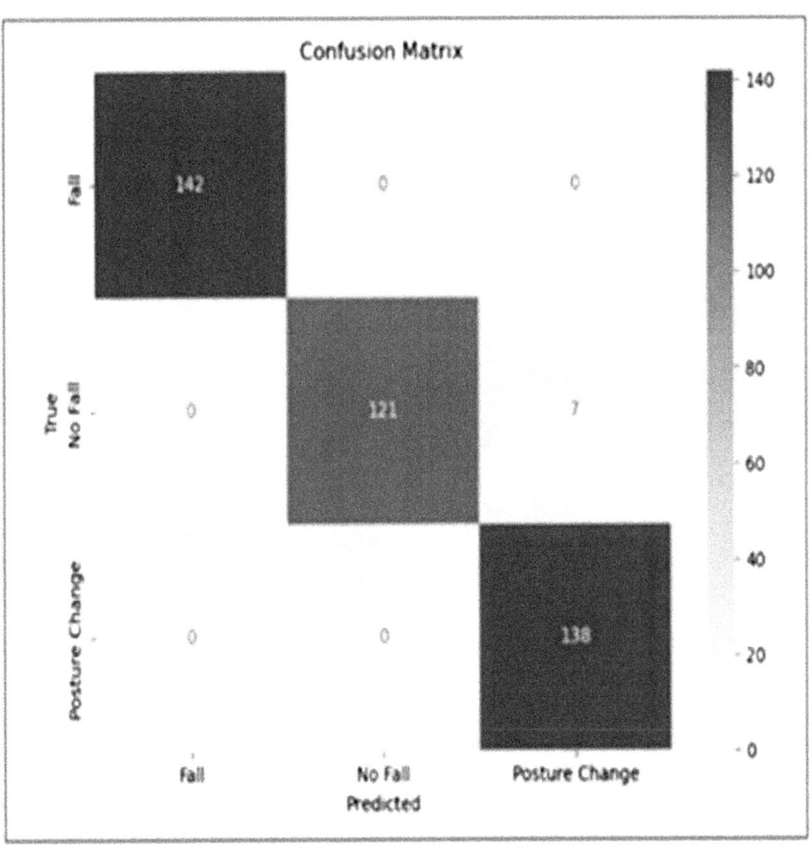

FIGURE 22.6 Confusion matrix.

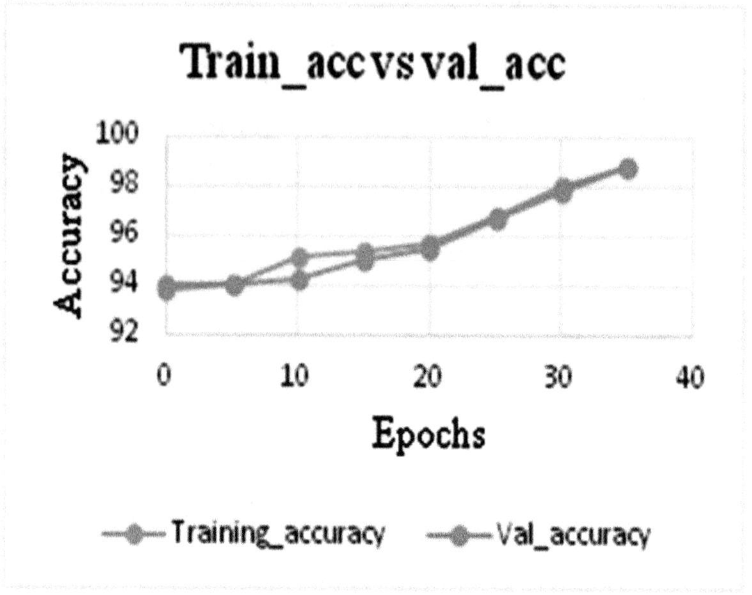

FIGURE 22.7 Training_acc vs Validation_accuracy.

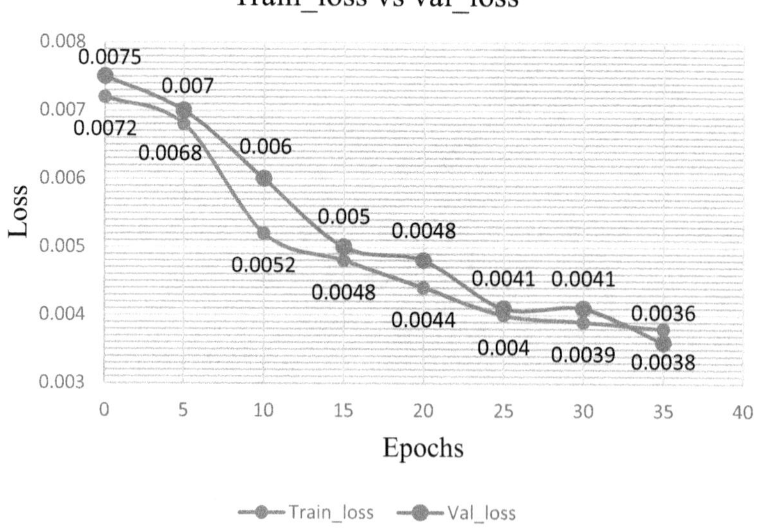

FIGURE 22.8 Training_loss vs validation_loss.

outcomes, confirming its capacity to consistently adapt to novel and unknown settings. This feature establishes the model as a dependable and adaptable instrument for improving safety, especially when it comes to elders by recognizing and reducing the risks connected to falls and environmental difficulties.

22.5 CONCLUSION AND FUTURE ENHANCEMENT

The CNN model's effectiveness in this particular application acts as a starting point for future developments in technology-enabled elderly care. It paves the way for more study and creativity that could improve and broaden the scope of fall detection systems. This CNN model serves as an example of how artificial intelligence and healthcare can come together to change the way that aged care is provided and make ageing populations feel safer and more secure. To sum up, the remarkable performance of the CNN model represents more than just a numerical accomplishment; it is a major step towards a future in which technology is critical to ensuring the safety of our elderly. The benefits of such developments in fall detection technology on the quality of life of older people are immeasurable. To further increase the accuracy of fall detection systems, future improvements may concentrate on improving the CNN model, investigating cutting-edge sensor tools, and integrating real-time information analytics.

REFERENCES

Abou, L., Fliflet, A., Presti, P., Sosnoff, J. J., Mahajan, H. P., Frechette, M. L., and Rice, L. A. (2023). Fall detection from a manual wheelchair: Preliminary findings based on accelerometers using machine learning techniques. *Assistive Technology*, 1–9.

Al Husaini, Y. N., Al Nuaimi, M., and Sherimon, P. C. (2022, October). Remote monitoring of elders using internet of things. In *AIP Conference Proceedings* (Vol. 2519, No. 1). New York: AIP Publishing.

Anitha, A. (2017a, November). Garbage monitoring system using IoT. In *IOP Conference Series: Materials Science and Engineering* (Vol. 263, No. 4, p. 042027). New York: IOP Publishing.

Anitha, A. (2017b, November). Home security system using internet of things. In *IOP Conference Series: Materials Science and Engineering* (Vol. 263, No. 4, p. 042026). New York: IOP Publishing.

Anitha, A., Shivakumara, P., Jain, S., and Agarwal, V. (2023). Convolution neural network and auto-encoder hybrid scheme for automatic colorization of grayscale images. In *Smart Computer Vision* (pp. 253–271). Cham: Springer International Publishing.

Bakshi, P., Bhambri, P., & Thapar, V. (2021). A review paper on wireless sensor network techniques in Internet of Things (IoT). *Wesleyan Journal of Research, 14*(7), 147–160. Retrieved from http://www.wesleyanjournal.in/

Chowdhary, S. K., Hassan, B. U., and Sharma, T. (2023). Monitoring senior citizens using IoT and ML. In *Computational Intelligence: Select Proceedings of InCITe 2022* (pp. 777–789). Singapore: Springer Nature.

Gatti, R., Avinash, J. L., Nataraja, N., Poornima, G. R., Kumar, S. S., and Kumar, K. S. (2020, November). Design and implementation of vision module for visually impaired people. In *2020 International Conference on Recent Trends on Electronics, Information, Communication & Technology (RTEICT)* (pp. 373–377). New York: IEEE.

Haritha, T., and Anitha, A. (2023). Multi-level security in healthcare by integrating lattice-based access control and blockchain-based smart contracts system. *IEEE Access*. https://ui.adsabs.harvard.edu/abs/2023IEEEA.11k4322H/abstract

Hu, C. L., Bamrung, C., Kamintra, W., Ruengittinun, S., Mongkolwat, P., Hui, L., and Lo, S. H. (2019, October). Using camera array to detect elderly falling and distribute alerting media for smart home care. In *2019 8th International Conference on Innovation, Communication and Engineering (ICICE)* (pp. 98–101). New York: IEEE.

Jeyashree, G., Padmavathi, S., and Shanthini, D. (2022, August). An explainable deep learning model for vision-based human fall detection system. In *2022 Third International*

Conference on Intelligent Computing Instrumentation and Control Technologies (ICICICT) (pp. 1223–1229). New York: IEEE.

Kaur, J., and Bhambri, P. (2019). Design of paddy crop prediction technique based on K-mean, Naïve Bayes, KNN and SVM classifiers. I.K. Gujral Punjab Technical University, Jalandhar (M.Tech. thesis).

Kumar, E. S., Sachin, P., Vignesh, B. P., and Ahmed, M. R. (2017, June). Architecture for IOT based geriatric care fall detection and prevention. In *2017 International Conference on Intelligent Computing and Control Systems (ICICCS)* (pp. 1099–1104). New York: IEEE.

Manna, T., and Anitha, A. (2022, December). Forecasting air quality index based on stacked LSTM. In *2022 IEEE 7th International Conference on Recent Advances and Innovations in Engineering (ICRAIE)* (Vol. 7, pp. 326–330). New York: IEEE.

Manna, T., and Anitha, A. (2023a). Deep ensemble-based approach using randomized low-rank approximation for sustainable groundwater level prediction. *Applied Sciences, 13*(5), 3210.

Manna, T., and Anitha, A. (2023b). Precipitation prediction by integrating rough set on fuzzy approximation space with deep learning techniques. *Applied Soft Computing, 139*, 110253.

Mrozek, D., Koczur, A., and Małysiak-Mrozek, B. (2020). Fall detection in older adults with mobile IoT devices and machine learning in the cloud and on the edge. *Information Sciences, 537*, 132–147.

Nandhini, N., and Anitha, A. (2023, March). Seasonal-wise occupational accident analysis using deep learning paradigms. In *International Conference on Machine Learning, IoT and Big Data* (pp. 183–193). Singapore: Springer Nature.

Nguyen, T. Q., Young, J. H., Rodriguez, A., Zupancic, S., and Lie, D. Y. (2019). Differentiation of patients with balance insufficiency (vestibular hypofunction) versus normal subjects using a low-cost small wireless wearable gait sensor. *Biosensors, 9*(1), 29.

Papara, R., Buzura, L., and Galatus, R. (2021, October). Ultrasonic indoor navigation prototype for visual impaired users. In *2021 IEEE 27th International Symposium for Design and Technology in Electronic Packaging (SIITME)* (pp. 254–257). New York: IEEE.

Rachakonda, L., Mohanty, S. P., and Kougianos, E. (2021, November). cStick: A calm stick for fall prediction, detection and control in the IoMT framework. In *IFIP International Internet of Things Conference* (pp. 129–145). Cham: Springer International Publishing.

Rachna, C., and Bhambri, P. (2021). Various approaches and algorithms for monitoring energy efficiency of wireless sensor networks. *Lecture Notes in Civil Engineering, 113*, 761–770.

Rajagopalan, R., Litvan, I., and Jung, T. P. (2017). Fall prediction and prevention systems: Recent trends, challenges, and future research directions. *Sensors, 17*(11), 2509.

Sarowar, M. H., Khondakar, M. F. K., Roy, H. S., Ullah, H., Ahmed, R., and Hossain, Q. D. (2022). Internet of things based fall detection and heart rate monitoring system for senior citizens. *International Journal of Electrical and Computer Engineering (IJECE), 12*(3), 3204–3216.

Singh, M., Bhambri, P., Dhanoa, I. S., Jain, A., and Kaur, K. (2021). Data mining model for predicting diabetes. *Annals of the Romanian Society for Cell Biology, 25*(4), 6702–6712.

Škoda, P., Lipić, T., Srp, À., Rogina, B. M., Skala, K., and Vajda, F. (2011, May). Implementation framework for artificial neural networks on FPGA. In *2011 Proceedings of the 34th International Convention MIPRO* (pp. 274–278). New York: IEEE.

Song, W., Liao, J., and Han, J. (2021). A real-time human posture recognition system using internet of things (IoT) based on LoRa wireless network. In *Advances in Computer Science and Ubiquitous Computing: CSA-CUTE 2019* (pp. 379–385). Singapore: Springer.

Srinivasan, A., Natarajan, N., Karunakaran, R. V., Elangovan, R., Shankar, A., Sabharish, P. M., . . . Radha, S. (2020, December). Elder care system using IoT and machine learning in AWS cloud. In *2020 IEEE 17th International Conference on Smart Communities: Improving Quality of Life Using ICT, IoT and AI (HONET)* (pp. 92–98). New York: IEEE.

Sulzbachner, C., Humenberger, M., Srp, Á., and Vajda, F. (2012). Optimization of a neural network for computer vision based fall detection with fixed-point arithmetic. In *Neural Information Processing: 19th International Conference, ICONIP 2012, Doha, Qatar, November 12–15, 2012, Proceedings, Part IV 19* (pp. 18–26). Berlin, Heidelberg: Springer.

Sung, G. M., Wang, H. K., and Su, W. T. (2020, October). Smart home care system with fall detection based on the android platform. In *2020 IEEE International Conference on Systems, Man, and Cybernetics (SMC)* (pp. 3886–3890). New York: IEEE.

Thyagharajan, K. K. (2022, October). A patient-specific single sensor IoT-based wearable fall prediction and detection system using machine learning. In *AIP Conference Proceedings* (Vol. 2519, No. 1). New York: AIP Publishing.

Xu, J., Xia, H., Liu, Y., and Li, Z. (2021, July). Multi-functional smart E-glasses for vision-based indoor navigation. In *2021 6th IEEE International Conference on Advanced Robotics and Mechatronics (ICARM)* (pp. 267–272). New York: IEEE.

Yacchirema, D., de Puga, J. S., Palau, C., and Esteve, M. (2019). Fall detection system for elderly people using IoT and ensemble machine learning algorithm. *Personal and Ubiquitous Computing*, *23*(5), 801–817.

23 Is Rural India Forgoing the Benefits of Non-implementing AI-enabled Healthcare
A Prospective Analysis

Soumik Gangopadhyay, Arkaprava Chakrabarty and Amitava Ukil

23.1 INTRODUCTION

The tertiary care services sector in India is forecast to develop at a compound annual growth rate (CAGR) of 16%, with a projected value of USD 372 billion by 2022. This growth is attributed to the unexpected rise in non-communicable diseases among the population. However, the distribution of healthcare delivery in India's cities and rural areas is not uniform. The problem becomes more complicated when diseases predominate in different demographic groups. Changing patterns of disease dominance in India has caused health services to be more complex. Although, ischemic heart disease is top health diseases in 2009 and 2019, diarrheal diseases and neonatal disorders were the second and third ranked in 2009. COPD and stroke were ranked second and third health problem in 2019. Moreover, the emergence of COVID-19 pandemic has brought an unexpected shift in the global health landscape. Several countries have been forced to transition healthcare services from in-person to online in order to facilitate the rapid growth of the healthcare industry. However, the disparity in value across many domains serves as a compelling catalyst for advocating transformative measures. Affordable healthcare, patient's safety, security of information and patient's satisfaction are the top priorities to any healthcare service provider today. Management of big data, that is, information collection and data processing with respect to patient information, lab results, claims and insurance claims related data, patient appointment scheduling, prescription maintenances, etc., are some of the prime responsibilities of the healthcare organizations. Constraints can spur creativity.

With the changing paradigm of the industrial era, the health sector has marked its progressive step with the help of technology. Modern healthcare use technology, that includes artificial intelligence (AI), digital operations, e-services. diagnosis,

DOI: 10.1201/9781032698519-23

treatment and surgery are the subsections where fundamental changes have been observed. But, healthcare is a labour intensive service. Other than manpower shortage, variable cost, capital investment, depreciation and cost of maintenance can exaggerate the expenditure burden further. An efficiency analysis comparing manual versus AI-driven healthcare services might serve as a policy recommendation to guide future development. This chapter will analyze and compared the new AI-enabled option with the existing options in rural areas. It will further justify the relevance of the replacements.

23.2 INTERVENTION OF AI IN HEALTHCARE

Novel clinical practices includes design, functional and operational advancements, that is, digital healthcare, AI-based algorithms, targeting high-risk patients, medical decision support, telemedicine, etc., that can provide quality service at a reduced cost of therapy. It can ensure better integration of sub sectors and improve adaptability (ISRO, 2005). Moreover AI-assisted healthcare initiatives have also lowered numerous sector specific costs by the usage of remote nursing help, robot-guided surgery, administrative workflow assistance, medication error reduction, clinical trial participation identification, fraud detection. etc., (Mohammad, 2021; Euro.WHO, 2021). 'Elsa Science app', 'CroDiab' (a web-based diabetes data registry system), 'Niramai Health Analytics','Wyasa' (AI-enabled Chatbot), 'Health Hub', 'Medicine from the Sky' (drone assisted medicine delivery) and M-Health are few such alternative options to manage difficult accessibility to resources and serves the purpose of 'health', 'healthcare' and 'health policy'(Vidal-Alaball et al., 2020; Cremer and Kasparov, 2021; Mohammad, 2021; Khanna, 2020; Zhang and Zaman, 2020; Latif et al., 2017; Bokolo, 2021; Gram Vaani, 2012; Vidal-Alaball et al., 2020; Borges do Nascimento et al., 2021).

23.3 TRANSFORMATION OF HEALTH SECTOR IN INDIA

The healthcare delivery system of India is primarily divided into two primary categories: private and public. Primary healthcare centres (PHCs) of rural India primarily focus on providing fundamental healthcare for the residents, whereas a significant portion of secondary and tertiary healthcare facilities are basically committed to serving metropolitan cities, tier-I and tier-II cities (Anand and Bhambri, 2018). Indian health service sector comprises of a large set of segments like hospitals, medical equipment, pharmaceuticals, diagnostics, medical insurance, etc. Following the changing burden of disease, Indian health service approach has shifted its direction from reactive to proactive initiative (Subramanian, 2021). So, technology has a much-intensified role to achieve the objective.

National health portal (NHP), online services, hospital information system (HIS) and telemedicine, etc., were introduced for this purpose. The NHP2017 (National health policy) has given more emphasis on the use of digital modes to improve the holistic efficiency and effectiveness of the existing health system (Ministry of Health and Family Welfare, 2020). Eventually, it will focus the 'health for all' approach with better and easy access, improving quality of healthcare and minimizing the expenditure of healthcare service. It gives more emphasis on digital technology for health services (Bhambri et al., 2019). Moreover, National Digital Health Blue Print (NDHB) was prepared to fulfil the vision of NHP2017. Table 23.1 shows the five

TABLE 23.1
Framework of Digital Health Services in India

Layers	Particulars
Layer-1 Infrastructure	Secure Health Network: Strong data link through high bandwidth network system. Application: Tele-health, Tele-radiology, etc. Health Cloud (H-cloud): Government Community Cloud (GCC) developed by MeitY. Application: Key data hub management Security and Privacy Operations Centre (SOC): Establishment of Privacy Operations Centre (POC) for 24/7 security surveillance. Application: Health Cloud and Heath Network
Layer-2 Data Hubs	Unique Health Identifier (UHID): Specific details including demography, location, family, relationship, contact details of an individual. Application: Generation of medical records Electronic Health Record (EHR): General and aggregate digital health records. Application: Multiple users can exchange heath data for the treatment Health Directories and Health Registers (HDHR): Master data of various entities which are sub divided as Facility, Doctors, Nurses and Paramedical, Health Workers and Allied Professional Directory.
Layer-3 Technology Building Blocks	Anonymizer: Collect data from 'Health Locker' or other data sets, provides anonymized data to the users after removing personally identifiable information for better security purposes. Consent Manager: The electronic consent framework specified by 'MeitY' to be used prior to use of health records. Health Locker: It helps to create longitudinal health record from the various links it stores and provide EHR to the users. Health Information Exchange: Real-time data exchange mechanism is applied and subject to authorization and authentication for every data exchange. Health Analytics: Helps to decision making support in the areas of quality of care, quality of data, wellness, public health, fraud detection, policy making, etc.
Layer-4 GIS/Visualization	Take the data set from the health analytics system and produce output as per the queries like nearest hospital with specialty, disease incidence in a geographic area etc.
Layer-5 Access and delivery	Call Centres: Provide telephonic supports to the residents of India. Health Portal: Multi language portal for digital health services. Social Media: Information, education and communication, etc. MyHealthApps: Several apps can be designed by open market.

Source: National Digital Health Blueprint, MOH and FW, GOI

layered system consisting of: Infrastructure, Data Hubs, Technology and Building, GIS/Visualization and Access and Delivery. In 2015, the Indian health administration initiative launched a 'Digital India' campaign to ensure electronic access of healthcare to the people. It has been argued that e-health, or digital health, promotion will lead to major improvements in the provision of public healthcare.

Recent initiative of September 2021, 'Ayushman Bharat Digital Mission' is a mind-blowing approach to enlist every citizen by creating a digital health ID and retain their digital health record for future. 'Dig doctor', a digital registry of clinicians has been designed to fulfil this purpose (Ministry of Health and Family Welfare, 2021). Additionally, the orientation of National Digital Health has been created by e-hospital software, the "mCessation (Tobacco)"/"mDiabetes" program, "MeraAspataal," telemedicine software by Apollo Group of Hospitals, "AarogyaSetu," "CoWIN," and "Live Health" management information system (Nautiyal, 2022; Paul et al., 2018; Theo, 2021).

23.4 RURAL HEALTHCARE IN INDIA

The rural parts of India are home to the majority of the population (66%), while urban areas make up only 33% of India's overall population. The proportion of older rural residents who are 60 years of age or older increased from 6% to 8.3% between 1991 and 2016. The rural population has a percentage of 28.6% belonging to the age group of zero through 14 years, whereas the urban region has a lower percentage of 23.6%. It suggests that those who live in cities have a higher relative risk of contracting infectious diseases. People in rural areas are more likely to be unemployed than in urban areas, which increases their vulnerability to costs. Six point nine percent of Indian rural population is either widowed/divorced or separated. The neonatal and under five mortality rate of rural India is comparatively higher than urban India (Ministry of Statistics and Programme Implementation, 2019). Average rural life expectancy is 62 years at birth as compared to 68 years of Indian urban population. The three-tier Indian rural health care system is a support of 155,404 sub centers, 24,918 PHC (Primary health centers) and 5,183 CHC (Community health centers) (Ministry of Statistics and Programme Implementation, 2019; Mohammad, 2021). However, a majority of the clinicians (67%) serve in urban areas and only 33% serve in rural areas (Paul et al., 2018). Each sub-centre, PHC and CHC covers the healthcare need of 300–5000, 20000–30000 and 80000–120000 population, respectively. Each unit covers 2.51 km (4 villages), 6.28 km (27 villages) and 13.77 km (128 villages) radial distance consecutively for sub-centre, PHC and CHC (Ministry of Statistics and Programme Implementation, 2019). As of 31st March 2020, there is a 2% shortfall of health workers and auxiliary nursing matrons whereas, 6.8% shortfall of physicians. Moreover 63.3% of the specialists at CHCs are yet to be recruited. Overall, 78.9% of surgeons, 78.2% of physicians, 78.2% of pediatricians, 69.7% of obstetricians and gynecologists are yet to be recruited. Overall, there is a shortage of 76.1% specialists at the CHCs. Table 23.2 shows the shortage of qualified medical professionals like doctors, nurses, lab technicians, health assistants, health workers in sub-centres, primary and community health centres in rural areas as of March 2020.

TABLE 23.2
Manpower Status in Rural Areas in India as of 31–03–2020

Sl. No.	Particulars	Sub-Centres		PHCs		CHCs	
		Required (in Nos.)	Shortfall (in Nos.)	Required (in Nos.)	Shortfall (in Nos.)	Required (in Nos.)	Shortfall (in Nos.)
1	Health Workers (Female)	155404	6038	24918	5066	–	–
2	Health Workers (male)	155404	101828	–	–	–	–
3	Health Assistant	–	–	49836	35824	–	–
4	Doctors	–	–	24918	1704	–	–
5	Specialists [Surgeons, OB and GY, Physicians and Pediatricians]	–	–	–	–	20732	15775
6	AYUSH Specialist	–	–	–	–	5183	3922
7	Radiographers	–	–	–	–	5183	2884
8	General Duty Medical Officers	–	–	–	–	10366	355
9	Pharmacists	–	–	24918	6240	5183	249
10	Lab Technicians	–	–	24918	12098	5183	284
11	Staff Nurses	–	–	24918	5772	36281	3334

Source: Rural Health Statistics 2019–20

For an estimated mid-year rural population of 890329000, there is an infrastructural shortfall of 24% sub-centres, 29% PHCs and 38% CHCs which indicates the overload on existing facilities. Moreover, lack of infrastructure facilities like diagnostic centres, modern equipment, poor connectivity, etc., are also serious issues for providing good quality, easy accessibility, better affordability and equity in healthcare services in rural India (Gangopadhyay and Ukil, 2022).

23.5 SCOPE OF ALTERNATIVE APPROACH

Healthcare systems effectiveness is a function of resource allocation. This leads to high costs of operations and slow processing. Leveraging the support of AI and RPA, healthcare operation can achieve highest precision as it can automate many manual functions. More e-health is being used by developing countries to properly allocate health budgets within their GDP, which may increase their reliance on e-health (Bhambri and Gupta, 2018). Disease dynamics of rural India has a complex scenario as it is not only flooded with infectious diseases but also with non-communicable diseases. After the emergence of COVID-19, the situation is more critical. Advanced facilities and diagnostic services are the need of the hour (Goel and Khera, 2015). Moreover, poor accessibility and affordability of legitimate healthcare is a function of social disparity (Singh and Badaya, 2014). Lack of awareness, inadequate transportation and shortage in medical and paramedical professionals have increassed the problem further (Devarakonda, 2016). Existing health facilities are in absolute dilemma to fix several burning issues, that is, shortage in skilled manpower, inadequate infrastructure, zero preventive option, non-availability of guaranteed treatment, high mortality, etc. But solving the issues are a huge undertaking. Rural India has only 33% of Indian doctors (Paul et al., 2018). So, it is time for both quality and quantity (Barik and Thorat, 2015). But, it is impossible to transform the primary healthcare of India within a short period (Kumar et al., 2020). Smart design of healthcare can help to balance the legitimate uniformity in medical facility allocation, push the process of health reform, promote the strategic diseases prevention campaigns and reduce mass medical costs (Xiang et al., 2016). Rapid advancement in AI is a game changer, even in healthcare. It is a cost saving option (Reddy et al., 2019). Healthcare access and quality score of India has improved its position from 24.7% in 1990 to 41.2% in 2016 due to change in policy. Healthcare is becoming more affordable now with the help of health insurance. Replacement of human with AI application is highly contextual and conditional (Dick, 2020). But, hybrid intelligence has sector specific application (Dellermann et al., 2019). Moreover, emotional intelligence is a missing component in AI driven applications (Shabbir and Anwer, 2018). Further, introduction of AI is best suitable for system augmentation rather than replacing human (Cremer and Kasparov, 2021; Jarrahi, 2018).

Indian population is overburdened with the out-of-pocket health expenditure that can be eased by accelerating public spending 2.5–3% which may lower down the current OOP from 60% to 30% (Subramanian, 2021). Fifty-six percent of the rural healthcare problem is infrastructural deficiency which is followed by distance and connectivity (28%), staff condition (8%), quality of care (5%) and medicine and vaccine (3%) (Gram Vaani, 2012). Digital healthcare can reduce the gap of healthcare facility access across urban and rural residents of India (Mohan and Kumar, 2019). In a clinical establishment, clinicians are normally engaged in patient care, administrative activities and professional activities. Further, in the United States, physicians spend one sixth of their total daily duty hours for administrative tasks (Woolhandler and Himmelstein, 2014). For surgeons, these tasks are one-third of their total working hours (Di Pietro Martinelli et al., 2022). This percentage varied between 22.6–33% in related studies (Medscape.com, 2014; Merritt, 2022). It is more interesting in a country like India with a low doctor-to-patient ratio structure. Thus, AI can assist in relieving the administrative burden (Mesko, 2021). Patient-related documentation also piles up as an administrative load among physicians. But, electronic medical records were not always found as a time saver. In Europe, billing and insurance related paper work are 4.9% of total working hours of a physician (Kahn et al., 2005). Further, emergence of COVID-19 pandemic has changed the workplace dynamics and lifestyle of clinicians and healthcare workers. Use of AI can even justify the areas of cost aversion.

On the other hand, the salary of doctors and medical staff contributes to 50% of total expenditure of a hospital (Dutta, 2018). Expenditure related to human resource is the principle cost for both district and tertiary care hospitals followed by capital cost and material for operational cost (Chatterjee et al., 2013). The 85% of radiodiagnostic business in India is highly fragmented, with one radiologist for every lakh people (Nautiyal, 2022). A radiologist's eight-hour shift entails analyzing a fresh image every three to four seconds, increasing the likelihood of an error. Over 500 hospital diagnostic centres are using an AI, natural language and computer vision based solution developed by Synapsica that may help to achieve better precision and high efficiency. Similar facilities could contribute to providing a greater level of service to the rural population of India. In rural areas, the risk of spreading sexually transmitted diseases can be reduced by using chatbot and voice assisted mechanisms where the patient can privately receive the right medical support when discussing their problems. Currently, the Indian rural sector is developing with artificial intelligence, particularly machine learning. AI, which is the application of computer software with preprogrammed functions to replace human brains, has revolutionized the healthcare sector. However, these new technologies are renovating the infrastructure and lowering the one-time treatment expenses in the rural sector. As the utilization of AI decreases risk, the accuracy in treatment increases which indirectly improves profit due to the reduction of total costs. New ML or other AI technologies are a solution for age-old rural health problems such as quality healthcare, inadequate ratio of skilled clinicians to patients (Bhambri et al., 2019). If these technological developments can be implemented in the Indian rural sector, the cost minimization can make a huge impact to the developing economy of a country like India that spends approximately 2.1% of India's GDP for the healthcare sector. In India, cost modelling, treatment variability and drug discovery are the healthcare sectors where the application of artificial intelligence is profitable by improving both quality and cost. But application of AI in healthcare involves a few risks and challenges, like quality, safety, governance, privacy, consent and ownership, etc. Therefore, prototype testing will justify the significance of AI oriented activity. Requisite training must be conducted at a reasonable or feasible cost to increase the potential of the infrastructure. Also, other related issues like spontaneous electricity and high-speed network with dedicated server, are necessary for the successful implementation of AI in rural India which can increase the technological development costs. Hence, wishful thinking and willful action is a prerequisite.

23.6 OPPORTUNITY COST

Measuring the cost of replacement is a proactive step to consolidate any health plan. The scope of healthcare development in a country like India is mounting everyday because of the enhancement of innovative capacities and infrastructural sustainability. But, in this sector, inequalities in the distribution of funds by the government and other financial institutions, and lack of properly trained or equipped health workers are of major concern (Paresh et al., 2019). Costs of facilities are a key driver in this industry in spite of getting internet connections and smartphones in the hands of participants of the healthcare. The financial investments in healthcare of India are divided in two levels, that is, public and private (Kaur and Bhambri, 2019). The objectives of Indian public sector healthcare investments levels are to find out the cost ratio between total government funded healthcare and the expenditures for the financially weak people. Presently, India is spending around 8% of GDP in public healthcare which is more than China and Africa but less than Thailand. To justify the investments, the government of India now encourages PPP models in this sector where better facilities can be provided by the support of corporate funds through CSR (Anand and Bhambri,

2018). This technique has helped the Voluntary Health Service Association of India's "Khoj" programs and CMC Vellore, Tamil Nadu's rural health projects work well in this nation. In developing countries like India, it is very difficult to increase public health costs rapidly, the non-doctor-based healthcare approach becomes popular these days. In this, treatment or facilities are provided through nurses, medical practitioners and physician assistants. They have been selected, prepared, and trained for the rural areas under the guidance or recommendation of a licensed medical professional. The majority of the time, individuals choose to treat themselves at their own expense using community-based healthcare services and indigenous medicines to provide affordable healthcare to rural areas of India (Srinivisan, 2020).

Table 23.3 presents the distribution of individuals' health expenditure in urban and rural areas, regardless of their inclusion in insurance coverage. Mean healthcare expenses (in Rs.) per instance of hospitalization for public and private hospital of rural area is 5000 and 28000, respectively. For urban India the cost are Rs. 6000 and Rs. 40000, respectively. With the application of AI, the cost can be Rs. 20000 irrespective of the demography to which the hospital belongs. Unit costs for radiology, pharmacy, NICU, eye OT, IPP OT, dialysis unit, labor ward, laboratory, pharmacy, physiotherapy, ICU, and 6539, 2365, 3380, 186, 13, 160, 7845, 7861, 2223, and 1222 are as follows. 255, 232, 296, 202, 642, 531, 1103, 502, 11431, 3520, 62, 139, 22, 269, 314, 399, 98512, 11763, 22240, 17338, 15578, 8287, 4127, and so on are the average prices of medication for private teaching hospitals and tertiary care hospitals, respectively. cardiology, outpatient department, and surgery Outside Patient Division, ocular Orthopedics outpatient department medication, out-of-patient department In-patient surgical unitEye in the Patient Department Orthopedics outpatient department (Chatterjee et al., 2013) Out-of-patient department; orthopedics operating room; emergency room; all laboratories; microbiology lab; biochemistry lab; pathology lab; radiography; physiotherapy; private hospital; CTOT; SICU; CTICU; RICU; MICU; ICCU; dialysis unit.

TABLE 23.3

Distribution of Individuals by Type of Health Expenditure Coverage, Expressed as a Percentage Breakdown

		% of persons covered by					
Sector	% of persons not covered	Government-funded insurance program	Govt./PSU as an employer	Private health insurance provided by employers (excluding government or public sector)	Arranged by household with insurance companies	Other	All
Rural	85.9	12.9	0.6	0.3	0.2	0.1	100
Urban	80.9	8.9	3.3	2.9	3.8	0.2	100

Source: Ministry of Statistics and Programme Implementation (MOSPI), (2019)

The Indian healthcare industry is divided in various sectors. In these sectors, the implementation of artificial intelligence is playing a pivotal role. The players who have been benefitted include hospitals, drugs, diagnostics centres, medical equipment manufacturers, suppliers and medical insurance institutions (Paul et al., 2018). It is obvious that in country like India, rural healthcare services delivered by the private sector undertakings have not grown so much. The reason behind it is that the service is not supported by the per capita income of the rural people. Various surveys have demonstrated that private care accounts for approximately two-thirds to three-quarters of all medical expenses in each household, amounting to roughly 10% of the yearly household expenditures. Currently, the nation must increase its investment in the healthcare service sector in order to achieve hypothetical savings (Srinivisan, 2020).

23.6.1 Cost of AI in Healthcare in India

According to (Netscribes India Pvt Ltd, 2019), the investment in AI in Indian healthcare was Rs. 432 billion in 2021 at growth of approximately 40% to 2020. If this growth increases, the doctor-patient ratio in India will be increased to 7:1000 in 2023 from 4.8:1000 in 2017. This ratio can change the dimension of the healthcare industry of India. Respiratory, infectious diseases and cardiac diseases are presently dominating in rural areas which need emergency but costly treatment (Kuzhaloli et al., 2020). AI-supported healthcare services, that is, automated analysis of pathological tests, automated predictive diagnosis with the help of screening and monitoring equipment and sensor driven devices, are expected to revolutionize medical care and treatment in India (Netscribes India Pvt Ltd, 2019). Table 23.4 shows the average medical expenditure during hospital stay.

TABLE 23.4
Average Medical Expenditure During Hospital Stay

	Average medical expenditure (Rs.)/hospitalization case		
Category of Ailment	**Public hospitals**	**Private hospitals**	**All Hospitals**
Cancer cases	22,520	93,305	61,216
Neurological and Psychiatric cases	7,235	41,239	26,843
Cardio-vascular casess	6,635	54,970	36,001
Musculo-skeletal cases	5,716	46,365	32,066
Genito-Urinary cases	5,345	33,409	24,770
Gastro-intestinal cases	3,847	29,870	19,821
Respiratory cases	3,346	24,049	13,905
Eye diseases	2,605	18,767	10,912
Infections	2,054	15,208	9,064
Other diseases	4,452	31,845	20,135

Source: Ministry of Statistics and Programme Implementation (MOSPI), (2019)

23.6.2 Cost of Healthcare Before Implementation of AI

The operational indirect cost of OPD, IPD, emergency, OT in a district hospital is respectively 6%, 18%, 51% and 8% of the total treatment cost. For a tertiary-care hospital it is 15%, 15%, 26% and 17%. The expense of human resources rises for vital healthcare, and scientific reason might not allow this to happen (Coye et al., 2009).

23.6.3 Cost of Healthcare After Implementation of AI

Table 23.5 shows the components of medical expenditure (hospitalization) per case of hospitalization, post-AI implementation. Table 23.6 shows the elements of healthcare spending (outside of hospitals) following the introduction of AI. Table 23.7 shows the opportunity cost of medical expenditure in India.

The Table 23.7 shows a fundamental reduction of expenditure of treatment incurred by a rural patient, that is, 12.7% and 29.55%, respectively, in public and private hospital. Hospitals can even reach to their breakeven level faster due to minimum manpower dependence, larger scale of service reach, time saving and low depreciation cost. Accessibility and the scarcity of labor are two side benefits of AI-enabled healthcare. More administrative work will free up medical and paramedical personnel to concentrate on their primary duties.

23.7 PROPOSED MODEL

Designing a robust healthcare system for the Indian rural sector demands not only reducing cost and enhancing service quality, but also scale of operations and

TABLE 23.5
Components of Medical Expenditure (Hospitalization) Per Case of Hospitalization, Post-AI Implementation

	Average medical expenses (Rs.) during hospital stay per case of hospitalization in			
Component of medical expenditure	**Public Hospital**		**Private Hospital**	
	Rural area	Urban area	Rural area	Urban area
Package component	427	867	6,631	15,380
Fees of clinician	172	197	5,340	6,284
Drugs/Medicaments	2,220	2,100	6,818	7,035
Diagnosis	800	770	2,802	3,403
Bed charge	118	152	3,377	4,176
Other	553	752	2,379	2,544
Total	4,290	4,837	27,347	38,822

Source: Ministry of Statistics and Programme Implementation, (2019)

TABLE 23.6

Elements of Healthcare Spending (Outside of Hospitals) Following the Introduction of AI

Component of healthcare spending	% share of medical spending				
	Healthcare service provider				
	Public Hospital	Private Hospital	Charitable/NGO/ trust-run hospital	Private doctor/ clinic	All (incl. informal healthcare provider)
Medicines	82.2	64.3	54.1	70.1	70.3
Pathological test	10.9	15.7	28.8	10.9	12.6
Fee of Doctor	2.4	14.2	14.3	17.1	13.3
Other	4.5	5.8	2.8	1.9	3.8
All	**100**	**100**	**100**	**100**	**100**

Source: Ministry of Statistics and Programme Implementation, (2019)

TABLE 23.7

Opportunity Cost of Medical Expenditure in India

Description of medical expenditure	Average savings of medical expenditure (INR) during treatment stay/case			
	Public hospital		Private hospital	
	Rural	Urban	Rural	Urban
Capital Expenditure Save				
Human resources	24%	22%	21%	20%
Material	12%	14%	17%	17%
Building infrastructure	3%	1%	2%	1%
Land	3%	0.50%	0.90%	0.70%
Equipment	11%	11%	13%	12%
Indirect cost	10%	9%	8%	7%
Revenue Expenditure Save				
Package component	17%	15%	11%	11%
Doctor's/surgeon's fee	2%	3%	2%	3%
Medicines	8%	6%	7%	6%
Diagnostic tests	1%	0.50%	0.90%	1.10%
Bed charges	11%	12%	12%	11%

Source: Author's analysis

affordability of service. It must be used across the clinical establishment of India. Thus, three objectives of AI integrated rural healthcare service is basically a 3R approach, that is, Replace-Rationing-Resurge.

- Replace

Replacement of manual processes with AI based technologies can improve the performance, perfection and productivity of rural healthcare. Moreover, it is a solution without trading off the time of service and price. One time investment is 'value for money'.

- Rationing

Every alternative may not be a good fit. It is not conceptual, rather highly contextual. Many areas of healthcare service need a humanistic approach with deep empathy. These functions can't be replaced by a machine. A rationalized approach needs to be tested by a prototype. Minimum recurring cost justifies optimum utilization of resources.

- Resurge

An AI based system is automated. Hence, an existing facility can explore its inorganic capacity to cope with the 38% shortage in infrastructure. Even the current force of clinical and paramedical employees could function more effectively in terms of administration.

23.8 CONCLUSION

Time of service is the essence of good healthcare. Disparity in gap of reach in healthcare facilities is an age-old reality of rural India. The progressive status of this gap has further widened by the emergence of COVID-19 pandemic. The disease burden of Indian rural areas is not shifting its pattern fast. But the challenges are more confined to deficiency in structure, manpower, facility and access. Structural advancement and systematic delivery of service are the fundamental changes imminent to upgrade healthcare delivery geography. It is not an overnight affair. Opportunity is there to fill the gaps. Therefore, AI integrated health service approach can be a dependable solution. Further, it can provide legitimate benefit to the residents of rural India.

Technology cannot serve as a replacement for medical and paramedical personnel. However, it can assist medical practitioners in expanding their reach to a larger number of patients in underdeveloped regions where the availability of high-quality healthcare is still a challenge. The issue of staff shortage can be temporarily alleviated for less urgent cases. The utilization of AI in conjunction with other technologies can render remote clinical monitoring, chronic illness management and preventative care viable possibilities. Therefore, harnessing the untapped potential of AI can facilitate the development and prosperity of rural India. Otherwise, the healthcare administration will continue to be overshadowed by the financial burden of rural healthcare.

REFERENCES

Anand, A., & Bhambri, P. (2018). Rotation, Scale and Translation Invariant Character Recognition System using Neural Network. Punjab Technical University, Jalandhar (M.Tech. thesis).

Barik, D., & Thorat, A. (2015). Issues of Unequal Access to Public Health in India. *Frontiers in Public Health*, *3*, 245.

Bhambri, P., & Gupta, O. P. (2018). Implementing Machine Learning Algorithms for Distance based Phylogenetic Trees. I.K.Gujral Punjab Technical University, Jalandhar (Ph.D. thesis).

Bhambri, P., Sinha, V. K., & Jaiswal, M. (2019). Change in Iris Dimensions as a Potential Human Consciousness Level Indicator. In *International Conference on Innovations in Communication, Computing and Sciences*, *8*(9S), 517–525. https://www.ijitee.org/wp-content/uploads/papers/v8i9S/I10820789S19.pdf

Bokolo, A. J. (2021). Application of Telemedicine and eHealth Technology for Clinical Services in Response to COVID-19 Pandemic. *Health and Technology*, *11*(2), 359–366.

Borges do Nascimento, I. J., Marcolino, M. S., Abdulazeem, H. M., Weerasekara, I., Azzopardi-Muscat, N., Gonçalves, M. A., & Novillo-Ortiz, D. (2021). Impact of big data analytics on people's health: Overview of systematic reviews and recommendations for future studies. *Journal of Medical Internet Research*, *23*(4), e27275.

Chatterjee, S., Levin, C., & Laxminarayan, R. (2013). Unit Cost of Medical Services at Different Hospitals in India. *PLoS One*, *8*(7), 69728.

Coye, M. J., Haselkorn, A., & DeMello, S. (2009). Remote Patient Management: Technology-Enabled Innovation and Evolving Business Models for Chronic Disease Care. *Health Affairs (Project Hope)*, *28*(1), 126–135.

Cremer, D. D., & Kasparov, G. (2021). AI Should Augment Human Intelligence, Not Replace It. *Harvard Business Review*. https://hbr.org/2021/03/ai-should-augment-human-intelligence-not-replace-it.

Dellermann, D., Ebel, P., Söllner, M., & Leimeister, J. M. (2019). Hybrid Intelligence. *Business and Information Systems Engineering*, *61*(5), 637–643.

Devarakonda, S. (2016). Hub and Spoke Model: Making Rural Healthcare in India Affordable, Available and Accessible. *Rural and Remote Health*, *16*(1), 3476.

Di Pietro Martinelli, C., Haltmeier, T., Lavanchy, J. L., Perrodin, S. F., Candinas, D., & Schnüriger, B. (2022). Work Characteristics of Acute Care Surgeons at a Swiss Tertiary Care Hospital: A Prospective One-Month Snapshot Study. *World Journal of Surgery*, *46*(2), 330–336.

Dick, S. (2020). Artificial Intelligence. *Harvard Dta Science Review*, *1*, 102–129.

Dutta, S. S. (2018). Private Hospitals Spend 50 Per Cent of Operational Costs on Salaries of Medical Staff, Including Doctors Report. *The New Indian Express*. www.newindianexpress.com/nation/2018/jun/16/private-hospitals-spend-50-per-cent-of-operational-costs-on-salaries-of-medical-staff-including-doc-1829098.html.

Euro.WHO. (2021). *Artificial Intelligence and Data Technology Provide Smarter Healthcare for Solutions that have Made a difference for Noncommunicable Diseases*. Noncommunicable Diseases. www.euro.who.int/en/health-topics/noncommunicable-diseases/pages/news/news/2021/12/.

Gangopadhyay, S., & Ukil, A. (2022). Being Resilient to Deal with Attrition of Nurses in Private COVID-19 Hospitals: Critical Analysis with Respect to the Crisis in Kolkata,

India. In Garg, L., Chakraborty, C., Mahmoudi, S., & Sohmen, V. S. (eds) *Healthcare Informatics for Fighting COVID-19 and Future Epidemics. EAI/Springer Innovations in Communication and Computing*. Cham: Springer, 353–363. https://doi.org/10.1007/978-3-030-72752-9_18.

Goel, K., & Khera, R. (2015). Public Health Facilities in North India. *Economic & Political Weekly*, 53–54.

Gram Vaani. (2012). *Rural Healthcare: Towards a Healthy Rural India*. Ministry of Health, Govt of India. https://gramvaani.org/rural-health-care-towards-a-healthy-rural-india/#:~:text=In rural India%2C where the,largest number of maternity deaths.

ISRO. (2005). Telemedicine Healing Touch Through Space: Enabling Specialty Healthcare to the Rural and Remote Population of India. In *Publications and Public Relations Unit, ISRO*. https://doi.org/10.1109/ICTTA.2008.4529925.

Jarrahi, M. H. (2018). Artificial Intelligence and the Future of Work: Human-AI Symbiosis in Organizational Decision Making. *Business Horizons*, *61*(4), 577–586.

Kahn, J. G., Kronick, R., Kreger, M., & Gans, D. N. (2005). The Cost of Health Insurance Administration in California: Estimates for Insurers, Physicians, and Hospitals. *Health Affairs (Project Hope)*, *24*(6), 1629–1639.

Kaur, J., & Bhambri, P. (2019). Design of Paddy Crop Prediction Technique Based on K-Mean, Naïve Bayes, KNN and SVM Classifiers. I.K. Gujral Punjab Technical University, Jalandhar (M.Tech. thesis).

Khanna, M. (2020). Three School Kids Try To Solve Healthcare Problem In Rural India With AI. *India Times*. www.indiatimes.com/technology/news/healthcare-without-doctors-ibm-cbse-healthhub-521402.html.

Kumar, A., Rajasekharan Nayar, K., & Koya, S. F. (2020). COVID-19: Challenges and Its Consequences for Rural Health Care in India. *Public Health in Practice (Oxford, England)*, *1*, 100009.

Kuzhaloli, S., Devaneyan, P., Sitaraman, N., Periyathanbi, P., Gurusamy, M., & Bhambri, P. (2020). IoT Based Smart Kitchen Application for Gas Leakage Monitoring. IN Patent App. 202,041,049,866 A.

Latif, S., Rana, R., Qadir, J., Ali, A., Imran, M. A., & Younis, M. S. (2017). Mobile Health in the Developing World: Review of Literature and Lessons from a Case Study. *IEEE Access*, *5*, 11540–11556.

Medscape.com. (2014). *Medscape Physicians' Compensation Report 2012 & 2013*. www.medscape.com/features/slideshow/compensation/2013/public.

Merritt, H. (2022). *A Survey of America's Physicians: Practice Patterns and Perspectives*. www.physiciansfoundation.org/uploads/default/Physicians_Foundation_2012_Biennial_Survey.pdf.

Mesko, B. (2021). 5 Reasons Why Artificial Intelligence Won't Replace Physicians. In *The Medical Futurist*. https://medicalfuturist.com/5-reasons-artificial-intelligence-wont-replace-physicians/#.

Ministry of Health and Family Welfare, G. of I. (2020). *Rural Health Statistics 2019–20*. https://main.mohfw.gov.in/sites/default/files/RHS 2019–20_2.pdf.

Ministry of Health and Family Welfare, G. of I. (2021). *e-Hospital*. Govt of India. https://dashboard.ehospital.gov.in/dashboard-testing2/#.

Ministry of Statistics and Programme Implementation (MOSPI), G. og I. (2019). *Key Indicators of Social Consumption in India: Health*. National Sample Survey Organisation. http://mail.mospi.gov.in/index.php/catalog/161/download/1949; www.mospi.gov.in/sites/default/files/publication_reports/KI_Health_75th_Final.pdf.

Mohammad, S. (2021). Telangana Launches 'Medicine from the Sky' Project to Drone-Deliver Vaccines, Medicines to Remote Areas. *The Hindu*. www.thehindu.com/news/national/telangana/telangana-launches-medicine-from-the-sky-project-to-drone-deliver-vaccines-medicines-to-remote-areas/article36401406.ece.

Mohan, P., & Kumar, R. (2019). Strengthening Primary Care in Rural India: Lessons from Indian and Global Evidence and Experience. *Journal of Family Medicine and Primary Care*, *8*(7), 2169–2172.

Nautiyal, S. (2022). *Artificial Intelligence Can Significantly Improve Radiology Reporting: Meenkashi Singh, Synapsica*. Financial Express Health Care. www.financialexpress.com/healthcare/diagnostic/artificial-intelligence-can-significantly-improve-radiology-reporting-meenkashi-singh-synapsica/2427544/.

Netscribes (India) Pvt Ltd. (2019). Artificial Intelligence (AI) in Healthcare Market in India (2018–2023). In *Research and Markets*. https://doi.org/4787271.

Paresh, S. S., Greco, T. L., & Rohr-Kirchgraber, T. (2019). The Sex and Gender Influence on Hypertension. *Health Management The Journal*, *19*(5), 420–422.

Paul, Y., Hickok, E., Sinha, A., Tiwari, U., Mohandas, S., Ray, S., Hickok, E., & Bidare, P. M. (2018). Artificial Intelligence in the Healthcare Industry in India. In *The Centre for Internet and Society*. https://news.medgenera.com/12-artificial-intelligence-health care-startups-india-ai/.

Reddy, S., Fox, J., & Purohit, M. P. (2019). Artificial Intelligence-Enabled Healthcare Delivery. *Journal of the Royal Society of Medicine*, *112*(1), 22–28.

Shabbir, J., & Anwer, T. (2018). Artificial Intelligence and its Role in Near Future. *14*(8), 1–11.

Singh, S., & Badaya, S. (2014). Health Care in Rural India: A Lack between Need and Feed. *South Asian Journal of Cancer*, *3*(2), 143–144. https://doi.org/10.48550/arXiv.1804.01396

Srinivisan, R. (2020). *Health Care in India-vision 2020*. https://api.semanticscholar.org/CorpusID:50295456.

Subramanian, K. (2021). Economic Survey Takes Aim at Out-of-Pocket Spend, High Private Healthcare Costs. *The Wire Staff*. https://thewire.in/health/economic-survey-takes-aim-at-out-of-pocket-spend-high-private-healthcare-costs.

Theo, S. (2021). Artificial Intelligence In Healthcare: Will AI Replace Doctors? *Electronicsforu.Com*. www.electronicsforu.com/technology-trends/tech-focus/artificial-intelligence-healthcare-replace-doctors.

Vidal-Alaball, J., Acosta-Roja, R., Pastor Hernández, N., Sanchez Luque, U., Morrison, D., Narejos Pérez, S., Perez-Llano, J., Salvador Vèrges, A., & López Seguí, F. (2020). Telemedicine in the Face of the COVID-19 Pandemic. *Atencion Primaria*, *52*(6), 418–422.

Woolhandler, S., & Himmelstein, D. U. (2014). Administrative Work Consumes One-Sixth of U.S. Physicians' Working Hours and Lowers Their Career Satisfaction. *International Journal of Health Services : Planning, Administration, Evaluation*, *44*(4), 635–642.

Xiang, G.-Y., Zeng, Z., & Shen, Y.-J. (2016). Present Situation and Development Trend of China's Intelligent Medical Construction. *Chinese General Practice*, *19*, 2998–3000.

Zhang, X., & Zaman, B. U. (2020). Adoption Mechanism of Telemedicine in Underdeveloped Country. *Health Informatics Journal*, *26*(2), 1088–1103.

24 A Review Study of Machine Learning Algorithms for Diabetic Prediction Using PIMA Dataset in Cloud Computing

S. Lakshmi Narayanan, S. Krithika, P. Geetha and R.K. Kapila Vani

24.1 INTRODUCTION

High glucose levels are a steady component of diabetes. It happens when the body does not use insulin duly or the pancreas does not make enough insulin. Insulin is a molecule that regulates blood sugar levels by facilitating the body's complete conversion of glucose to energy within the cells. To reduce complications and improve the well-being of those who have diabetes, the disease should be identified and managed from the outset. Diabetes treatment, diagnosis, and expectations are determined by medical care professionals. Artificial intelligence (AI) computations are being employed more frequently to improve the viability and accuracy of diabetes diagnosis and treatment. Large datasets of clinical data can be utilized to prepare AI calculations to find patterns and hazard factors.

Predicting diabetes in a person can be challenging, as there are many factors that contribute to the increase of diabetes. Predicting diabetes in a person requires a comprehensive assessment of their medical history, family history, lifestyle, and other factors (Rattan et al., 2005). Regular monitoring of blood sugar levels and other indicators of diabetes can also help identify people who are at risk of developing the condition. The technique for creating a prediction model based on inputs regarding the person's health conditions is described in this paper. The quantity of pregnancies, pulse, skin thickness, insulin level, this article uses age, body mass index (BMI), and diabetes family capability as some of the elements to determine a person's diabetes status. Cloud computing services are provided by external vendors who manage and maintain the infrastructure required to execute these services, as opposed to enabling these services on private PCs or local servers.

DOI: 10.1201/9781032698519-24

In order to make diagnosis more accurate and efficient in the treatment for diabetes, machine learning algorithms are being utilized more and more frequently (Singh et al., 2004). To find trends and characteristics related to diabetes, machine learning models can be trained on massive datasets of medical records. There are numerous benefits to using machine learning models to diagnose diabetes. AI calculations can handle a tremendous amount of information, including electronic medical records and clinical imaging, to distinguish examples and chance factors that medical care experts may not know about. This can lead to more accurate diabetes diagnosis and personalized treatment plans. Utilizing machine-learning models to diagnose diabetes has numerous advantages, including improved accuracy, earlier detection, individualized treatment, efficiency, and decision-making that is more objective. Diabetes management and health outcomes can be improved by taking advantage of these benefits (Jain and Bhambri, 2005). Age, blood pressure, blood sugar, skin thickness, insulin level, number of pregnancies, diabetes pedigree function, and body mass index (BMI) are all included in the dataset. A completely managed platform for delivering web apps, APIs, and background workers—including machine learning models—is offered by the cloud platform Render. In this research paper, Render has been used to deploy ML models. Five models (Random Forest classifier, K-Neighbors classifier, Gaussian Naive Bayes (GaussianNB), Decision Tree classifier, and Support Vector classifier (SVC)) were used to analyze the dataset and determine whether the person had diabetes or not. This study report demonstrates that the Decision Tree classifier is the best algorithm since it generates results that are more accurate. In this study report, the accuracy of each machine learning model used is discussed. It is discovered which machine learning model diagnoses diabetes the best. The three main components of the process are cloud computing, big data analytics, and machine-learning models.

24.2 REVIEW STUDY

According to Bhatia et al., three metrics—accuracy, score, and error—have been assessed for each model and are suggested as measures for diagnosing diabetes.

The primary focus of the review, according to Neha Prerna et al., is the use of AI calculations to predict the risk of Type 2 diabetes based on lifestyle and family history, much like a correlation of the practicality of various AI calculations in this way. After gathering social event data from 952 participants using an online and disconnected poll, the inventor used a variety of artificial intelligence computations to determine the likelihood of developing diabetes. The review made use of a dataset that included data on a number of factors, such as age, sexual orientation, and diabetes family history, as well as information on blood pressure, skin thickness, insulin levels, glucose levels, and circulatory strain. In both the collected dataset and the PIMA Indian Diabetes data set, the investigation discovered that the Arbitrary Woods classifier calculation played out the best in foreseeing diabetes risk. The study found that individuals could use machine learning algorithms to determine their own risk of developing diabetes. Subsequently, diabetes and its confusions can be recognized and treated before. In view of way of life and family ancestry, six particular

AI calculations were utilized in the review to anticipate the risk of Type 2 Diabetes. Six calculations, including Strategic Relapse (precision 74%), K-Closest Neighbor (exactness 70%), Backing Vector Machine (precision 74%) Guileless Bayes classifier (exactness 69%) Choice Tree (exactness 70%), and Arbitrary Woods classifier (exactness 75%), are utilized in this review.

Muhammad Exell et al., the use of supervised machine learning to predict diabetes is the focus of this paper, which also stresses the significance of early disease detection and treatment to prevent serious complications. The authors described how the key diabetes-causing factors are incorporated into the machine learning model. The study's findings demonstrate that the model accurately predicts diabetes. The authors concluded that healthcare professionals could use machine learning to prevent and manage diabetes. The study mentions that different machine learning algorithms were compared to see how accurate they were at classifying similar data. Additionally, the authors claim that the Pima Indians Diabetes Database, a Kaggle-accessible public dataset, provided the study's data. Consequently, it is likely that k-nearest neighbors, decision trees, logistic regression, support vector machines (SVMs), and other machine learning methods were utilized to classify the diabetes data in the study. The study's suggested model classification makes use of the Pima Indians Diabetes Database dataset, which predicts diabetes based on a variety of health characteristics using two machine learning algorithms—k-nearest neighbor (k-NN) and Naive Bayes. The authors compare the accuracy, precision, and recall of these two algorithms and conclude that Naive Bayes performs better than k-NN in all three areas.

Huma Naz et al., the author addresses the need for early diabetes detection and lifestyle interventions to mitigate its devastating consequences. In order to build a system for diabetes prediction utilizing the PIMA dataset, this research uses advanced machine-learning techniques to leverage healthcare data, including electronic health records and omics data. The results show that classifiers like Artificial Neural Networks (ANN), Naive Bayes (NB), Decision Trees (DT), and Deep Learning (DL) have outstanding accuracy rates ranging from 90% to 98%. Notably, DL has the best accuracy (98.07%), which gives healthcare providers access to a potent predictive tool. These discoveries open the door for the creation of a robotic early detection system.

Jordan et al. explained the benefits to scientific research and to individual and public health.

Priyanka Sonar et al. explained that diabetes is a deadly condition that can cause heart failure, blindness, kidney disease, and other conditions. Traditional diagnostic methods require patients to visit a center, which is both time-consuming and costly (Febrian et al., 2023). Machine learning methods have emerged as a solution to this problem, using data processing to predict the presence of diabetes. A system that accurately predicts a patient's level of diabetic risk is the goal of this research. The model utilizes characterization strategies, including Decision Tree, Artificial Neural Network (ANN), Naive Bayes, and Support Vector Machine (SVM) algorithms. Then the results indicate that the Decision Tree model achieved an 85% precision rate, Naive Bayes achieved 77%, and SVM reached 77.3%. These outcomes demonstrate the significant accuracy of these methods in predicting diabetic risk levels.

Rishab Bothra et al., the application of Big Data Analytics plays a crucial role in locating valuable insights, hidden patterns, and correlations in the data in the healthcare industry, which relies heavily on large databases. This paper presents a diabetes expectation model outfit through AI calculations, pointed toward further developing grouping exactness. Through rigorous experimentation, various machine learning algorithms were evaluated, with Random Forest emerging as the frontrunner, boasting an impressive classification accuracy of 90%. The study further scrutinized algorithm performance by comparing confusion matrices, with a specific focus on minimizing False Negative values. This research not only enhances our understanding of diabetes prediction but also opens doors to the prospect of foreseeing the risk of diabetes in non-diabetic individuals in the years to come. The accuracy results of different algorithms used in this paper like Random Forest (accuracy 90%), Logistic Regression (accuracy 73%), XGBoost (accuracy 80%), SVM (accuracy 74%), KNN (accuracy 89%).

Kotsiantis et al. proposes a symmetrical approach is to parcel the information, staying away from the need to run calculations on exceptionally enormous datasets.

Yang et al. calculated the initial phase of diabetes risk and assisted them in obtaining expectations for future blood glucose increase levels. For diabetic arrangement and expectation, MLP and LSTM are adjusted.

24.3 PROPOSED WORK

Generally, women are more prone to diabetes than men for several reasons. Chemicals assume a critical part in the development of diabetes, and ladies experience hormonal changes all through their lifetime that can influence their glucose levels (Singh et al., 2005). For example, during puberty, menstrual cycles, pregnancy, and menopause, women may experience fluctuations in their hormones that can affect their insulin sensitivity and glucose metabolism. Women often carry more body fat than men, which can increase their risk of developing insulin resistance and diabetes. Furthermore, people who experience gestational diabetes during pregnancy are at a higher risk of developing diabetes sometime down the road. Certain studies have suggested that women may be more vulnerable than men to the harmful effects of high-sugar diets and obesity. Overall, the increased risk of diabetes in women is likely due to a combination of hormonal, physiological, and behavioral factors, and highlights the importance of diabetes prevention and management strategies targeted specifically towards women. Therefore, the number of pregnancies is considered as a factor to predict diabetes. For men, it is denoted as zero.

Since diabetes is depicted by high glucose levels, glucose levels are a critical marker. A fasting blood glucose level of 126 mg/dL or higher commonly demonstrates diabetes. A blood glucose level of 200 mg/dL or higher that is sporadic and higher two hours subsequent to completing a refreshment high in glucose are likewise side effects of diabetes. Because hypertension (high blood pressure) is a common diabetes comorbidity, blood pressure is an important factor to consider when predicting diabetes. Diabetes patients are more likely to develop hypertension, which can make them more vulnerable to cardiovascular disease and its complications (Naz and Ahuja, 2020). Diabetes patients are advised to maintain a blood pressure reading of less than 140/90 mmHg in order to reduce their risk of complications. In general, a blood pressure reading of 130/80 mmHg or higher is indicative of hypertension. In order to provide a more comprehensive assessment of an individual's risk of developing diabetes, blood pressure is frequently taken into consideration in conjunction with other risk factors, such as age, family history, BMI, glucose levels, and lifestyle factors. Skin thickness can be a useful diagnostic tool for evaluating certain diabetes complications like diabetic neuropathy and skin ulcers. A type of nerve damage known as diabetic neuropathy can occur in diabetics, particularly those whose glucose levels are not adequately controlled. Damage to the skin's nerves might cause numbness or unexpected feelings as chewing or trembling. Because insulin production is insufficient in people with Type 1 diabetes, blood insulin levels can be a useful marker. Insulin opposition is a typical side effect of Type 2 diabetes, which can bring about raised insulin levels. BMI (Body Mass Index) is a generally elaborate figure predicting diabetes, particularly Type 2 diabetes. BMI is a measurement of a person's muscle to fat ratio based on their weight and height; it is not fixed by dividing a person's weight in kilograms by the square of their height in meters. A few tests have revealed significant positive correlations between BMI and the chance of getting type 2 diabetes. People with higher BMIs are generally more likely than those with lower BMIs to develop type 2 diabetes.

The Diabetes Pedigree Function (DPF) is used in diabetes prediction, particularly in the case of Type 2 diabetes (Kotsiantis et al., 2007). The DPF is a measure of the genetic risk for developing diabetes based on family history of the individual. The DPF calculated by assigning points to each family member with diabetes, based on their degree of relatedness to the individual who is being evaluated. A higher score is given to first-degree relatives—parents, siblings, and children—than to second-degree relatives—grandparents, aunts, uncles, and nieces/nephews (Jordan and Mitchell, 2015). The average DPF score is then divided by the total number of relatives. A greater genetic risk of developing diabetes is indicated by a DPF score that is higher. Age is a huge calculate diabetes forecast, especially because of Type 2 diabetes. This is because the risk of developing Type 2 diabetes increases with age. As people age, their body's capacity to utilize insulin can diminish, prompting raised blood glucose levels and an expanded risk of developing diabetes.

In this proposed work, pre-processing of PIMA datasets use the "pandas", "NumPy", "matplotlib" tools. Numpy is used to calculate the size of a data collection (Bothra, 2021). It enables quick arithmetic computations on groups and vectors for the user. Pandas, the most used machine learning system or module, enables us to provide a short overview of the methods used to collect the data. It offers simple tools that make machine learning's intricacy and depth more understandable. With Pandas, it's simple to play with various machine learning concepts. Pandas are coded as follows: bring in Pandas as pd. Matplotlib is a Python library used for creating visualizations such as plots, charts, and graphs. It provides a range of customizable options to create high-quality and interactive visualizations.

i. Model Splitting (80:20)—80:20 is the most typical division percentage. Overall, 80% of the data is utilized as the preparation set, and 20% is utilized as the testing set. Ensure the data is sizable enough prior to partitioning

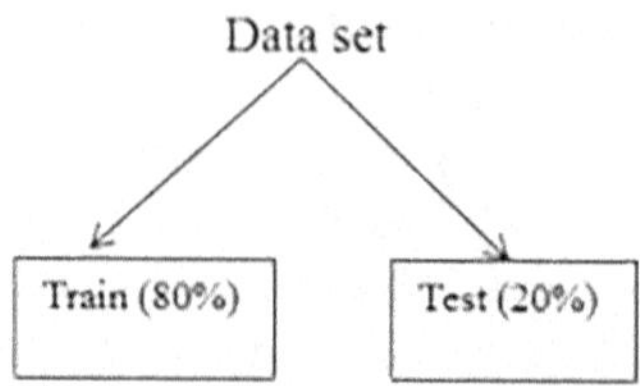

FIGURE 24.1 Model splitting

it. Enormous datasets answer well to prepare/test parting. Figure 24.1 shows the model splitting.

ii. Gathering of Data: A PIMA dataset with 1769 data samples has been used in this research paper to predict diabetes. In this research paper, a dataset with 1769 data samples was used to predict diabetes. The dataset likely incorporates a scope of factors, for example, number of pregnancies, glucose level, circulatory strain, skin thickness, insulin level, BMI, diabetes family capability and age, that might be pertinent to diabetes expectation. The use of a dataset with a large number of data samples is beneficial for several reasons. Firstly, a larger dataset allows for more accurate and robust modeling of the underlying relationships between the variables and the outcome of interest, in this case, diabetes. This increased accuracy and robustness can lead to more reliable and valid predictions. Secondly, a larger dataset provides greater representativeness and generalizability of the findings (Bhatia et al., 2020). This is particularly important in healthcare research, where the findings need to be applicable to a broader population of patients. The use of a larger dataset helps to reduce bias and improve the external validity of the results.

iii. A well-liked machine learning algorithm known as the Random Forest classifier is utilized for classification tasks such as disease prediction. Data pre-processing, random sampling, building decision trees, combining decision trees, and prediction are the steps involved in this algorithm. There are two formulas were used in the random forest classifier. First, one, Gini impurity formula is used here to compare the probabilities of two classes in a binary classification. Second, information gained in decision tree formula is used for optimal split. It will decide the highest value of information gain at a node in decision tree is used as the best feature for splitting the node. Then calculate the average weighted Gini impurities of both the nodes whether it may be above or below.

The weight of a node is based on the number of samples involved divided by the total number of samples. The class probability and accuracy are also calculated in Random Forest classifier algorithm.

The formula for calculating the class probabilities for a given data point:

Class Probability = (# of trees predicting the class for the data point)/(total number of trees)

The overall accuracy formula for the random forest classifier algorithm:

Accuracy = (number of predicted data after corrections)/ (total number of data)

iv. K-Nearest neighbors (KNN) classifier algorithm is also used for classifying the tasks, including diabetes prediction. Data pre-processing, splitting the data, determining the value of K, calculating the distance, nearest neighbors, majority voting, and prediction are the steps involved in this algorithm. Here are some formulas commonly used in diabetes prevention using KNN classifier. In this KNN classifier algorithm is used to find the Euclidean distance between two points in the n-dimensional space and Manhattan distance is used to find the distance between two points measured along the axes at right angles based on the features of first point to the second point. In KNN, Minkowski distance is also used to find the generalized form of Euclidean and Manhattan distances that depends on a parameter p as a positive integer. Finally, in KNN classifier algorithm is to find the accuracy based upon the overall performance based on the test data.

v. Gaussian Naive Bayes classifiers used Bayes hypothesis, which expects that the presence of a specific component in a class is free of the presence of different elements. It also makes a naive assumption of feature independence. It is widely used for classification problems in natural language processing, document classification, and spam filtering. Data pre-processing, split the data, compute class probabilities, calculate conditional probability, and make predictions are the steps involved. The formulas commonly used in the Gaussian Naive Bayes algorithm:

Prior Probability: It is the probability of a particular class in the training dataset. Prior probability = (Number of instances of class C/Total number of instances)

Conditional Probability: It is the probability of a feature given a class in the training dataset.

$$P\left(Xi|C\right)=\left(1/\left(sqrt\left(2*pi\right)*sigmaCi\right)\right)*\exp\left(-\left(\left(Xi-meanCi\right)^{\wedge}2/\left(2*sigmaCi^{\wedge}2\right)\right)\right) \tag{1}$$

where Xi is the value of the ith feature, mean Ci is the mean of the ith feature for class C, sigma Ci is the standard deviation of the ith feature for class C, and pi is the constant value 3.14159265359.

Posterior Probability: It is the probability of a class given a feature in the test dataset.

$$\boldsymbol{P}(C|X)=P\left(C\right)*P(X1\,|\,C)*P(X2|C)*...*P(Xn|C) \tag{2}$$

where C is the class label, X is the vector of feature values in the test dataset, and n is the number of features.

vi. Decision tree classifier algorithm is for classification and regression problems. It makes a choice tree that recursively parts the dataset into more modest subsets in view of the main highlights, utilizing factual measures like Gini pollution or data gain, to accomplish most extreme immaculateness and homogeneity in every subset. Choice tree classifier calculation begins with gathering and pre-processing the dataset, trailed by parting it into preparing and testing sets. The model is then prepared on the preparation set by building a choice tree utilizing the main highlights and factual measures like Gini pollution or data gain. At last, the prepared model is utilized to make expectations on new information by crossing the choice tree and doling out a class mark to each instance.

Gini impurity measures the degree of impurity or disorder of a set of instances in a binary classification problem, where p(i|t) is the probability of an instance belonging to class i in a subset t.

$$Gini(t) = 1 - Sum\left(p(i|t)^2\right) \quad (3)$$

Information gain is to find the reduction in entropy or degree of uncertainty of a set of instances in a binary classification problem, where p(i|t) is the probability of an instance belonging to class i in a subset t.

$$Information\,Gain = Entropy(parent) - Weighted\ Average\left(Entropy(children)\right) \quad (4)$$

Entropy measures the degree of uncertainty or randomness of a set of instances in a binary classification problem, where p(i) is the probability of an instance belonging to class i.

$$\text{Entropy} = -\text{Sum}\left(\text{p}(\text{i}) * \log 2\left(\text{p}(\text{i})\right)\right) \quad (5)$$

Splitting criteria, the measure used to select the most significant feature and the split point to create the child nodes based on Gini impurity or information gain.

vii. SVC stands for Support Vector classifier algorithm and is used for classification problems. It finds the hyperplane that boosts the edge between the classes in a high-layered space by changing the information into another space utilizing bit capabilities. The calculation begins with gathering and pre-handling the dataset, trailed by parting it into preparing and testing sets. Include scaling is then performed to keep away from predisposition towards high-change highlights. The model is then prepared on the preparation set by finding the hyperplane that amplifies the edge between the classes in the changed element space utilizing portion capabilities. The hyper parameters of the model are tweaked utilizing cross-approval and framework search, and the exhibition of the model is assessed on the test set. At last, the prepared model is utilized to make expectations on new information by changing the elements into the changed component space and foreseeing the class name in light of the position comparative with the hyperplane. In this SVC, the decision function for the linear kernel is given by:

$$f(x) = w^T x + b \tag{6}$$

where w is the weight vector perpendicular to the hyperplane, b is the bias term, and x is the feature vector. The decision function for the non-linear kernel is also calculated and the hinge loss function is used as the objective function to minimize in the SVC.

In summary, the SVC algorithm uses the decision function for the linear or non-linear kernel, the hinge loss function as the objective function to minimize, and the regularization parameter C to control the trade-off between maximizing the margin and minimizing the classification error. Scores of different ML algorithms are shown in Table 24.1.

24.4 PERFORMANCE RESULTS OF ML MODELS

The table contains the following information of algorithms:

- **Outcome of zero (Non-diabetic):** The probability of the model predicting the outcome as zero or non-diabetic.
- **Outcome of one (Diabetic):** The probability of the model predicting the outcome as one or diabetic.
- **Actual Outcome:** The true outcome of the data point.

For example, the Random Forest classifier has a probability of 0.12 of predicting the outcome as zero or non-diabetic, and a probability of 0.88 of predicting the outcome as one or diabetic, and the actual outcome in the dataset is one or diabetic. Similarly, for the other models, we can see their probabilities of predicting the outcome as zero or one and how well they match with the actual outcome in the dataset.

TABLE 24.1
Scores of Different ML Algorithms

Machine Learning Model	Outcome of getting 0 (Non-diabetic)	Outcome of getting 1 (Diabetic)	Actual Outcome
Random Forest Classifier	0.12	0.88	1(Diabetic)
K-Neighbors Classifier	0.4	0.6	1(Diabetic)
Gaussian NB Classifier	0.29	0.70	1(Diabetic)
Decision Tree Classifier	0.0	1.0	1(Diabetic)
SVC Classifier	0.380	0.619	1(Diabetic)

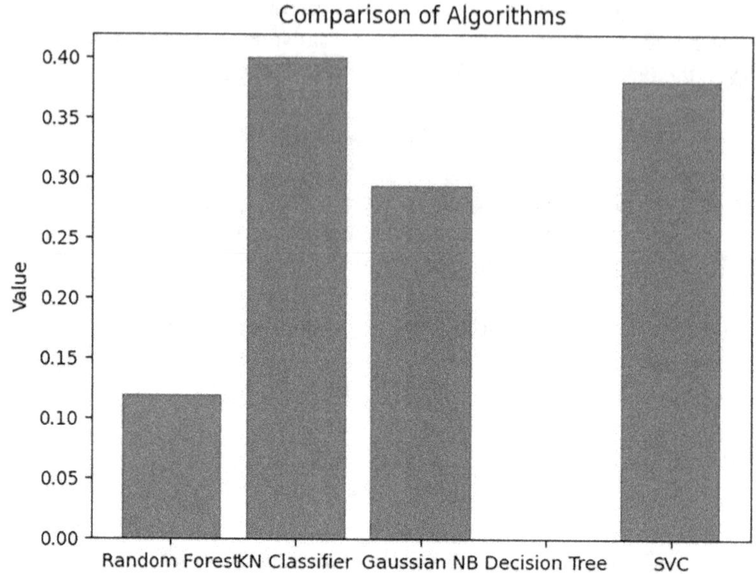

FIGURE 24.2 Graphical representation of the models getting output as zero.

From Table 24.1, it is inferred that the decision tree classifier is the best algorithm to predict diseases as the outcome is very precise and accurate. Figure 24.2 shows the graphical representation of the models getting output as zero. Figure 24.3 shows the graphical representation of the models getting output as one. Figure 24.4 shows the result of accuracy and prediction of patient is diabetic or not.

i. Cloud Computing: Render is a cloud platform that provides a fully managed platform for deploying web applications, APIs, and background workers, including machine learning models. In this research paper, Render has been used to deploy machine learning models.

In this research, ML deployment in the cloud has several advantages. One of the most significant advantages is the ability to scale the model's resources according to the research requirements. This scalability allows researchers to handle large datasets and complex models without the need for expensive hardware and infrastructure.

Additionally, ML deployment in the cloud enables researchers to collaborate more easily. It allows researchers to share code and data, and work on the same model from different locations simultaneously. This collaboration can lead to more effective research outcomes and accelerate the development of new and innovative approaches.

Moreover, ML deployment in the cloud provides researchers with a high level of security and reliability. Overall, ML deployment in the cloud can significantly improve research outcomes and accelerate the development of new and innovative approaches. It provides researchers with access to powerful tools and resources, facilitates collaboration, and ensures the security and reliability of the data. As such,

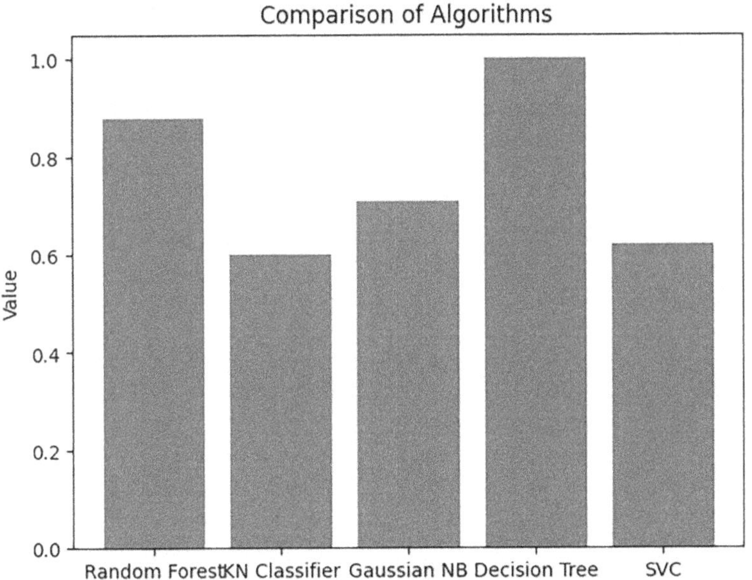

FIGURE 24.3 Graphical representation of the models getting output as one.

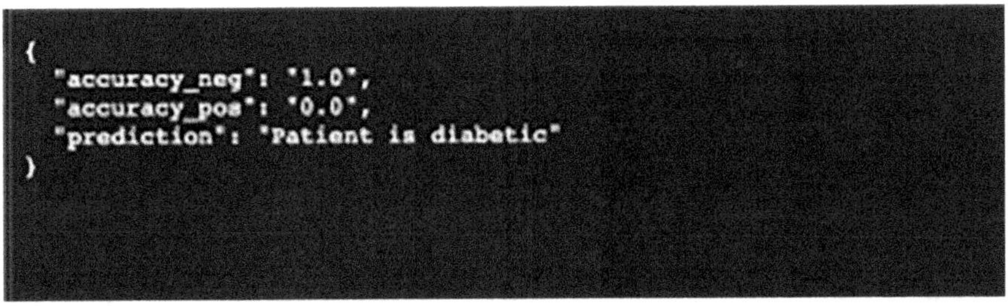

```
{
  "accuracy_neg": "1.0",
  "accuracy_pos": "0.0",
  "prediction": "Patient is diabetic"
}
```


FIGURE 24.4 Prediction score.

it is an essential step for researchers looking to leverage the power of machine learning in their research projects.

24.5 CONCLUSION

Big data analytics and cloud computing techniques have been used together along with machine learning models to predict diabetes. It is concluded that decision tree classifier is the best algorithm to predict diseases as the outcome is very precise and accurate. A dataset with 1769 data samples has been used in this research paper to predict diabetes. Render, a cloud platform that provides a fully managed platform for deploying web applications, APIs, and background workers, including machine learning models has been used in this research paper. Render provides the appropriate output when the input is provided. In conclusion, big data analysis on healthcare using cloud computing for diabetic prediction is a critical area of research with tremendous potential to improve patient care and outcomes. By leveraging the power of big data analytics and cloud computing, healthcare organizations can process and analyze vast amounts of patient data, leading to more personalized treatments and better decision-making.

The deployment of machine learning models in the cloud can enable healthcare organizations to accurately predict the onset of diabetes, identify patients at high-risk of developing the disease, and provide targeted interventions. The scalability and flexibility of cloud computing can also enable healthcare organizations to overcome the challenges associated with handling large and complex datasets.

REFERENCES

Bhatia, R., Gera, M., and Singh, A. (2020). Diabetes prediction using big data analytics on cloud computing. *Journal of Medical Systems*, *44*(9), 1–11.

Bothra, R. (2021). Diabetes prediction using machine learning algorithms. *International Journal of Engineering Applied Sciences and Technology*, *6*(5), 151–154. ISSN No. 2455–2143.

Febrian, M. E., Ferdinan, F. X., Sendani, G. P., Suryanigruma, K. M., and Yunanda, R. (2023). Diabetes prediction using supervised machine learning. *7th International Conference on Computer Science and Computational Intelligence 2022, Procedia Computer Science*, *216*(2023), 21–30.

Jain, V. K., and Bhambri, P. (2005). *Fundamentals of Information Technology & Computer Programming*. KATSONS.

Jordan, M. I., and Mitchell, T. M. (2015). Machine learning: Trends, perspectives, and prospects. *Science*, *349*(6245), 255–260.

Kotsiantis, S. B., Zaharakis, I. D., and Pintelas, P. E. (2007). Supervised machine learning: A review of classification techniques. *Emerging Artificial Intelligence Applications in Computer Engineering*, 160–183.

Naz, H., and Ahuja, S. (2020, April 14). Deep learning approach for diabetes prediction using PIMA Indian dataset. *Journal of Diabetes and Metabolic Disorders*, *19*(1), 391–403.

Rattan, M., Bhambri, P., and Shaifali, R. (2005). Information retrieval using soft computing techniques. In *National Conference on Bio-informatics Computing* (pp. 58–60). TIET.

Singh, P., Singh, M., and Bhambri, P. (2004, November). Interoperability: A problem of component reusability. In *International Conference on Emerging Technologies in IT Industry* (p. 60). PCTE.

Singh, P., Singh, M., and Bhambri, P. (2005, January). Embedded systems. In *Seminar on Embedded Systems* (pp. 10–15). KMV.

Index

S

V

W

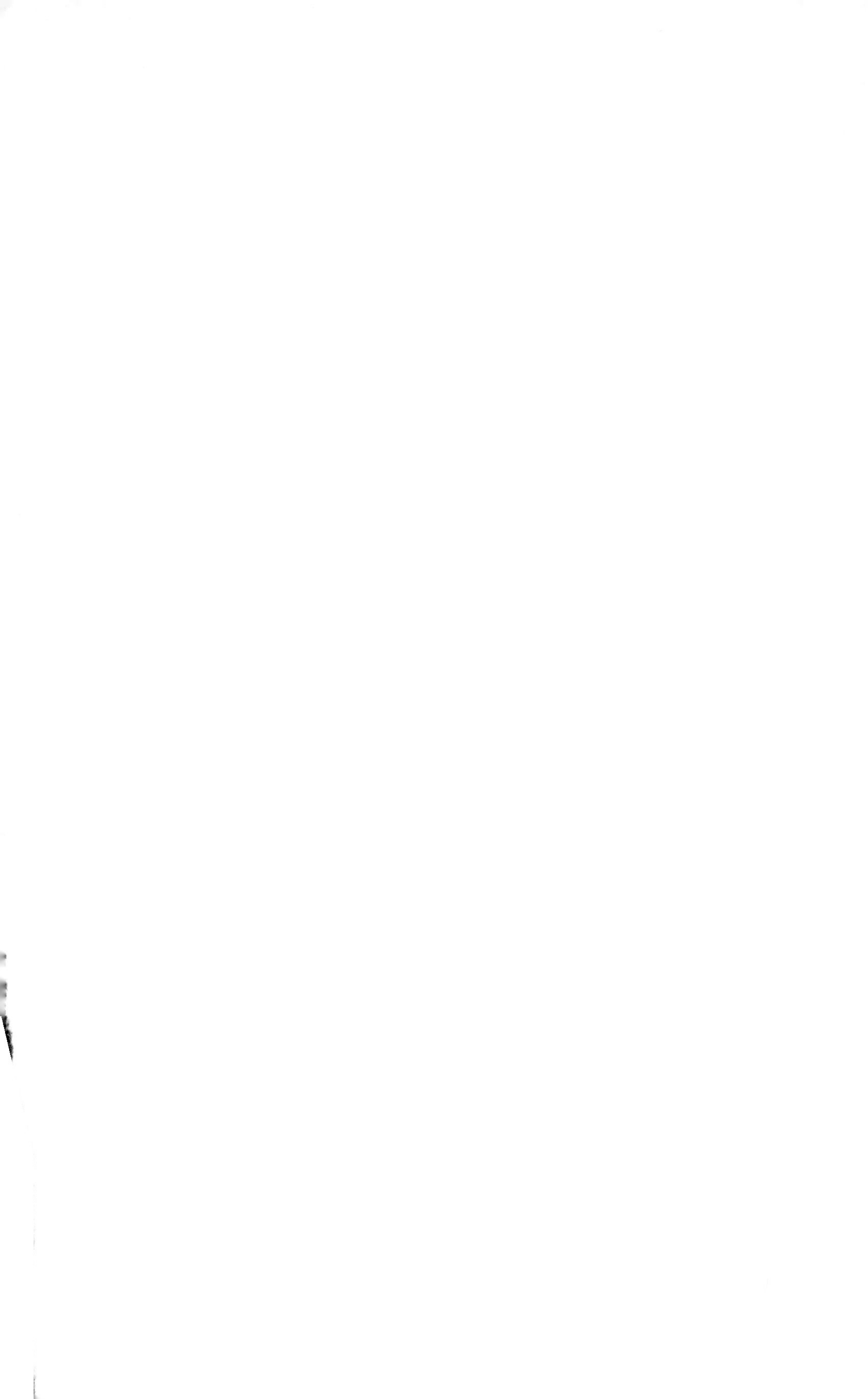

For Product Safety Concerns and Information please contact our EU representative GPSR@taylorandfrancis.com
Taylor & Francis Verlag GmbH, Kaufingerstraße 24, 80331 München, Germany

www.ingramcontent.com/pod-product-compliance
Lightning Source LLC
LaVergne TN
LVHW020608110826
845149LV00002B/401

* 9 7 8 1 0 3 2 6 9 8 5 0 2 *